URBAN HEALTH & DEVELOPMENT

A practical manual for use in developing countries

Beverley E. Booth
Kiran Martin
Ted Lankester

MACMILLAN

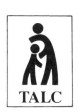
TALC

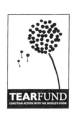
TEARFUND
CHRISTIAN ACTION WITH THE WORLD'S POOR

Macmillan Education
Between Towns Road, Oxford OX4 3PP
A division of Macmillan Publishers Limited
Companies and representatives throughout the world

www.macmillan-africa.com

ISBN 0 333 67934 2

Illustrated by David Gifford

Cover illustrations courtesy of Panos Pictures

The authors and publishers would like to thank the following
for permission to reproduce their photographs:
ASHA for: Figures 2.1, 2.2, 2.3, 2.5, 3.2, 3.4, 4.3, 5.2, 5.3, 5.4, 7.2, 7.4, 8.3,
8.7, 9.1, 9.4, 9.9, 10.4, 10.6, 12.2, 13.1, 15.1, 15.5, 16.3, 16.6, 16.9, 17.2, 17.3.
Tearfund for: Figures 1.1, 1.5, 1.7, 1.8, 7.3, 8.4, 15.7, 17.4.
WHO for: Figure 14.4

The publishers have made every effort to trace the copyright holders, but if
they have inadvertantly overlooked any, they will be pleased to make the
necessary arrangements at the first opportunity.

Printed in China

2005 2004 2003 2002 2001
10 9 8 7 6 5 4 3 2

Contents

Acknowledgements

The writing and publication of this book were only possible through the help and support of many people.

We would first like to thank the staff of ASHA and the people living in the communities that share its vision and who have taken the responsibility of improving their own lives. We thank them for teaching us so much about how to work successfully in partnership with the urban poor. We also thank colleagues with whom we have worked in other countries, including Africa, the Philippines, Nepal, Bangladesh and Mexico. We have also visited people working in urban community health and development in several countries, including Thailand, Hong Kong, Ethiopia, Nepal, Kenya, Brazil, Mexico, Bangladesh and the Philippines. We would especially like to thank Ms Jackie Pullinger in Hong Kong; Sr. Joan in Bangkok; Rev. Janet Gruyer in Chiang Mai; Ms Debbie Dortzbach in Nairobi; Ms Marty Rajandran in New Delhi; Fr. Dominic George in southern India; Ms Maria Medina in Mexico; Ms Christine Preston in Nepal; Ms Jember Teferra, Addis Ababa, Ethiopia; Mr Giridhar Vaswani, Baroda, India; Mr Paulo Machado, Curitiba, Brazil; Dr Nirai Chatterjee, Ahmedabad, India; Undugu Society of Kenya, Kenya; Mr Vijay Pavamani, Calcutta; Favela Barrio Programme, Rio De Janiero, Brazil; Pastor Antonio Jose da Silva, Sao Paulo, Brazil; and Dr Tesfaye Yacob, Ethiopia for their time and willingness to share their experiences with us. We have acknowledged shared experiences and contributions, where known, at appropriate places in the text.

We thank Dr David Morley for his review of the manuscript and very helpful suggestions, and Dr Raj Arole, Dr Carl Taylor and Dr Dan Fountain for their input and encouragement. We also thank Dr Betty Cowan for her inspiration and wisdom. We thank Mr Lalchuangliana of the Emmanuel Hospital Association for his undying encouragement.

We would also like to thank our respective families and friends for their support, encouragement and forbearance during the writing of this book.

We are grateful to TEAR Fund and Presbyterian Church (USA) for their financial support and encouragement for the publication of this book. We thank TALC for its interest and support. We are especially indebted to Ms Shirley Hamber, freelance publisher at Macmillan whose patience was sorely tested during the writing of this book by three authors on different continents.

Authors to reader

We hope you won't be put off by the size of this book. It has to be large because it is trying to cover such a huge topic. In practice not many of us will be doing more than a few of the things mentioned in this book. Most people wanting to start a programme, or expand one that has already started, will be wanting to concentrate on just a few activities, and doing these effectively before going on to something else.

In urban development we face a great many challenges but there are just three we would like to mention.

The first challenge is the sheer size of the task we face. Huge numbers of people, all needy, and most of them each facing not just one but many problems. Where do we start? There is a proverb which says that if you want to eat an elephant you need to decide where to start and then eat just a little bit at a time. It's the same with urban health. We need to start with one or two improvements that the community needs and wants, which we can achieve with them. Then when these improvements are achieved, we can move on to other things. It will take time, but each small thing we do will enrich the lives of a few people in a few ways – and knowing that will be our reward.

The second challenge is discouragement. Even the simplest thing we try to do will run into obstacles. Community members won't agree about what needs to be done or how to do it. When they do, there will then be all the bureaucracy and 'red tape' we have to face. The very people who could help – who have the power and the influence – may not be interested at all, or at least not until they see how they can also gain from any success. Meeting and overcoming discouragements is part of our job description. They will happen and these challenges can become positive things for us. Often they will help to unite us, and when the battles are won – even small battles – we will feel good. That will help to empower us for the next task we take on.

The third challenge is ourselves. We will be involved in urban development for a whole range of different reasons. For some of us it will arise from a desire to help our fellow human beings. For others it will spring from religious conviction – either because we feel God is meaning us to do it, or because we feel moved with compassion to do something when we are confronted with the poverty and misery on our doorstep. But whatever our motivation we will all become deeply affected by the experiences we go through. We will all become discouraged but we must try to stop this from making us cynical or despairing. We will all get tired out, but we must guard against this leading us into permanent exhaustion or burn-out. Many of us may feel envy at our friends getting well-paid jobs. Some of us will have so many ideas about what we would like to do that we try to do too much without enough thought or planning: we will make a lot of noise but not much progress – rather like fireworks going off in a suitcase.

One way we can help ourselves is to take time out to reflect, and perhaps pray, about what we are doing. To have regular time off so we can get refreshed and do something completely different. To get away from our slum community and even from our city to somewhere completely different, where we can rest, relax and have fun. Unless we look after our own health – physically, emotionally and spiritually we will find the job becomes too much for us.

This book is separated into five parts:

1. **Introduction to the urban poor:** provides an introduction to slums and their problems.
2. **Working with the community:** discusses how to work with communities towards empowerment and sustainable development.
3. **Health care:** discusses the health problems of slum communities and how to deal with them.
4. **Environmental improvements:** provides a step-wise process to assist the community.
5. **Important project management issues:** discusses the issues of sustainability, relationships and working with donor agencies.

We very much hope you will find this book useful and practical. It is the first edition and there may be things we have missed out and probably some things you will disagree with. We hope there will be a chance later to revise this book and we need your help for this. Please send us your comments, your experiences and your ideas so that these can help to make the next edition better than this one.

May God give you wisdom and strength as you identify with the poor and work with them. There is nothing more important that we could ever do.

The authors.

Dedication

This book is dedicated to the staff and community health workers of the ASHA Community Health and Development Project.

Part 1

INTRODUCTION TO THE URBAN POOR

1 Introduction

In downtown Nairobi you can stand on a hill and look across the valley, and all you can see is the hot sun beating down on the tin roofs of the huts of Nairobi's largest slum. They seem to go on forever. This slum has an estimated population of over 450,000 people. People say that in Nairobi, 95% of the people live on 5% of the land...

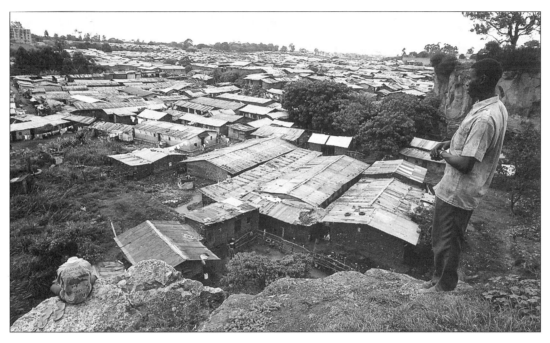

Figure 1.1   Mathare, one of the largest slums in Nairobi, Kenya. (Tearfund)

The plight – and survival – of the urban poor is one of the major worldwide challenges of the new millennium. WHO estimates that as of the year 2000, more than 1 billion people will be living in urban poverty. In the developing world, particularly Africa, cities are growing faster than ever before (Table 1.1). In some African countries, the urban population will likely increase three-fold in the 25-year period between 2000 and 2025 (Figure 1.2). According to WHO, 50% of people living in cities in developing countries live in conditions of extreme poverty with poor housing, pollution and lack of basic water and sanitation.

There are the two main reasons why cities are growing:

1. **High fertility rates**. Most people migrating to cities are young adults. They often bring young families with them and within the city will quickly produce children. This high fertility accounts for about 40–60% of the increase in urban population.
2. **The push and pull factors** – see box on page 4.

Table 1.1 Increase in urban population by region				
Region	Year		Increase	
	2000	2025	No.	Magnitude
Africa	309,651,000	752,082,000	442,431,000	2.4
Asia	1,386,721,000	2,507,732,000	1,121,011,000	1.8
Latin America	387,869,000	566,448,000	178,579,000	1.5
Oceania	21,180,000	29,892,000	8,712,000	1.4
North America	238,271,000	307,356,000	69,085,000	1.3
Europe	221,435,000	227,486,000	6,051,000	1.0

Source: DESIPA, United Nations, 1996 figures.

Life in a slum

Ahmed hadn't wanted to leave his village. The only skill he knew was working the land. He owned no land himself, and had been able to earn just enough money to feed his family by tilling the soil of the headman in his village. But in recent years the rains had been less. In this past year they had failed altogether and now there was no work. Ahmed watched his four children become thinner and thinner. In desperation he moved his family to Dhaka, hoping to find work so that his family wouldn't starve. For the first few days after they arrived the family slept on the street until they found the slum where relatives were living. Ahmed and his family moved in with two of his nephews. Eventually he was able to get a job delivering new furniture. He was then able to rent a small hut in the same slum. His wife and older daughter became rag-pickers, going through garbage looking for recyclable items that they could sell. Their younger daughter took care of the baby while their older son went to school. (Bangladesh)

Push and Pull

Why do people move from the countryside to the city?

They are **pushed** from their rural homes because:

- There is not enough land to earn a livelihood for all family members.
- There is not enough food to feed the family because of flood, drought, war or other disaster.

They are **pulled** to the city because:

- They believe jobs will be available and they can earn more for themselves and their family.
- There may be better health care, education and entertainment.
- For some people, especially youth, there is the 'glamour factor' of city life.

Source: DESIPA, United Nations, 1994 figures

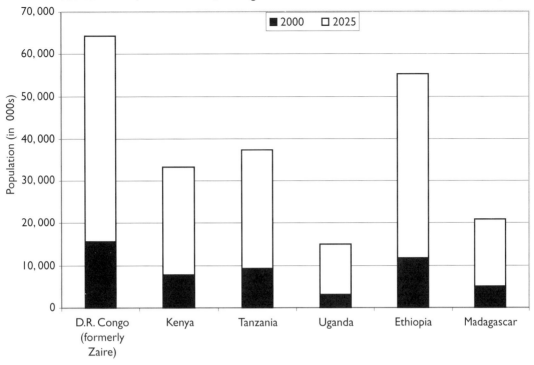

Figure 1.2   Increase in urban population 1994–2025.

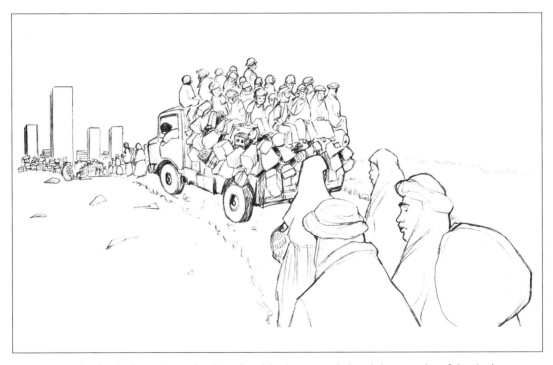

Figure 1.3   The flood of people coming into the cities has overwhelmed the capacity of developing countries to provide housing and essential civic services.

What is the definition of a slum?

There are many and varied ways of describing a slum. One helpful approach is to define four features that are usually present in a slum community:

1. The housing is substandard, and often made of discarded materials that provide some shelter.
2. The residents have limited access, or no access at all, to civic services such as water, sanitation and electricity.
3. Houses are usually small and crowded together.
4. The land is often occupied without the owner's consent.

How do slums come into being?

Cities in developing countries are not able to provide enough jobs, housing and civic services for their rapidly growing populations. Slums result from this rapid growth of population, coupled with the government's inability to accommodate them. Slums represent a minimal level of existence for the urban poor, whose poverty gives them no choice of living in areas which are better provided with good quality housing, piped water, sanitation and other services.

In many cases people who live in slums originally migrated to the cities in search of work, like Ahmed and his family. But the work that is available for these unskilled workers usually provides only enough income for mere survival. In order to obtain shelter for themselves and their families, they set up house illegally on unoccupied pieces of land that are convenient for transportation and employment. They also choose sites where they hope they will not be evicted, even if this means paying a bribe to the local police or landowner. Eventually, as others join them, the area

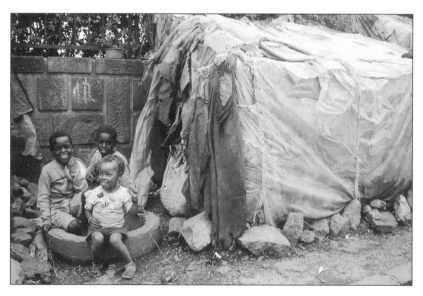

*Figure 1.4   Slum dwellings are often made of materials that others throw away.
(Jennifer Loughlin/ Tearfund)*

Slums are often located in dangerous and unhealthy areas such as next to railway tracks, on a steep hillside (for example the *favelas* of Rio de Janeiro) or on riverbanks that periodically flood. This is because these are open areas with no other use. Healthier sites are already occupied.

develops the semi-permanence of a slum. Later arrivals, often the family or friends of those already settled, may rent a dwelling that is already there, or construct a new one. Sometimes, when the government announces some scheme that will benefit slum-dwellers, there is a sudden influx of people, as more relatives are summoned from elsewhere to take advantage of the scheme.

Although people may come and go, most slums are not temporary. Some slums may exist for more than a generation so that people can be born in a slum, live their entire life there, and finally die in the same sordid conditions.

How do slum dwellers manage to stay on the land they occupy?

Slums can usually only exist because either the government or private landowners grudgingly allow it. In practice this means that in order to survive, a slum must not threaten the interests of the government or wealthy landowners sufficiently to risk eviction or demolition. In fact, sometimes private landowners, police or politicians, may actually benefit from illegal rentals, sales or bribes making the existence of the slum a shadowy benefit to all concerned. Slums are also tolerated because they are a source of cheap labour for the informal sector.

Residents may pay rent to a fellow slum-dweller, usually a slum landlord, who 'owns' the land. In turn he will usually pay off officials or police, or gain the support and protection of a local politician. In practice many slum-dwellers are both dependent and in fear of slum landlords who may demand their loyalty – and votes – in return for offering them security.

Occasionally slums gain legal status, often after lengthy negotiation or bargaining with the government, to establish a community on that land. This is most likely to be the case when the government has no use for the land for the foreseeable future. Such land is occasionally provided to residents free of cost, or more usually at a very low rent.

In practice city bureaucracy is often so chaotic that the various municipal agencies don't really know which agency is responsible for a particular piece of land. Sometimes the land is marginal or dangerous, with no clear ownership. In both these instances slums may exist and grow on the land without interference.

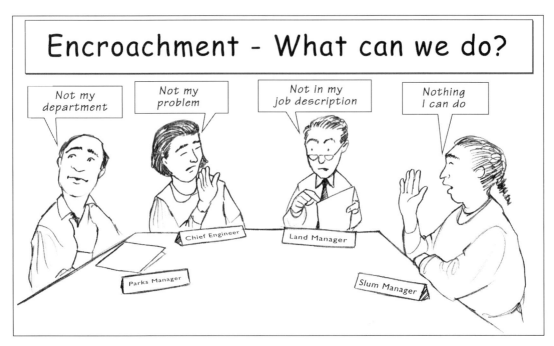

Figure 1.6   Sometimes the government does not know which agency holds responsibility for a piece of land.

Sometimes slums develop on open land that is privately owned. This may occur in two ways:

1 Slum residents may encroach on the land without the permission of the owner and usually without paying rent. They may pay bribes or gain the support of local politicians or police to prevent eviction or delay it indefinitely.

2 The owner sells or rents plots to people who then move in. The colony is often illegal in that permission was not obtained for the purpose of providing small plots of land for residential use.

Why are slums unhealthy?

Inadequate water and sanitation

In most cities in developing countries, the majority of upper or middle income neighbourhoods have reasonable water, sanitation and other civic services. These are usually provided by the government and delivered to each household. Although residents contribute to the costs, these services are usually subsidised by the government from local taxes.

The urban poor, however, usually have no sanitation services from the government, and water, if provided, is usually inadequate in amount and poor in quality. With the large numbers of new residents, added to the lack of funds, bureaucratic red tape, inflexibility, inefficiency, corruption and the rigid restrictions of rules, standards and regulations, it is easy to see why governments are often hostile to the needs of slum residents. Not surprisingly, governments often respond to the situation by denying the rights of slum dwellers to receive any services. An exception may come during election time, when the concentrated block of potential votes is very attractive, and politicians will be quick to take a real or pretended interest in the problems of slum dwellers.

Sometimes, the government may be willing to construct or improve facilities but the technical problems are too great. A simple example would be the construction of tube wells, when the slum lanes are too narrow to let drilling trucks reach their sites.

The net effect of all these problems is that slum residents often must resort to private providers of water, and may end up paying much more and receiving a far inferior service than those living in richer neighbourhoods. But because water is a necessity, over a period of time, each slum will find a way to obtain enough water to sustain existence, even though it will be at great expense in time and effort.

In the case of sanitation, which may be less of a felt priority than a water supply, disposal of human waste, wastewater and solid waste may be non-existent. The level of services may be less than in a refugee camp, and rarely of high enough quality to prevent diseases associated with poor sanitation, such as diarrhoea, hepatitis, worm infestations and schistosomiasis.

Environmental pollution and hazards

In addition to health hazards directly due to inadequate water and sanitation, the environment poses other major health risks.

- **Air pollution**. Smoke from indoor cooking fires and cigarettes reaches high levels in small, poorly-ventilated dwellings of the urban poor. In addition, slums are often located in areas where outdoor air pollution is severe, such as near major roads or factories that release pollutants into the air.

- **Industrial pollutants**. Many slums are located around factories that employ large numbers of unskilled labourers. Often these factories release noxious gases or discharge poisonous chemicals into nearby bodies of water. Slum dwellers may use this water for bathing or even for drinking. Some slum dwellers do piecework in their own homes, which can expose households to dangerous chemicals or equipment, especially if not stored away when not in use.

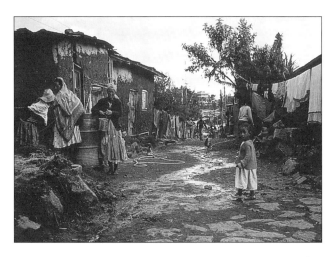

- **Hazards**. Slums are often located close to roads, railways and canals. In addition to the air and noise pollution, their location also

Figure 1.6   Poor drainage is a common problem in slums. (Tearfund)

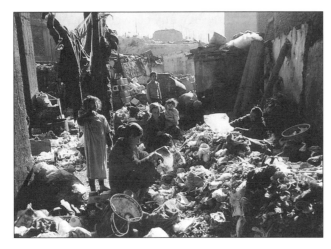

increases the risk of road and rail accidents, and drowning. Illegal electricity connections make fire and electrocution real dangers. Small children and those abusing drugs or alcohol are at particular risk.

Figure 1.7   Slum dwellers sorting garbage for saleable items: a very hazardous occupation. (Tearfund)

Lack of security

Slum dwellers feel insecure. Usually they will be occupying land illegally, so that demolition of their homes is at the whim of the authorities. This insecurity of tenure makes residents reluctant to invest money in improving their homes or environment. At times of threat or crisis they have few advocates among people of influence, such as politicians, government bureaucrats or influential neighbours. Employers often exploit them, knowing that slum dwellers have little choice for alternative employment and no advocates to speak for them. In addition to the environmentally-associated illnesses, stress, physical and sexual abuse can be consequences of the lack of security.

Decline of the traditional social structure

Slum communities are radically different from traditional village societies. In a single slum colony, people of different tribes, castes, religions, occupations, geographical area and ethnic origin are living side-by-side in over-crowded and stressful circumstances. A community of such diversity rarely provides the level of support needed in times of stress, illness or unemployment. Indeed the very diversity can spark off tension and violence.

Also the three-generation extended family is less common in slums than in rural areas. Nuclear families and female-headed households lack the resilience of the extended family during difficult times. Women themselves must take on multiple roles, as wage-earners, housekeepers and child carers. Changing attitudes towards marriage and sexuality contribute to social instability. Men are frequently absent, meaning women and children receive less care and protection. A culture of 'street children' quickly develops.

This combination of factors increases the risk of child abuse and neglect, mental stress, domestic violence, sexually transmitted diseases and substance abuse, especially alcoholism. AIDS, in particular, is a huge problem among the urban poor in sub-Saharan African cities, and is becoming so in Asian cities.

Life in a slum

Rosie and her husband had come with their three young children from their small village in the interior of Mexico to Reynosa, a small city on the US–Mexican border. Her husband Able slips across the river and finds migrant agricultural work in the US for many months each year. Now that the children are older and in school, Rosie is able to work in a small factory that makes cheap momentos for tourists. Rosie's husband's brother often stays with them in their small one-room shack. He is not married, is not inclined to work and drinks too much alcohol. One afternoon, when Rosie was at work, he raped Rosie's 12-year-old daughter, Ruby. Ruby and her 10-year-old sister now go to an after-school programme run by a local NGO until her mother comes home from work. (Mexico)

Dual risk from infectious illnesses and the diseases of city life

Poverty, ignorance and poor nutrition lock the urban poor in an environment where infectious diseases, such as pneumonia, diarrhoea and TB, are rife.

At the same time they are continually exposed to new temptations and addictions, both through their immediate environment and through the media. Abuse of alcohol, drugs and tobacco and the risk of acquiring sexually transmitted disease including HIV/AIDS are all increased. With less healthy eating, greater environmental pollution and less exercise, heart disease, diabetes and certain forms of cancer become more common. There is a rise in mental illness. Accidents and violence are common. These factors mean that the urban poor have greater health risks than the rural poor.

> **From the field**: The urban poor have greater health risks than their richer neighbours in their own city. Studies in Accra, Ghana and Sao Paulo, Brazil showed that in the urban poor, mortality from infectious and parasitic diseases was double that for the urban rich in their own city. This is not surprising given the poor water and sanitation conditions. But surprisingly, the urban poor were also twice as likely as the urban rich to die of heart diseases caused by unhealthy lifestyles associated with a city life.
>
> **Lesson learned**: The urban poor are at great risk for infectious illnesses as well as the diseases of city life.
>
> **Source**: Wilkinson, 1994.

It is not hard to see how this range of problems poses a huge challenge to the community, and to the community health and development programmes that work with them.

Chapter summary

Slum colonies result from rapid urbanisation and the government's inability to cope with the huge influxes of people, many of them young with high fertility rates. Slums represent a minimal existence for the urban poor, whose income is too low to permit them the option of living in areas of the city with better civic services such as water, sanitation, and electricity. Most slum colonies are illegal and are situated on land owned either by the government or by private landowners. Their presence is tolerated either because the land has no other use, or because of rentals and bribes paid by residents to landowners, politicians and police often through slum-landlords.

Slums are unhealthy places to live for various reasons: inadequate water supply and sanitary disposal of waste: exposure to air pollution and other environmental hazards, lack of security; decline of traditional social structure; and the dual health problems of infectious diseases, including TB and HIV disease, and other risks associated with city living, including accidents, violence and substance abuse.

Resources

1. *Health and Environment in Sustainable Development*. WHO, 1997. A comprehensive review of the effects of the environment on health with many mini-case studies.

2. *A City for All: Valuing Difference and Working with Diversity*. J Beall, (ed). Zed Books, 1997. Good discussions of the impact of urban life on women.

3. *An Urbanizing World: Global Report on Human Settlements 1996*. United Nations Centre for Human Settlements, Oxford University Press, 1996. A very extensive and detailed discussion of housing of the urban poor, including the various ways land and housing come into being and the effects on health.

4. *Urbanization: A Global Health Problem. Proceedings of a WHO Symposium, Kobe, 18–20 March 1996*. WHO, 1996. Overview of urbanisation, including case studies from industrialised countries.

5. *The Urban Health Crisis*. WHO, 1993. A good review of the effect of urbanization on health.

6. *The Poor Die Young: Housing and Health in Third World Cities*. JE Hardoy, S Cairncross, B Satterwaite. Earthscan Publications, 1990. Good review with many case studies.

Part 2

WORKING WITH THE COMMUNITY

2 Working with the community

This chapter is largely about partnership – partnership between the slum community and the Community Health and Development Programme (CHDP). Before looking at how this partnership works it is helpful to look at some of the key characteristics of a CHDP, whether it is organised by an NGO or the government, or is community-based or not.

What should be some key characteristics of a CHDP?

A CHDP is an organisation that works with one or more communities to improve their health and environment.

An effective CHDP shows the following characteristics:

1. It works in partnership with the community: partnership becomes the basis for all programme activities.

2. It acknowledges that the community is responsible for its own health and development; that the CHDP's role is to enable the community to carry out its activities most effectively. The CHDP is therefore acting as facilitator and catalyst, not controlling body.

3. It works by empowering community members and building the community's capacity to bring about effective change.

4. It encourages social equity and justice by focusing its efforts on the most marginalised groups, including women, children, the elderly and the disabled.

5. It aims to use a holistic, multi-sectoral approach.

6. It encourages active collaboration between the community and the government, other NGOs and agencies.

Partnership: the essential relationship between CHDP and the community

When a CHDP begins to work with a community, the easiest path may go something like this. The CHDP evaluates the community, determines and prioritises the problems, decides on a plan of action, implements the programme, then evaluates the results. Unfortunately, the evaluation will usually spell failure. When a CHDP uses this controlling top-down model, it seldom leads to a lasting, positive change. Why is this?

- **It promotes a sense of powerlessness, passivity and fatalism** – the very responses already common in poor communities.

- **It promotes dependency and discourages self-reliance**. Since community members expect things to be given **to** them and done **for** them, they do not learn to do things for themselves.

- **It does not transfer essential skills and knowledge to community members.** If the CHDP ceases to function for any reason, members of the community won't have the skills or experience to carry on and maintain the changes that have started.
- **It does not promote ownership.** Community members participate as beneficiaries of the project. But since they do not contribute to the planning or implementation of project activities, they feel no ownership. They don't experience the sense of accomplishment and the growth in confidence which doing the job brings about.

An overall goal of any CHDP working with the urban poor must be to help community members take on the responsibility of improving their own health – and that of their family and community. The community must come to see that making improvements is the community's responsibility, not the CHDP's. This concept does not come easily to the urban poor who have come to expect handouts from politicians before elections – and from misguided NGOs.

Levels of participation of communities in their own health and development

No Participation

1. As beneficiaries	Attend clinics, accept food packages
2. As sources of information	Through surveys, interviews, group discussions and focus groups.
4. As contributors	Through fee for service, labour for building school, volunteers
5. As local decision-makers	Through prioritising needs, planning, implementing, monitoring and evaluating activities
6. Self-mobilisation	Through local decision-making and finding resources

Full Participation – Ownership

What are the benefits of a genuine partnership?

Partnership promotes sustainable development

Development is a positive change in people's health and environment and their ability to make choices that improve their lives. It is **sustainable** when people identify and prioritise their own problems, and then act in community to solve them. **Empowerment** is the process of gaining vision, knowledge, skills and confidence that prepares people to carry out sustainable development.

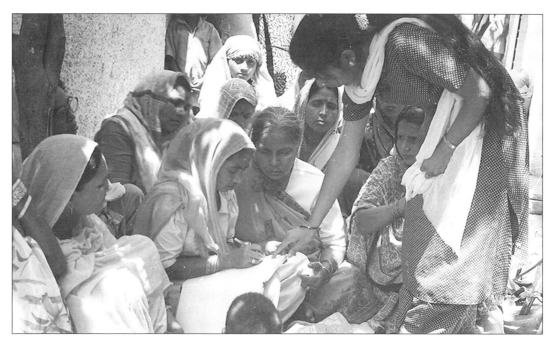

Figure 2.1   Empowerment of community members means giving them new skills. (Godfrey Martin/ASHA)

- **Genuine partnership allows the poor to make choices about their lives.** When the community chooses which problems to address, and how to tackle them, the decisions taken are likely to be culturally appropriate, acceptable to the community and affordable, important factors for sustainability.

- **Genuine partnership prepares the community to make lasting changes**. Community members gain skills, knowledge, changes in attitudes and experience that empower them not only to make permanent improvements now, but in the future to recognise areas that need improvements and understand the process for bringing them about.

> The term partnership can be misused. For example cost-savings through volunteer community labour, in the absence of training or joint planning, is not partnership. It will not result in empowerment and permanent change in the community.

- **Genuine partnership protects against exploitation**. When community members are armed with knowledge and self-confidence, they can protect themselves against:
  - police who demand bribes,
  - politicians who make empty promises,
  - quacks who recommend unnecessary and expensive medicines,
  - exorbitant money lenders (loan sharks).

From the field: A CHDP in Brazil noted that many in the community were buying expensive inappropriate drugs or useless tonics from chemist shops for illnesses which clean water and good diet might prevent or which traditional herbal remedies could alleviate. In addition to health education, project staff encouraged the older residents to share their knowledge about herbal medicines and to grow plants and herbs around their homes. Herbal dispensaries have been set up and patients are becoming increasingly confident about these forms of treatment. Apart from herbal remedies being cheaper, more accessible and often more effective, their use re-enforces peoples beliefs in their traditional values.

Source: Author visit.

- **Genuine partnership brings about improvements in health**. Health only improves permanently as a result of behavioural change – both in the individual and in the community. An effective way of bringing about this change is for people to analyse problems and participate in finding solutions. If this is ignored, no progress is made.

From the field: In Addis Ababa, a dry waste disposal system was being implemented with the help of a CDHP. Large neighbourhood garbage bins were placed for households to dump their household dry waste. But community members thought that they were far too nice to be used for garbage and began to store grain in them! This experience taught the CHDP the importance of participatory management, health education and awareness building.

Source: Harpham *et al.*, 1988.

Partnership saves money

- Resources (manpower, materials and money) are least expensive when provided by the community. A community that participates in partnership is more likely to provide resources.
- A community in partnership is also more likely to have a sense of ownership and responsibility. It will take better care of facilities and equipment, now seen as belonging to them rather than to somebody else.

Partnership encourages others

- People empowered to act themselves and who have been bringing about change in their own community are proud to share their accomplishments with people in neighbouring communities.
- Similarly, people nearby who see these changes will want the same progress for themselves.

What problems is partnership likely to bring?

Although partnership is the best model, it can have problems. In fact running a project with the community as beneficiaries is in many ways easier. There is less discussion and everything can move ahead faster.

Unfortunately it fails to bring lasting benefits, and can make genuine partnership harder to establish later. Many of the problems listed below have arisen because of top-down approaches used by projects in the past.

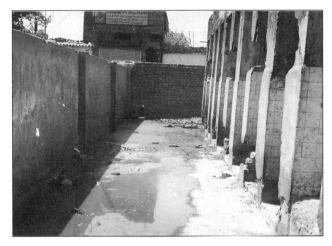

Figure 2.2   *Government installed and 'maintained' latrines: unless the community has 'ownership', latrines fall into disuse. (Godfrey Matin/ASHA)*

Problems that can occur in the beginning

- **Dependency mind set**. Politicians, government agencies and NGOs frequently offer to provide slum dwellers with certain services, or to enrol them in some scheme. Over time, the people begin to feel it is the responsibility of these agencies to solve their problems. Therefore when a CHDP comes in and encourages the people to solve their own problems, they show no interest, resist, or may even be hostile.

- **Fatalism**. People who live in slums often feel that nothing can be done to improve their state. They accept the situation as their fate and are reluctant to set about changing things. At least they have learnt to cope with the way things are. How can they know that change will actually bring any benefit?

- **Distrust**. Politicians, government agencies and even NGOs often make empty promises to slum dwellers. Thus they are suspicious when approached by yet another organisation that makes promises.

- **Need for immediate results**. People who live in slums are living on the edge of survival. For many of them, each day brings the challenge of getting enough food for the family. They have trouble participating in a venture when they cannot see the immediate benefits to them.

- **Lack of time**. People who live in slums, especially women who often must be wage-earner, homemaker and mother, don't have time for a new activity. In the cash economy of the city, time lost is considered money lost.

- **Absence of community spirit**. As we have seen, slums are diverse, composed of a wide range of people, with little in common. These differences can breed mutual distrust and dislike. The process of uniting them into a cohesive, functional group can be very difficult.

- **Those in power feel threatened and try to interfere**. Formal and informal slum leaders generally want to maintain the status quo. When an NGO comes in with intent to organise the community and empower the poor, leaders and others who benefit by suppressing the poor, will obviously feel threatened.

Problems that can occur when partnership has been established

- **Disagreements**. Disagreements can divide the community, paralyse progress and cause discouragement.
- **Rival groups fighting for control**. Political, tribal or other groups often fight for power – usually for the control of decision-making or use of resources.
- **Individuals join the programme for the wrong reasons**. They may want benefits for their family or have political ambitions.
- **Marginalised groups are ignored**. The concerns and needs of marginalised groups such as women, the elderly, and minority religious or tribal groups are not addressed.
- **Lack of interest**. After initial enthusiasm, interest and participation may collapse especially if there is no evidence of progress, or immediate result.
- **Poor decision-making**. One cost of partnership is the risk of allowing others to learn by experience, frequently through making wrong decisions. Sometimes this leads to delay – occasionally to outright failure.

How do we prepare ourselves for partnership?

Here are some suggestions:

1. **We must understand and be committed to partnership**. This is the first and most important step in working with the community.
2. **We must be willing to give up control to the community**. This includes decision-making and finances.
3. **We must be ready to share skills, knowledge and power with the community. We must be flexible and open to alternatives**. For example, it is likely that the community will **prioritise** its problems in a different order from the CHDP. For example, what we consider to be important health problems may not seem so to the community.
4. **We must be willing to accept the slow pace of progress**. Changing attitudes and behaviour can rarely happen fast.
5. **We must be prepared to remain committed for the long-term**. We must be prepared for failures and setbacks, seeing these as an inevitable part of the process.

Sometimes the largest blocks to partnership can be within ourselves, whether we are the programme director, team leader, or other member of the team. We may not want to give up control. We may like the idea of partnership in theory but be frustrated by the problems that arise. At an early stage we will need to take a long hard look at ourselves – and at our attitudes.

Because so much of this personal preparation is to do with our attitudes, and with factors which have formed our personality it is sometimes helpful to bring in an outside facilitator. Games, group discussion, role play, prayer, meditation, and even psychometric testing can all help us to better understand ourselves and others, and can aid us in our own process of behavioural change. Some of the resources at the end of this chapter contain group exercises that can help CHDP staff to develop essential skills needed to work in genuine partnership with communities.

How do we prepare the community for partnership?

1. **We must build relationships between the CHDP and the community, especially with community leaders**. We must keep them informed and involved in the process. This may involve frequent visits, joining in with community activities, eating, celebrating and mourning with community members, spending time building friendships or joining a community sports team. We can invite community members to join in our activities such as a birthday party or act of worship.

2. **We must develop trust by making CHDP aims clear and transparent**. We must help the community to understand who we are, and where we have come from.

3. **We should fight fatalism and encourage the development of self-reliance through facilitating a success experience**. One way of doing this is to help the community to address a felt need that can achieve a quick result with a high chance of success.

4. **Identify a common goal**. We have already highlighted the great diversity in background and beliefs within a slum colony. We should help the community to identify factors that can unite the colony, such as a simple improvement that will benefit all. Then work on this together.

Community groups: the vehicle of partnership

If members of the community are to be genuine participants in a programme, and not merely beneficiaries, there needs to be a Community Action Group (CAG). The CAG will plan, implement, maintain, and monitor the activities. A community is likely to wield more power, and be able to influence outcomes far more effectively, if it acts in a unified, organised and thoughtful fashion.

In fact, low-income communities are not an unorganised mass of people, as might appear to an outsider. Community organisations nearly always exist already. Examples might be:

- political parties,
- welfare or residents' associations,
- labour unions,
- cultural or religious societies,
- women or youth groups,
- burial or festivity societies.

Before deciding whether to work through a pre-existing group or to set up a new one, the CHDP must carefully weigh the advantages and disadvantages of each approach.

Advantages of working with an existing group

- It saves time.
- The group has (presumably) already proved itself able to function within the social dynamics of the community.
- The community will be familiar with the group so may be less suspicious if the CHDP works through it.
- Formal and informal community leaders are often members of these groups and may be useful entry points for outside organisations.
- These groups may already have considerable influence in the community.

Disadvantages of working with an existing group

- It may appear that the CHDP is aligning itself with a specific group in the community.
- The CHDP may not be aware of problems that the group is having with other members of the community.
- The group often is composed of the rich and powerful and does not usually have representatives from the entire community. The poorest and most marginalised may not be represented at all.
- Usually the work of existing groups is only for the benefit of its members and not for the community as a whole.
- The needs of marginalised groups, especially the very poor and women, are unlikely to be addressed.

What types of Community Action Group can be formed?

Often the disadvantages outweigh the advantages of working with an existing group, and it is necessary to form a new CAG.

There are several different types of CAG that can be formed. The particular type varies with the situation. Often there can be more than one group in a community.

> When forming a new group, do not ignore existing groups. Keep them informed and include them in activities, utilising their resources and gifts.

It may be useful to organise the community into relatively small neighbourhood groups, each represented by a committee. Each neighbourhood committee in turn provides a member to form a community-wide welfare committee, which can represent the needs of the community as a whole. The neighbourhood committees can become the main organising groups for the construction and maintenance phases of projects. This can be especially helpful when community-wide environmental improvements like drains or piped household water supply are being considered.

What should the main functions of a CAG be?

Although the goals and activities of each CAG will vary, most CAGs will have the following functions:

1. To **initiate** action and **lead** the process forward.
2. To **consult** the community, making sure that the voice of minority groups is heard.
3. To **represent** the community in its contact with outside agencies, including government, lending institutions and other NGOs.
4. To **motivate** and **mobilise** the community for action.

Table 2.1   Some Community Action Groups: advantages and disadvantages

Women's CAG

Advantages

- More likely to address the problems of at least one marginalised group (women)
- Women are motivated to work for improvements since they bear the brunt of the existing problems
- Women are more likely to work for better conditions for their family and their community than men are

Disadvantages

- Community leaders are not members and may feel threatened
- Men, especially husbands, may feel threatened
- Women are less mobile and so are less able to go out of the community on group business
- Women are less likely to have needed skills such as literacy and numeracy
- Women have less time to spare than men

Youth CAG

Advantages

- Often have free time
- Gives them something constructive to do
- Have energy and enthusiasm for the task
- More likely to be educated
- Relatively flexible and open to new ideas
- Prepares future leadership

Disadvantages

- Do not have much power in the community
- Lack of maturity
- Lack of interest or commitment

General CAG

Advantages

- Includes community leaders
- Includes men and women

Disadvantages

- More likely to work to the advantage of a few (community leaders)
- Men may monopolise meetings and women might be hesitant to speak out
- Men are less interested and more difficult to motivate, yet have the power

> **From the field**: The Integrated Holistic Approach Urban Development Project (IHAUDP) in Addis Ababa has organised a poor urban area (total population 36,373) into neighbourhood groups of about 25 households which have a neighbourhood committee of 15 people (about 10% of the neighbourhood population). This committee is responsible for the decision-making, implementation and management of the project. Community priorities have determined project activities, even when project staff have thought priorities should be otherwise. Water supply and sanitation have been improved dramatically. The community pays for and maintains the improvements. The sense of ownership by the community was demonstrated during riots in the area when all public or community buildings were destroyed except the project offices. (Ethiopia)
>
> **Lesson learned**: The formation of local neighbourhood groups can take advantage of the sense of community that neighbours have, their interest, concern and loyalties for each other – and also the strength of peer pressure when a neighbour is unco-operative.
>
> **Source**: Jarman, 1997.

⑤ To **inform** community members of progress towards community-set goals.

⑥ To **act** as troubleshooter and arbitrator in minor disputes.

> Don't call the group a community health committee. The term 'health' may unnecessarily tend to narrow the scope of activities to medical care. Other names such as 'welfare' or 'development' are less restrictive.

Women's community action groups: agents of change

In many countries of the world women's groups have proved to be very effective vehicles for partnership. They have helped projects to bring lasting improvements. However, women in many parts of the world can be particularly fatalistic because they have been oppressed for so long and have rarely had control over their own lives. This section discusses women's CAGs in more detail. Much of this section also applies to other types of CAGs, or can be easily adapted to them.

The five steps in setting up a women's Community Action Group

Step 1. Begin slowly and informally

Start by walking around the community and talking with women singly or in small groups. This gives the community and CHDP staff a chance to get to know each other. It also gives staff the chance to look out for women with potential leadership skills.

It is important at this time to develop good relationships with community leaders. We should minimise their suspicion by explaining who we are, why we have come and involving them whenever there is a chance.

In many cultures it is inappropriate for women to speak with outsiders. Be sensitive to such customs. We can minimise this problem by developing the confidence and trust of men and community leaders first, and by using female staff to work with community women.

Step 2. Identify a felt need of women in the community

An effective way to mobilise people is to address a concern that is important to most of them. Motivation will follow if they can see that solving this problem will bring real benefits, and that by acting together a solution is within reach. It is important that this first problem is relatively easy and quick to solve, so that women can experience a success. Examples might be to have a drain covered over, or to get a handpump fixed.

Step 3. Empower women to tackle the problem through increasing awareness, knowledge and skills

The women will need to have certain skills and knowledge in order to tackle the problem they have chosen. For example they must know:

● the cause of the problem,

● how to solve the problem,

● how to prevent the problem from recurring.

Key to this process is for women to learn specific skills. Examples include how to write effective letters, how to meet government officials and present their case, and technical skills needed for example in maintaining a water pump. This is also an opportunity for women to learn about how common illnesses can be cured and prevented.

As the programme develops the CHDP can start teaching women about serious problems they may not be familiar with. Often communities have serious health issues they are not fully aware of, or feel they can do little about: HIV/AIDS, child malnutrition, measles epidemics, tuberculosis. As the women learn more about health and illness in their community they can start to tackle these problems.

A women's meeting is a good way of introducing new ideas, as it reaches many people with relatively little effort. Face-to-face follow-up meetings in women's homes are very valuable. They can be especially helpful for women who were too shy to speak at a public meeting (often widows, the marginalised or very poor), but who have concerns to share or interests they want to take forward.

In women's meetings, include action and activities as well as discussion. Make sure meetings are fun, interesting and interactive. Dramas, puppet shows, videos, and role-play are effective ways of raising issues, changing attitudes and motivating for change. Demonstrations can be very effective, for example: dipping a child's hand into a glass of water, and rubbing off the dirt, shows very effectively just how dirty the hand is. Placing two drops of water under a microscope, one from a deep bore hole and the other from standing water in the community shows the huge difference between the two – and the likelihood of infection.

Leaflets too can be useful, especially for explaining how improvements work, how they are constructed, and the various options. They need to be clear, relevant, and should address an issue that is both important and interesting. Designs should be field tested before printing.

Working with women often gives a natural opportunity to work with children as well. Include school children whenever possible – they will then take new ideas into their homes – and into the future.

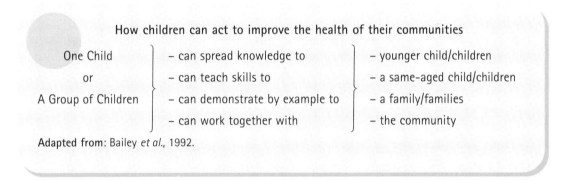

How children can act to improve the health of their communities

One Child	– can spread knowledge to	– younger child/children
or	– can teach skills to	– a same-aged child/children
A Group of Children	– can demonstrate by example to	– a family/families
	– can work together with	– the community

Adapted from: Bailey *et al.*, 1992.

Step 4. Motivate women to take action

The following approaches help in motivation:

❶ Talk about the benefits a particular activity or intervention can bring:
- in health and safety benefits,
- in convenience and comfort benefits,
- in increased property value resulting from a community improvement,
- in cost-effectiveness of an intervention.

From the field: A CHDP convinced a community about the value of using mosquito nets by showing that they were cost-effective. At a community meeting, project staff asked people how many episodes of malaria had occurred in their household during the last malaria season. Then they asked how much money was spent on treatment, and how much was lost through days absent from work. They multiplied the average number of cases per household by the amount of money lost per episode. The average cost of malaria per household during the previous malaria season came out to be twice the cost of a mosquito net. The people attending were persuaded that mosquito nets were worth buying.

Source: Authors.

❷ Set up a demonstration model for smokeless cookers, pit latrines, etc.

③ Take a group of community members to visit another slum where they can see successful changes that have already taken place.

④ Build trust. Most community members will have heard endless promises to be made, only to be broken, both by politicians and by outside enthusiasts.

Motivating a community to call on its own resources to make changes in health practice can be very rewarding. People start to see that they themselves can take steps to improve their family's health. Success then brings a sense of pride and self-worth, and with it a change in attitude. People realise that even though resources are limited, they have some control over their lives and surroundings.

From the field: In Bamako, Mali, the community identified blocked and overflowing local drains as its most pressing sanitation problem. Further discussion led to the cause: garbage was not collected from the community collection site often enough so it was over-flowing most of the time. Therefore, women didn't bother taking their household garbage to the collection site, instead dumping it in drains nearby their houses. After discussing the problem with local authorities, garbage collection was contracted out to private contractors, including a women's co-operative. Garbage from the community collection site was collected regularly and the community women began to carry their household garbage to the collection site.

Lesson learned: We should look for the reasons for unhealthy behaviour. Sometimes health education and awareness are not enough.

Source: Narayan, 1993.

Table 2.2 Factors that can affect mobilisation of the urban poor*	
Help mobilisation	**Hinder mobilisation**
1. The people may be more aware of health as a need and a right, because health care is more accessible in urban areas	1. The people may have an attitude of dependency from previous interactions with other groups or government agencies
2. The people may be more informed about programmes, schemes, etc., of other urban communities through proximity and greater access to media	2. The community is likely to be more heterogeneous than a rural population – from different regions, religions, castes/tribes. Thus less sense of community may exist than in rural communities
3. The community is more likely to be educated	3. Tenure is insecure, land/house is not theirs, therefore people may have less interest in working to improve surroundings
	4. Livelihoods are likely to be more varied
	5. The economy is likely to be based on cash; people may be reluctant or unable to devote time without pay

*Compared with rural poor

Step 5. Over time, organise the women's Community Action Group more formally

Set aims and choose activities

As women's CAGs grow in understanding and confidence they can increase their range of aims and activities. It is helpful to look at some of the specific ways in which women's CAGs can directly help to improve health care in the community, and the environment. CAGs should choose one or two activities they can carry out effectively, which bring success and increase their own self-confidence and standing in the community. Then they can add in other activities. Here is a 'menu' of possible activities:

Improve health in the community:

1. Monitor the health of the community, including frequency of serious illnesses such as TB and AIDS and the frequency and cause of death in young children.
2. Monitor the activities of the community health volunteer.
3. Assure that pregnant women, young children and the elderly receive health care.
4. Encourage women to be delivered by a trained birth attendant.
5. Encourage and train CAG members to serve as lane health visitors to provide health education, detect illness early, promote the use of oral rehydration solution and motivate for family planning.
6. Promote family planning.
7. Address social issues in the community such as domestic violence, alcoholism and drug abuse, etc.
8. Organise vocational training and income generation projects for women.
9. Encourage and facilitate all school-age children to attend school.
10. Spread awareness health and social issues to other slum communities and assist them in setting up their own women's groups.
11. Network with other women's groups and other organisations to fight for common causes.
12. Resolve conflicts and disputes within the community.

Life in the slum

In one slum community, illicit alcohol was being made and sold. Drunkenness and domestic violence were becoming a growing problem. When young boys started drinking alcohol, the women's group decided to do something about it. So they went to the local policeman. But those who were making the alcohol were paying him a bribe so he would do nothing. So the women stormed the office of the superintendent of police demanding action. The police raided the community, destroyed the equipment and arrested the owners. Now the women act as soon as they become aware of someone selling illicit alcohol. Recently there has been no problem because word has spread about the action the women take. (India)

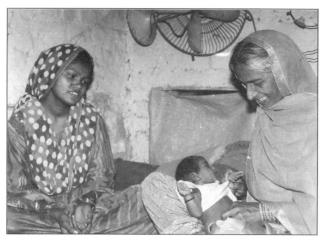

Figure 2.3   *Lady lane visitor checking on a new mother and new-born baby. Because she is a neighbour, the CAG female health visitor knows quickly when a baby is born. (Godfrey Martin/ASHA)*

Improve the community environment:

1. Organise, supervise and monitor community drains, pathways and latrines, including repairs and cleaning.
2. Advocate for improved civic services.
3. Find solutions to inadequate water and sanitation problems.
4. Increase awareness about sanitation, hygiene, etc.
5. Stand up for citizen's rights and especially those of women.
6. Stand up against illegal actions by landowners, whether government or private.

Decide on membership criteria

Decide about:

- **Qualifications**: e.g., residency in the slum, age, etc.; who determines membership (president or managing committee, etc.).
- **Obligations**: payment of dues, meeting attendance, degree of involvement in group activities, probationary period.
- **Grounds for termination of membership**: non-payment of dues, actions contrary to the group's aims, etc.

Set meetings protocol

- Frequency, time, length of meetings.
- Inclusive process for drawing up agenda, so member's concerns are considered.
- Method of reaching decisions (consensus, show of hands, secret ballot, etc.) Who chairs the meeting.
- Who keeps the minutes, emphasising actions.

Establish managing committee

The success of any women's CAG will depend in part on how fairly and effectively the organisation is set up. Key to this process will be the Managing Committee, which will need to be formed at an early stage, though not always at the very beginning.

Main areas to consider include the following:

- **Membership of the committee**: number and who is included.
- **Election of officers**: Process of nomination; quorum that is required to elect them; if more than one candidate, process of election (show of hands, etc.).
- **Term of office**: Length of office and how long before outgoing officers may be able to stand for re-election.

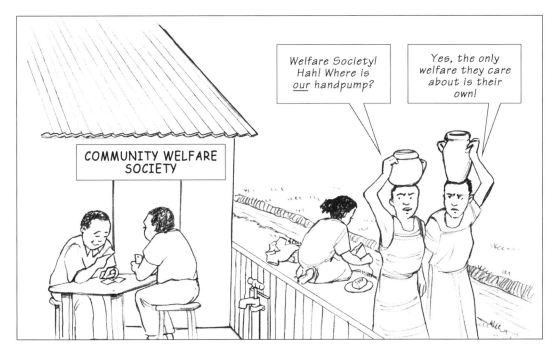

Figure 2.4   Ensure that marginalised groups are represented on the community committees.

Wherever possible, try to have officers selected by consensus rather than by vote. Voting can be divisive to the group, and if high profile, threatening to community leaders. Moving slowly is often appropriate, waiting for natural leaders to appear. Members selected through the joint consensus of the community and the CHDP are more likely to have the right characteristics, and less likely to represent powerful and vested interests. Sometimes however low-profile elections can be appropriate, as the following case shows.

Life in a slum

Miriam was elected president of the newly formed women's society. The women elected her because she was a widow and lived alone with her teenage son. They decided that she would be the best because she did not have a husband to control her. She would have less difficulty speaking out and visiting government agencies outside the community. The women also knew that this would help to increase her status within the community. (Ethiopia)

Set the duties of officers
President:

1. provides leadership,
2. chairs management and general meetings,
3. advises and supervises sub-committees,
4. implements the decisions of the managing committee and women's CAG,
5. ensures that meeting minutes are distributed.

Vice-president:

① performs the duties of the president when the president is not present.

Secretary:

① maintains all group records, including the membership register,

② takes minutes during meetings of managing committee and general body,

③ is responsible for correspondence.

Treasurer:

① maintains accounts, recording all money collected and spent,

② presents detailed accounts to the managing committee periodically, at least once or twice a year,

③ spends money only as sanctioned by the managing committee.

Establish relevant subcommittees

It may be helpful to have subcommittees that address areas of special interest to the women's CAG. Possibilities include:

- environmental improvements,
- health,
- education and income generation,
- culture and recreation.

The chairs of these sub-committees should be members of the managing committee.

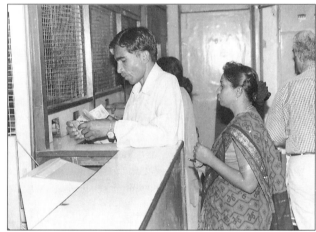

Figure 2.5   CAG treasurer making a deposit at the bank. Empowerment includes the development of new responsibilities. (Godfrey Martin/ASHA)

Establish a bank account in the name of the CAG

Determine who will be the signatories and how many signatures will be required. This must be minuted in a meeting of the managing committee.

What training do members of a CAG need?

It is important to train management committee members, especially the office bearers in management, administration and leadership. It will sometimes be helpful for this training to be open to other members of the CAG, so the group as a whole is empowered. Some of the specific skills needed include:

- Basic communication skills.
- How to run a meeting.

- How to take minutes and keep records.
- Basic accountancy skills.
- How to write letters to government agencies and others. In the case of government, letters should be addressed to the specific official who is in the highest position in the relevant department. Letters should be courteous, short and to the point.
- Details of their legal rights and mandated services etc.
- How to visit government and other agencies. Although the NGO may facilitate appointments with government officials, community members should be present at all meetings.

From the field: A women's group started a savings and loan scheme among its members. Within a few months members became worried that the person elected to keep accounts seemed to be keeping back part of the money. Her books did not agree with what the women felt they had contributed. This mistrust almost ruined the project. An NGO working with the community was called in to investigate. It discovered that the bookkeeper had no idea how to keep simple accounts and records. When she was taught these skills, the problem resolved. (Nepal)

Lesson learned: Prepare community members with the skills and knowledge they will need to carry out the tasks of project management.

Source: N. Gurung, 1999. CHDP, Kathmandu, Nepal.

Sometimes an officer or member may abuse her power contrary to the good of the community. For example, she may steal group funds, or give or receive bribes. In these situations, the managing committee should take appropriate action, aided by the CAG. The CHDP should only be called in at the specific invitation of the CAG, or if the situation gets out of control.

How can we maintain enthusiasm and motivation of a women's CAG?

Women face many barriers as they try to improve the health of their community. It is important that we do everything possible to maintain the enthusiasm and motivation of the women's CAG, as this will frequently be the primary agent of change within the slum community. Some ways to do this are:

- To give constant encouragement and praise.
- To acknowledge their efforts even when not yet successful.
- To invite government and other VIPs to visit and give encouragement.
- To arrange visits to other communities in which women's CAGs have made their communities healthier.

- To encourage unity and spirit through group functions such as picnics, trips to other colonies for mutual learning, and other team building activities.
- To stand with them and provide support during difficult times.

Chapter summary

Building a partnership between the CHDP and the community will form the basis for most programme activities. This is an effective model for achieving sustainable development. A variety of problems occur when we commit ourselves to partnership. They can be largely overcome if at an early stage we prepare both ourselves and the community for effective working relationships. This requires behavioural change in all committed to this approach.

A channel is needed for community action, and it is often helpful to set up a new Community Action Group (CAG). Often a CAG led by women is most effective. There are five steps in setting up an effective CAG: starting informally by getting to know the community; identifying a felt community need; empowering the community to tackle the problem through increasing people's awareness, knowledge and skills about relevant issues; motivating for action; and over a period of time formalising the structure and constitution of the CAG, in particular through setting up a managing committee. All members of a CAG need regular training and encouragement, as they will be the main agents of change within a slum community.

Resources

1. *Power, Process and Participation: Tools for Change*. R Slocum, L Wichhart, D Rocheleau, B Thomas-Slayter. Intermediate Technology Publications, 1998. Provides innovative tools for consciousness raising, information gathering, decision making, advocacy and action.

2. *Poverty and Health: Reaping a Richer Harvest*. M Feuerstein. Macmillan Education, 1997. An excellent review of poverty, its causes and effects, and practical suggestions on how to work with the poor, including the urban poor. (Available from TALC.)

3. *Partnerships for Social Development: A Casebook*. C Taylor *et al.* (eds). Future Generations, 1995. A series of case studies of community health and development programmes in which true partnership and empowerment with and of the community have been successfully implemented.

4. *Health Care Together: Training Exercises for Health Workers in Community Based Programmes*. MP Johnston, SB Rifkin. Macmillan Education, 1987. Many exercises that help health workers to develop the essential skills needed to work in genuine partnership with communities. (Available from TALC.)

5. *Facilitator's Guide to Participatory Decision-making*. S Kaner, L Lind, C Toldi, S Fisk, D Berger. New Society Publishers, 1996. Explains how to facilitate group participation. It has many activities that can help staff and community leaders to become better facilitators.

3 Initial activities

Select the community

One of the first decisions a CHDP has to make is which community or communities to work with. This can be a daunting decision. There are huge numbers of people, with limitless need on the one hand, but often suspicious of outside agencies on the other. At the same time the CHDP must take care only to select a community that will participate with enthusiasm and work in genuine partnership. Yet without gaining entry and starting to understand a community it is hard to know if the potential for partnership exists.

Approaching a new community

The urban poor are used to being exploited by outside groups. They may have received promises from politicians or from the government, which have never been kept. Especially in capital cities they may have had frequent visitors and numerous surveys. Not surprisingly they may be suspicious of outsiders. They may also have worked with other health or development programmes in the past which did things very differently, or for no obvious reason left without warning.

A new community may have heard already about the CHDP, perhaps from people living in a community in which the project is currently working. This new community may invite the project to work in the community. Sometimes, when the CHDP is well

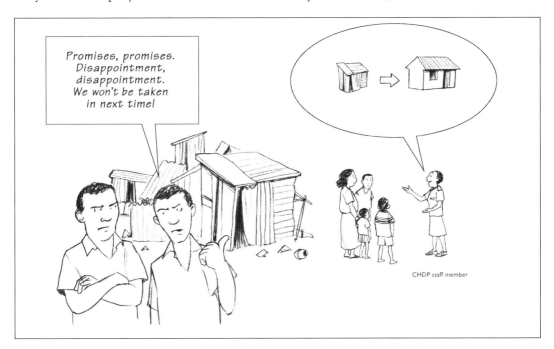

Figure 3.1   We must build trust and only raise expectations that we are sure can be met.

established and has a good reputation, the government may ask the CHDP to work with a particular community that has approached the government for help. Responding to such an invitation from the community is the ideal situation under which a good working relationship can be most readily established. But with the very first community, and sometimes later, the CHDP is the one that makes the initial overture by entering a community and talking with members and leaders of the community.

Life in a slum – a doctor's first experience in a slum

'It was during a cholera epidemic. I went into the slum – it was so dirty I could hardly walk. I naively thought that the slum dwellers would welcome me and appreciate that I had come to help. I met the slum leader. He was snobbish and arrogant and asked many questions – "Who are you? Why are you here? Where will the money come from?" Then he told me to come back in 2 weeks and at that time he would tell me whether I could work in the slum. I was very discouraged. The need was so great and the common people, especially the women, wanted me to come, but I was powerless. So I decided I had to develop a good relationship with the leader. I went to his house and met his wife and talked with her. I played with his child. After several visits and informal talks, I was invited to work in the slum. The slum leader offered his courtyard as the clinic site and his wife organised the use of her furniture. The answer is relationships. Develop a sincere relationship and people will change.' (India)

Factors to consider in the selection of a community

Size of the community

Slum communities vary greatly in size. There may be just a few households on a small patch of land whereas some slums may contain many thousands of households and extend for several kilometres. It is particularly difficult to work with large slums for several reasons:

- **Logistic problems of having to provide services to such a large number of people**. Instead of a single clinic site, several may be required in order to provide even the most basic services. Staffing needs can be too large to handle.

- **Political fighting**. Politicians are especially interested in winning the large block of votes in extensive colonies. This can lead to the dominance of party politics in the whole social structure of the colony.

- **Environmental improvements need to be co ordinated** and implemented so that one section of the community does not suffer or feel rejected when another section of the slum undergoes environmental improvements.

- **The state of water and sanitation is usually very poor in large slums because of the expense in providing civic services as well as the logistic problem of installing facilities in large, crowded slums with no road access.** Thus environmental improvement is the most pressing need and yet the most difficult problem to do something about.

The presence of these problems does not mean that a CHDPs should never work in large slums. It does mean however that they should start in smaller communities, and only work in larger slums when they have gathered experience, personnel, resources and government contacts.

It is usually impractical to work with only part of a large slum community for various reasons:

- **It is difficult to limit services to residents of a certain area of the slum**. Jealousy and resentment amongst those not being served will usually make the programme impossible to carry through.
- **Key environmental improvements, such as draining surface water cannot be limited to one area of the community**.
- **When government provides environmental improvements it usually considers the whole slum as a single unit**.

Political situation

It is important to find out about the basic political structure in the community, being careful not to be seen as supporting any one group. When party infighting is present, making any improvements is difficult. Groups may perceive the programme is allied to a rival party and may attempt to bring things to a halt. Ignorance and suspicion easily allow people to jump to wrong conclusions. A particularly difficult situation arises when the local and regional elected officials are from different parties.

From the field: A CHDP was helping a slum community of 10,000 people to upgrade their housing. On the day of the inauguration of the programme, the slum leader saw that the local politician from the opposition party was attending the function. The slum leader put a stop to the function and said that the community would not participate; so the upgrade was not done. The leader felt insecure and that the community was no longer dependent upon him. (Brazil)

Lesson learned: Community leaders have great power and can determine the success or failure of an activity. When possible, ensure that their authority is not threatened.

Source: Authors.

Community spirit

Progress towards sustainable development requires a basic degree of co-operation among community members. Although working towards a common goal can help to unite a community, major divisions tend to surface and undermine progress. It is important to assess whether divisions between rival groups whatever their origin, are so deep-rooted that it would be better to look for an alternative colony.

Existing services and health status

The health status of the community is directly related to a supply of safe water, adequate sanitation and access to health services. If these are present, the CHDP should consider working in more needy communities.

Presence of other agencies

If the government or another NGO is already doing effective work, even at an early stage, the CHDP should look for another site. An exception is if a CHDP has a particular area of expertise that is not provided by other agencies, and possibilities of working together clearly exist.

> **From the field:** The Undugu CHDP in Nairobi began to establish community-based health care in a slum community. They started by training a few community health volunteers, but they were not motivated and there was not much community support. There were other NGOs already working in the community that offered curative services and transport of sick people to the large government hospital. Thus community members saw no need to help themselves since outsiders were already providing health care services. The CHDP stopped their active work in the community, but kept in touch informally in case conditions changed. (Kenya)
>
> **Lesson learned:** NGOs have different philosophies. In many cases, the philosophies clash, making it difficult to progress.
>
> **Source:** Harpham *et al.*, 1988.

Location

The neediest slums are usually those most remote from good quality housing and facilities. Most NGOs tend to be located in more affluent areas of the city, and for reasons of time and economy prefer to work nearby. Consider therefore working in a remoter community, or one located in an industrial suburb, a satellite area of the city or an especially polluted location. Make sure the project has the resources to cope with the additional challenge.

Government co-operation

In some slums, the government is in the process of attempting to demolish the slum because it wants to use the land for another purpose, or the community is dangerously located such as on a piece of land subject to seasonal flooding. In such circumstances, the government is not willing to upgrade environmental services, and it may be fruitless for a CHDP that primarily assists communities to improve their water and sanitation to attempt working in such a colony.

An ideal situation is for local government to invite or encourage the CHDP to work in a particular community. When the government is an active partner lasting results are more likely to occur as the CHDP and community work together. It is worth making great efforts to develop good working relationships with government, even though this is always time-consuming and often takes great persistence. At an early stage it is helpful to draw up a working agreement which outlines the responsibilities of each partner.

After choosing a community in which to work, friendship and trust must be established before rushing into any activities. Community members will often have entirely different expectations about the way forwards. Commonly they will be expecting quick handouts, and the idea of solving problems together, with no guarantee of immediate solutions, can shake their interest and confidence.

> The key to successful partnership is to build friendships, establish trust and discuss issues openly and truthfully from the beginning. Members of the CHDP must be willing to listen and learn, and to treat community members with respect and humility.

Make a community diagnosis

Why should we involve the community?

Making a community diagnosis must be a joint activity between CHDP and slum members. It will often be the first activity they do together, and if done with sensitivity can help to build trust. But more importantly, it promotes initiative, responsibility and ownership by the community. Community members can make specific contributions such as:

- deciding which data is to be collected and how it is to be done;
- providing information and insights based on 'insider' knowledge;
- smoothing the way and facilitating co-operation by reluctant people;
- working on specific tasks, e.g. conducting a survey;
- drawing conclusions and suggesting solutions.

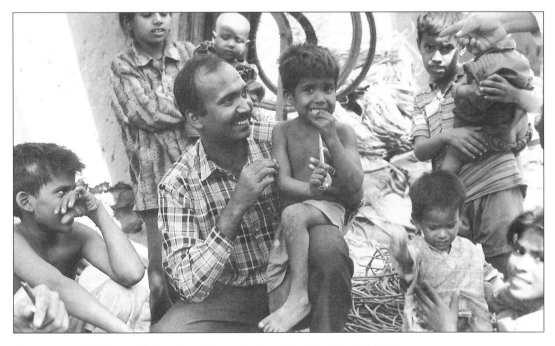

Figure 3.2   Holding a child can break down barriers. (Godfrey Martin/ASHA)

What is a community diagnosis?

Just as a health worker examines a patient to make a clinical diagnosis, the CHDP staff and some community members can do the same for their community. They gather information about the community – its structure, ways of functioning and the problems it faces. They tap into sources of information and ask questions. They try to identify the main problems and challenges that the community is facing.

Then they discuss their findings with the community at large, and start exploring solutions. That process leads on to making an action plan, which is described in the next chapter.

From the field: In the Klong Toey slum communities in Bangkok, Thailand, a women's group organised by a local NGO, the Human Resouece Centre, knew that AIDS was a serious problem. The women decided that they must learn more about HIV infection so that they could plan some effective action. They designed and completed a survey in their communities. Despite having to deal with fear and suspicion, the women were able to produce a comprehensive report that has been the basis of planning a focused AIDS care and education programme.

Lesson learned: When trying to get an accurate picture of sensitive problems such as AIDS, the active involvement of community members can help to reduce suspicion, and maximise results.

Source: Author visit.

Table 3.1 Similarities between making a patient and a community diagnosis	
Patient	**Community**
Step 1: Take a history	**Step 1: Gather information**
1. Find out symptoms from the patient	1. Find out about problems from the people
2. Review his past medical record	2. Review available records and data
3. Take a systematic history of the patient	3. Conduct a survey
Step 2: Conduct a physical examination	**Step 2: Inspect the community**
1. Examine the patient	1. Take a survey walk
	2. Map the community
Step 3: Make a diagnosis	**Step 3: Determine the problems**
1. Use what has been found in history and physical examination to make the diagnosis	1. Analyse the gathered data to determine the problems
2. Determine the cause	2. Find the root causes
Step 4: Discuss treatment with the patient	**Step 4: Discuss an action plan with the community**

What information do we want?

It is important for the community members and CHDP staff to decide clearly why we want the information and how we are going to use it. This helps us to know what we need to find out. Usually we will need information about:

- The main health and social problems in the community: what are the common problems, how common and how serious?
- The root causes of these problems: what are the underlying causes?
- Ways to solve the major problems, taking into consideration resources within and outside the community.
- Baseline conditions to help us monitor changes and improvements over time.

The tables at the end of this chapter contain lists of information important to health and environment, and the best ways of obtaining it. We can choose from this list, and also add other information that we need for our own community.

> Remember, we should only collect data that we need.

How do we obtain the data?

From the people

Hold discussions with key informants in the community

Key informants are people in the community who are particularly knowledgeable. As well as including elected leaders, they include the informal leadership, such as religious leaders, schoolteachers, women's group leaders, landlords, etc. Some key informants may be biased towards a particular community. An important group to meet with are health providers in the community: traditional healers, doctors, government health workers and owners of medicine shops.

Hold group discussions

Group discussions with members of the community give us the opportunity to get input from many people at one time. This is a useful method of learning about traditions, beliefs, customs, and practices. Often when we limit the group to a particular age or gender, such as youth or women, we are able to get more accurate information about sensitive issues such as sexual practices or domestic violence.

Talk to individuals

Informal discussions with community members will occur at various times, for example as we walk round the community and visit homes. During these discussions concerns and problems are often shared openly and the real daily concerns of people become more obvious. This is an opportunity for sensitive topics such as sexually transmitted diseases, domestic violence and substance abuse to be raised naturally.

From the field: In Lesotho, 11-year-old children from four villages were asked to draw a map of their villages, noting the main problems, resources, water sources and places of defecation. All four groups reported the same three main problems drunkenness, bad roads and low demand for sanitary latrines. They noted the different sources of water, defecation spots and garbage dumps. They listed the following resources: people, trees, VIP latrines; shops water supply, poultry and transport. They enjoyed the process and felt that part of the evaluation process.

Lesson learned: Children can contribute in making the community diagnosis. Participation at this stage can build a sense of ownership and lead to their contribution in working towards solutions.

Source: Narayan, 1993.

Lesson learned: Children can contribute in making the community diagnosis. Participation at this stage can build a sense of ownership and lead to their contribution in working towards solutions.

Source: Narayan, 1993.

From inspection of the community

Walk through the community

A walk through the community is an essential part of making a community diagnosis. It is an opportunity to get a general idea of health status, socio-economic levels, diversity of cultures, and good and bad behaviours and practices. It gives a chance to observe first hand, water, sanitation and housing conditions – and practices. It is also an opportunity to talk with ordinary community members from a wide range of backgrounds, and different areas of the slum.

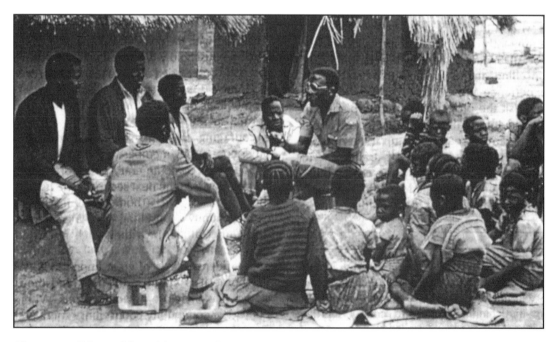

Figure 3.3   When talking with community groups, encourage discussion by making people feel at ease, gently encouraging shy people to contribute and showing appreciation of all comments.

Wealth ranking: a way for a community to assess the relative wealth of its own members.

1. A small group of 6–9 community members first makes a map of the community with each dwelling marked with the name of the head of household. Sometimes this map may already be available. It is unlikely to be fully accurate because of the rapid turnover of population: this is not important.

2. The group then decides how they would classify the community on a poverty scale. Specifically how many groups would there be? For example, very poor, poor, average, rich or very rich? Or maybe only 3 of those groups?

3. After they have decided on the number and names of the groupings, the group decides how to characterise each wealth group. Members of one community had four groups and defined them as follows:

People who are:

Rich	Average	Poor	Very poor
Get water from their own well	Get water from private vendor	Get water from river	Get water from river
Use household latrine	Use open defecation	Use open defecation	Use open defecation
Have electricity	Have electricity	Have electricity	Have no electricity
Own a motor scooter	Own a bike	Own no form of transport	Own no form of transport
Eat 3 meals per day	Eat 2 meals per day	Eat 2 meals per day	Eat 1–2 meals per day
Send their boys and girls to school	Send their boys and girls to school	Send boys, but not girls to school	Send neither boys nor girls to school
Wear leather/canvas shoes	Wear plastic/rubber sandals	Wear plastic/rubber sandals	Go barefoot

4. Then they assess each dwelling and mark the appropriate wealth grouping of the dwelling on the map. Sometimes a dwelling will not have all characteristics of one of the wealth categories. Such dwellings are given the category they fit best.

5. Then they can total up the number for each category and find the percentage for each category.

This exercise helps the community to identify and locate the poorest dwellings, which will need extra help and resources.

Before setting out on this walk it is helpful for team members to draw up a list of those aspects of slum life they particularly want to observe and study. Different team members can concentrate on particular aspects, e.g. some could look at the state of children (hygiene and nutrition), another at water points and human waste disposal (methods, practices and sites).

After the walk it is important to record information and impressions without delay. To avoid suspicion it is usually better not to take notes at the time.

Make a map of the community

Maps are very useful for assessing problem areas and resources within the community. It is important to visit and map the particular sites that are related to project goals. For example, if the project aims to improve drainage, then it is important to visit and map low-lying areas, existing drains, water points, etc.

A very useful exercise is to get community members to draw their own map of the colony, ideally in an open space, using the ground and various objects as symbols, e.g. stones for water points, bottles for liquor stores. Or, it may be drawn on paper, which can be saved and compared with later maps. This gives a good chance for participation and is an enjoyable way of building relationships. The map may reveal both facts about the colony, and/or people's perceptions about it. It can be especially revealing to compare and contrast maps made by different community groups such as men, women, youth and children.

The various techniques described above – including discussions, community walk and mapping, are special methods of assessing community needs usually known as PRA (Participatory Rapid Appraisal). The exact initials and terms used vary from country to country.

From review of available records

It can be very helpful to obtain relevant data from records within the community. For example, illness frequencies may be obtainable from health centre records, and the details of the drainage system from government engineers. Results of previous surveys or the work of other NGOs, or government programmes may be available.

Checking out these sources of information early on can sometimes save us from duplicating work already done.

From conducting a survey

This is an important part of making an accurate community diagnosis. The survey helps us:

- To find out about health and environmental problems in the community.
- To obtain baseline status to help us monitor and evaluate changes.
- To identify vulnerable community members such as young children, pregnant women, the disabled, people with AIDS, those with other serious illnesses such as TB, those at high social risk, from violence or abuse.

Conducting a detailed survey is not usually one of the very early activities since it is relatively expensive and time-consuming. It also requires the trust of the community.

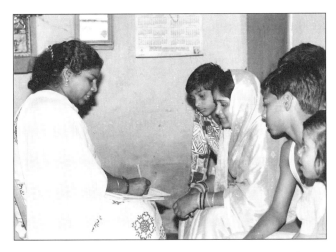

But there are other valuable add-ons:

- It informs community members about the project.
- It builds relationships.
- It dispels mistrust (providing the survey is done sensitively, and with full community participation).
- It starts the process of educating the community.

Figure 3.4   Surveys: an opportunity to make friends and to get to know the community better. (Godfrey Martin/ASHA)

Step 1. Make the survey questionnaire
The questionnaire should be:

- clearly and simply written in local language,
- short – less than 15 minutes required,
- designed for yes/no answers, numbers or ticks, with the minimum of written information: this makes analysis – and computerisation much simpler,
- field tested to ensure questions can be understood and do not cause offence.

Step 2. Decide which type of survey to do
There are two broad categories of surveys:

1. **House-to-house survey**: Every home is visited and data is collected about all household members.

    Advantages:
    - Since every household is visited, the survey can detect all people at risk (e.g. malnourished, pregnant, people with AIDS or tuberculosis, etc.).
    - If the project continues to visit houscholds regularly, at risk members can be regularly added or removed, so enabling the record to be an effective up-to-date management tool.
    - Full population data is known. If the project subsequently keeps track of births, deaths, and in- and out-migrations, an accurate database can be kept. A note of warning: in slum populations this information is difficult to maintain because of the rapid turnover of people: record keeping must not be allowed to dominate programme activities.

    Disadvantage:
    - It requires a large input of labour and time to collect, analyse, interpret and report the findings. Many slums are too large for house-to-house surveys.

❷ **Sample survey**: Only some of the homes are visited. Usually the sample is a randomised systematic sample in which the first house to be visited is chosen randomly and then each 2nd, 5th or 10th, etc., house from that first house is visited (systematic).

Advantages:
- It is quicker than a full house-to-house survey and gives equally valid information about the population.
- It is particularly useful when the target population is very large.

Disadvantages:
- Many at risk people will be missed unless detected in some other way.
- An accurate estimate of population and demographic changes cannot be maintained.

House-to-house survey or a sample survey – which should we do?

A house-to-house survey finds out which community members have a particular characteristic, such as malnutrition. The survey is time-consuming and costly. A sample survey finds out how common a problem such as malnutrition is in a community but not which community members have the problem. It is less costly and faster. In most cases, a sample survey is sufficient to make a community diagnosis.

Sometimes a combination of the two types of survey may be the most useful. Important data is collected from all households (such as notation of woman-headed households, nutritional status of young children, or presence of someone with AIDS or

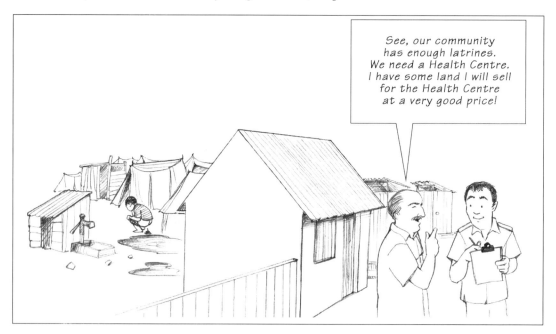

Figure 3.5   When planning a randomised sample survey ensure that the sample represents the total population.

TB, etc.). More detailed information (ages, sex, religion, socio-economic status, etc.) is collected on every 5th or 10th, etc., home.

Step 3. If a sample survey, decide how many households we need to survey

When doing a sample survey, it is important to include enough households to produce meaningful data, and not to include more households than necessary. There is a simple way to calculate the number we need:

❶ Decide which data is the most important. As an example, we will take the nutritional status of children under 3 years.

❷ If we do not know what proportion are severely malnourished, we make an informed guess. For example, we estimate that 25% of the children are severely malnourished (e.g. red on the mid-upper arm circumference band).

❸ Next, we estimate the likely proportion of children who will be malnourished after 3 years (or whenever we repeat the survey). Let's assume it will be about half the present rate, or 12%.

❹ Calculate the difference between the two proportions: 25% – 12% = 13%. Thus 13% is the expected difference.

❺ From Table 3.2, determine how many households need to be surveyed. Since 13% is the expected difference, then we would need a sample size of 195 households.

Step 4. If a sample survey, decide the interval between households

❶ Estimate the number of households in the community. (Often the slum leader or some other key informant can give a good estimate.) Let's say we estimate that there are 1500 households.

❷ Divide the total number of households by the number of households required for the sample. If we need 195 households, then 1500 divided by 195 = 7.6. We should always round off downward, so we need to survey every 7th household. The number 7 is then known as the interval number

Step 5. Prepare survey team members

Members of the survey team need training in two main areas:

❶ **How to interact with the community**. They will need to be:
  - good communicators, ideally being fluent in the local language;

Table 3.2 Sample size needed for sample surveys*					
Expected difference in percentage	2–4%	5–9%	10–14%	15–19%	20% or more
Sample size needed	4805	770	195	90	50

*Sample size based on the expected difference of proportions, extracted from Lwanga, SK and Lemeshow S, 1991, p. 34. Numbers rounded upward to an easily workable number.

- friendly so as to gain co-operation during the interviews and begin building relationship with families;
- tactful when asking questions;
- discrete so there is no gossiping about information discovered;
- patient and persistent to obtain the necessary information.

② **How to obtain information**. Members of the survey team must know:
- how to ask questions, including the precise wording – to obtain consistent information, all members of the survey team must ask the questions in the same way;
- how to record data – they must be familiar with the forms and how to fill them out;
- other special skills such as measuring mid upper-arm circumference.

Role-play is a good way to learn these skills. Interviewers should practise until they can conduct the survey without mistakes. When the team goes into the field it is important for a supervisor to review the completed forms regularly to detect mistakes. This is especially true at the beginning of the survey. Spot checks should be conducted from time to time during the survey. If mistakes are made, they should be corrected, if necessary by revisiting.

From the field: A health programme in Ludhiana, Punjab, India conducted a baseline survey in a new slum community. The results of the survey were surprising: the baseline immunisation coverage of young children was very high. Later on it became obvious that families had not reported truthfully. Only when the community developed trust for project staff did they confide that they had been suspicious. By saying that the children were fully immunised they had hoped the project would go elsewhere. (India)

Source: Authors.

Step 6. Conduct the survey

What time of day should the survey be conducted? In slum communities, adults, including women, often work outside the home. Therefore we should schedule activities when people are most likely to be at home, usually in the early morning or evening.

Numbering the houses. Slum houses are often already numbered for other reasons such as ration cards, voting registration or malaria or dengue prevention. Use those numbers to identify the household. Remember that sometimes a single house may have more than one number, which can lead to confusion. Identify and decide which numbers you will be using.

When households are not already numbered, it may be worthwhile making a metal number tag to attach to each house. If the project does number the houses, the purpose of this must be carefully explained to household members; otherwise they may become suspicious or misunderstand.

Life in a slum

One time a group of outsiders came into a slum where Faisal and his family lived and put a metal number tag on his house. The rumor was that a new government scheme would start soon in which families who lived in the slum would be given a small plot of land. Faisal and many others contacted their relatives in the village and told them to come quickly. Soon there were many extra families packing the slum. The group of outsiders was a CHDP that was simply numbering each household for their records. They had not explained their purpose. When community members finally understood, they became very angry at the CHDP because of the unnecessary expense that their village relatives had incurred by coming to the city for no reason. (Bangladesh)

If a sample survey, decide which household to start with. We should **NOT** start with the first house we come to because that is not a randomly chosen house. We need to select the first house randomly. To do this:

1. Take slips of paper and write a number on each slip from 1 up to the interval number. In our example, that number is 7, so we would have 7 slips of paper with a number written on each slip.

2. Fold the slips, mix them up and then choose a slip at random. Let's say we chose a slip with 6 on it.

3. From the first house, we count houses along the path until we get to the 6th house. We start the survey with this household.

4. After surveying the 6th household, we then survey every 7th household, starting from that house, i.e. 13th, 20th etc.

> When choosing which household to start with, it is helpful to explain what we are doing, and why we are starting with a particular house. Ask a community member, perhaps a child, to choose one of the pieces of paper with the numbers written on it. Then start with that house. This helps people to understand that their own house was not deliberately picked on – or ignored.

It is important that all survey team members agree on what actually constitutes a household. An often-used definition of household is: 'those people who generally eat from the same kitchen' – which in slums often means those who eat the same cooked meals. (Sometimes more than one family will be living in one house. So, those people should be counted as two households if the two families cook and eat meals separately.)

How do we convert the data we have collected into information?

By this stage, we will have collected a lot of data. Now we must convert it into information, which is data that has been converted into a useable form. We must always keep in mind the objective of the community diagnosis: to discover health problems, find their causes and construct solutions.

Using the methods just described, we will have collected two types of data:

- **Qualitative data** are descriptive or narrative, and cannot be tabulated so easily. Examples are observations made on places where children defaecate or breastfeeding practices. Most of the data from discussions and observations are qualitative data.
- **Quantitative data** are data that we can tabulate such as number of people, percentage of children who are malnourished, etc. Most data from the household survey are of this type.

Making qualitative data useful

We need to summarise relevant data that we gathered through discussions, the community walk and through community mapping. At this point we will have a great deal of data and can easily feel overwhelmed. We need to reduce and summarise the data. But sometimes it is hard to know how to organise the information. We must remember the purpose of making a community diagnosis. By this stage, we usually have an idea of what the major problems are, based on what we have seen and heard during the data collection process. If we answer the following questions about the problems, that will give us an idea of what information we need. Table 3.3 gives an example from one slum in which diarrhoea in young children was one of the major health problems in the community.

Making quantitative data useful

Quantitative data must also be summarised so that it can be used. To do this, we first tally up the number of households or household members that had a particular characteristic, e.g. how many households were rich, average, poor or very poor in the Wealth Ranking or how many children were malnourished (see examples below). Then we calculate what percentage of the households or household members had each characteristic.

Table 3.3 Problem: Many cases of diarrhoea in young children with deaths from dehydration	
Question	**Examples of relevant qualitative data**
What are the causes of the problem?	Infrequent hand washing
	Bottle feeding young infants
	Not enough water
	Unsafe water supply
What are the root causes?	Mothers work outside the home
	Caretakers do not know about the importance of hand washing
	Municipal water is supplied only twice a day and there is no storage tank
	Water pipes leak
	Other main source of water is shallow open wells

How do we discuss the diagnosis with the community?

Get the information to the right people at the right time and in the right way so that they can make the right decision!

It is important to present the findings to members of the community at large. We can do this at a community meeting. If the slum is very large, the findings can be presented to a smaller group of interested people, particularly women, who are most likely to take action.

We must present the findings in a way that can be understood. If the community is largely illiterate, we should use maps with symbols, and pictures rather than charts, tables and words.

Use money to convey the concept of percentage. For example, convert percents into cents per dollar or paisa per rupee.

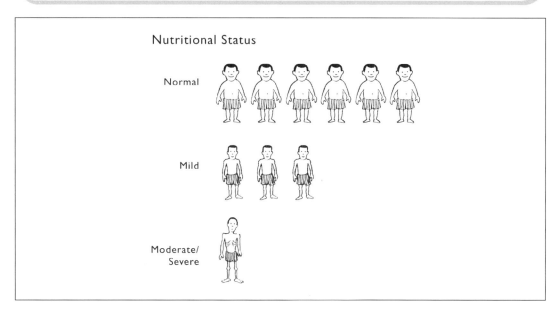

Figure 3.6   When presenting statistics to less educated groups, we can use pictures to convey percentages.

Data that may be helpful to a community health and development project: suggested methods of collection

Demographic data could include total population, age and sex distribution, cultural groups (language, religion, origin, etc.), literacy and school-going, number of households, number of female-headed households and number of people per household, and number of people in/out migrating. This data can be collected most readily through a survey.

Topics and methods of collection for **economic**, **social**, **environmental** and **health data** are shown in Tables 3.5, 3.6, 3.7 and 3.8.

Chapter summary

Many factors should be considered when choosing a community to work with: size, community spirit, political situation, existing services, health status, presence of other agencies, location and government co-operation. An early activity will be to make a community diagnosis in which we gather information about the slum, discover its problems and provide data to help guide solutions. A key way of collecting information is through a survey – either a house-to-house or sample survey. Group, individual and key informant discussions, along with community walks and mapping add further information. Basic to all these activities is training of the team and building relationships with the community.

Table 3.4	Analysis of household survey data: Tally, then convert to a percentage			

Example 1: Wealth ranking

Number of households = 60

House: Wealth category		Number	Calculation	%
Rich	⊞⊞ ⊞⊞	10	10/60 × 100	16.7%
Average	⊞⊞ ⊞⊞ ⊞⊞ ⊞⊞ ⊞⊞ ⊞⊞ I	31	31/60 × 100	51.7%
Poor	⊞⊞ ⊞⊞ II	12	12/60 × 100	20.0%
Very Poor	⊞⊞ II	7	7/60 × 100	11.6%
Total		60		100.0%

Example 2: Immunisation status

Number of children under 5 years of age = 50

Nutritional status

Malnutrition		Number	Calculation	%
None	⊞⊞ ⊞⊞ I	11	11/50 × 100	22.0%
Mild/moderate	⊞⊞ ⊞⊞ ⊞⊞ ⊞⊞ ⊞⊞ I	26	26/50 × 100	52.0%
Severe	⊞⊞ ⊞⊞ III	13	13/50 × 100	26.0%
Total		50		100.0%

Table 3.5 Economic data

Topic	Usual method of collection					
	Survey	Records	Survey walk/ observation	Mapping	Discussions with community members	Interview with key informants/experts
Housing: average size (area); building materials for walls, roofs	✓		✓		✓	✓
Occupation: of head of household; of other household members	✓				✓	✓
Seasonality: of work, availability of cash			✓		✓	✓
Presence of: television, radio, cassette player, fan, cooler, bicycle, computer/modem/internet, etc.	✓				✓	✓
Land: owned, rented, leased, encroached	✓				✓	✓
House: owned, rented		✓			✓	✓

Table 3.6   Social data

Topic	Usual method of collection					
	Survey	Records	Survey walk/ observation	Mapping	Discussions with community members	Interview with key informants/experts
Formal/informal organisations: objectives, effectiveness/achievements, activities, strengths and weaknesses, access and type of community representation					✓	✓
Formal/informal leaders: reason for being a leader (elected or appointed (by whom)), education, profession, landowner, landlord, religious leader, etc.; type of leadership			✓		✓	✓
Decision makers in the community: who makes decisions; who is consulted; role of community members; role of women and youth			✓		✓	✓
Marginalised groups with reasons (religion, origin, occupation, orphans, widows, female heads of households			✓		✓	✓
Disharmony in the community with reasons			✓		✓	✓
Day-care centres, recreational facilities, services for those dependent on alcohol or drugs, street or working children, or the homeless				✓	✓	✓

Table 3.7   Environmental data

Topic	Usual method of collection					
	Survey	Records	Survey walk/ observation	Mapping	Discussions with community members	Interview with key informants/experts
Terrain						
Area/population density	✓	✓	✓	✓		
Water						
Sources: surface, deep/shallow well, municipal; location			✓	✓	✓	✓
Delivery systems: surface, open/closed well, hand/electic pump, piped			✓	✓	✓	
Perceived benefits/disadvantages of various sources					✓	✓
Practices, rituals, beliefs			✓		✓	✓
Access: distance and social			✓	✓	✓	✓
Safety: opportunity for contamination, treated/not treated			✓		✓	✓
Household storage			✓		✓	
Adequacy: number of households dependent upon source, lines, flow rate and duration			✓		✓	
Reliability: breakdowns, dependency upon electricity, seasonality			✓			
Surface water disposal						
Drains (present/absent; covered/non-covered, gradient present?; blocked?; cleaned regularly?)			✓	✓	✓	✓

Table 3.7 Environmental data (continued)

Topic	Survey	Records	Survey walk/ observation	Mapping	Discussions with community members	Interview with key informants/experts
Paths: water/muddy/dry, sometimes/always			✓	✓	✓	
Pools of standing water			✓	✓	✓	
Excreta disposal						
Locations of latrines and open defecation areas			✓	✓	✓	
Latrines: community/group/household			✓	✓	✓	
Access: distance and social			✓		✓	✓
Use: by adult/child and sex			✓		✓	✓
Functioning?			✓	✓	✓	✓
Who maintains/operates/repairs?					✓	✓
Practices, rituals, beliefs, including taboos					✓	✓
Young children defecate in drains?			✓		✓	
Perceived advantages/disadvantages			✓		✓	✓
Solid waste disposal						
Household garbage (mode of disposal)			✓	✓	✓	✓
Community garbage (mode of disposal)			✓	✓	✓	✓
Roads: access for emergency vehicles			✓	✓	✓	✓
Electricity			✓		✓	✓
Schools, places of worship			✓	✓	✓	✓
Government facilities			✓	✓	✓	✓
Other NGOs			✓	✓	✓	✓

Usual method of collection

Table 3.8 Health data

Topic	Usual method of collection					
	Survey	Records	Survey walk/ observation	Mapping	Discussions with community members	Interview with key informants/experts
Common health problems						
Tuberculosis, sexually transmitted diseases (including AIDS), malaria and dengue fever	✓	✓	✓		✓	✓
In children: acute respiratory infection, diarrhoea, measles and malnutrition	✓	✓	✓		✓	✓
Maternal deaths	✓	✓				✓
Trauma, especially related to workplace, and accidental deaths due to burns, electric shock, drowning and road accidents	✓	✓			✓	✓
Domestic violence, alcoholism, drug abuse, prostitution and child labour?	✓	✓	✓		✓	✓
Personal hygiene						
Hand washing			✓		✓	✓
Food handling/storage			✓		✓	✓
Household waste disposal			✓	✓	✓	✓
Household cleanliness			✓		✓	✓
Bathing			✓			✓
Health services						
Health care providers: private/government; qualified doctors, traditional healers, quacks			✓		✓	✓

Table 3.8 Health data (continued)

Topic	Usual method of collection					
	Survey	Records	Survey walk/ observation	Mapping	Discussions with community members	Interview with key informants/experts
General curative		✓	✓	✓	✓	✓
Diagnostic and treatment services for tuberculosis		✓	✓	✓	✓	✓
Maternal and child health services (immunisations, vitamin A, antenatal care, etc.)	✓	✓	✓	✓	✓	✓
Trained birth attendants		✓			✓	✓
Deaths (infant, child, maternal, others)	✓	✓			✓	✓

Resources

1. *Power, Process and Participation: Tools for Change.* R Slocum, L Wichhart, D Rocheleau, B Thomas–Slayter. Intermediate Technology Publications, 1998. Provides many participative, innovative tools for information gathering.

2. *Managing for a Change: How to Run Community Development Projects.* A Davies. Intermediate Technology Publications, 1997. An excellent resource that guides through identifying problems and identifying solutions.

3. *Poverty and Health: Reaping a Richer Harvest.* M Feuerstein. Macmillan Education, 1997. Very good sections on ways to help the community analyse its situation in a participatory way. (Available from TALC.)

4. *Guidelines for Rapid Participatory Appraisals to Assess Community Health Needs: A Focus on Health Improvements for Low-income Urban and Rural Areas.* H Annett, SB Rifkin. WHO, 1995. Very practical stepwise presentation of planning and conducting rapid participatory appraisals.

5. *Community Assessment: Guidelines for Developing Countries.* D Stockman. Intermediate Technology Publications, 1994. Systematic step-wise discussion of how to do a community assessment.

6. *Health Care Together: Training Exercises for Health Workers in Community Based Programmes.* MP Johnston, SB Rifkin. Macmillan Education, 1987. Many exercises that help health workers to develop the essential skills needed to work in genuine partnership with communities. (Available from TALC.)

7. *Planning Urban Community Health.* TALC, 1987. A set of slides about assessing health and other problems in a slum community

8. *Supporting Development Action: From Identification to Evaluation.* E Beaudoux, G de Combrugghe, F Douchamps, M-C Gueneau, M Nieukirk. Macmillan Education, 1992. A set of guidelines for development projects.

9. *A Trainer's Guide for Participatory Learning and Action.* JN Pretty, I Guijt, I Scoones, J Thompson. International Institute for Environment and Development, 1995. Comprehensive review containing many games and exercises for use in training and in the field.

4 Making an action plan

What is an action plan?

An **action plan** is a tool that helps the community and CHDP to plan and carry out activities towards meeting the overall goals.

How does an action plan help?

An action plan helps both the community and the CHDP:

1. To have a sense of direction and purpose.
2. To remain 'on course' and make progress towards defined objectives.
3. To monitor progress towards meeting those objectives.
4. To manage its activities.
5. To motivate community members and staff. When the community and staff participate in making the action plan, they will understand and feel ownership of the activities.
6. To inform others (e.g. donors and other partners) of future plans.

> When there is no clear action plan that is understood and owned by both staff and community, everyone involved slips into a monotonous routine, staff become demotivated and the community loses interest.

When do we make an action plan?

Normally an action plan arises naturally from the results of the community diagnosis. If action plans are made earlier, at the insistence of donors and without community involvement, the programme is unlikely to be community-based or sustainable.

Each year, through regular monitoring, action plans can be refined and developed. Every 3 or 5 years after more major evaluations they can be revised or rewritten – but always as a joint exercise of the CHDP and the community.

Goals, objectives and plans

It is helpful to understand the different terms: goals (or aims), objectives and action plans.

The overall **goal** or **aim** of a CHDP project is a broad statement about why the project exists. Goals are the desired end-result of project activities. An example might be: 'To improve the health of slum colonies in active partnership with their members.' The goals of smaller CHDP projects, or those concentrating on particular aspects of health and development may be more specific. For example: 'To improve water and sanitation facilities in colony X', or 'To improve the overall health of children under

5 years of age.' Goals may have been included in the overall mission statement at the very start of the project. But often a project may never have formally stated its goals. If that is the case it is worth taking time to do that now – before developing an action plan, as all plans must fit in with project goals.

The goal is then broken down into specific **objectives**, which are statements of what the project and the community intend to achieve within a period of time. Examples might be: 'To provide seven deep bore wells in community X within 3 years' or 'To reduce the incidence of malaria by 50% within one year in community Y'. Step 2 starting on page 64 looks at setting objectives in more detail.

An **action plan** describes the process by which each objective is fulfilled.

In practice overall goals are often defined before much community work starts – any CHDP has to be aware of its own skills, capabilities and purpose before sharing in detail with community members. Objectives and action plans however must always arise from joint partnership with the community. The community diagnosis is an essential part of this process.

What steps are used in making an action plan?

Step 1. Prioritise the problems

As we analyse information gathered from the community diagnosis, a number of problems will come to light. Since the community cannot deal with all these problems at once, we will need to have a system of prioritising them. This process is made much easier if we answer these four simple questions:

1. **Is the problem serious**? For example, does the problem cause death or serious illness in young children or during pregnancy?

2. **Is the problem common**? Does it affect most community members? When resources are limited, they should be targeted for doing the most good for the most people.

3. **Can the problem be reduced or eliminated relatively easily** (e.g. in terms of cost, time, political will, etc.)? We will only know this if we first discover the causes of the problems. Only then can we assess how easily a problem can be solved. (A SWOT analysis as shown in Table 4.2 below is a helpful tool in doing this.)

4. **Is the community interested** in reducing or eliminating the problem? The problem must be a felt need in the community, or if it isn't we can create awareness to generate a strong commitment to do something about it.

A ranking table is helpful to prioritise problems. List each problem in the first column and the four criteria for ranking described above in the other column heads. Then in each column for each problem give scores from 1 to 3, with 1 being the least serious or least common etc., and 3 being the most. Then add up the scores for each problem. The problem with the highest score has the highest priority – in the example in Table 4.1 in adequate water supply comes out top.

Table 4.1	Ranking table for prioritising problems				
Problem	Serious ?	Common ?	Relatively easy solutions ?	Community interest?	Total Score
People with AIDS have no care-takers	3	1	2	1	7
Water supply is inadequate	3	3	2	3	11
Men drink too much alcohol	2	2	1	1	6
Measles epidemics	3	2	3	1	9

A SWOT analysis is a useful tool for working out how easy (or difficult) it is to solve a particular problem. SWOT stands for Strengths (S) and Weaknesses (W) – within the community; and Opportunities (O) and Threats (T) – from outside the community. An effective approach takes advantage of Strengths and Opportunities, and aims to overcome Weaknesses and Threats. This technique helps to determine the best strategy to incorporate into our action plans. An example is given in Table 4.2 about a community that is considering a community latrine complex.

Table 4.2 A SWOT analysis for a proposed community latrine complex		
SWOT	Strategy	Plan
Strength: Community has several divorced or widowed women who are doing unskilled construction work	• Train women in skills needed for latrine construction	• Identify women • Arrange training • Use them as resources when building latrines
Weakness: Land is too marshy so pit latrines cannot be used	• Persuade government to permit connection to municipal system • Determine site that is close to municipal sewer lines	• Visit government officials, agencies and politicians • Locate places where the sewer system runs closest to the community
Opportunity: International funding agency is willing to provide training for making latrine slabs from locally available materials	• Empower women's group to be responsible for making low-cost slabs for sale to community	• Motivate women's' group • Find production space
Threat: Latrines will become dirty and then people will stop using them if government appoints and poorly supervises outside agency to maintain latrines	• Community will hire cleaners, attendant and supervisor • CAG will supervise • Small user fee will be charged to cover expenses	• Inform community; increase awareness of need for income to pay for cleaners, etc. • Hire latrine staff • Train latrine staff • Monitor that latrines are clean and working

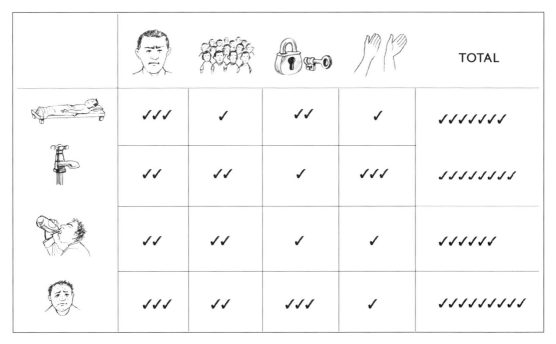

					TOTAL
	✓✓✓	✓	✓✓	✓	✓✓✓✓✓✓
	✓✓	✓✓	✓	✓✓✓	✓✓✓✓✓✓✓
	✓✓	✓✓	✓	✓	✓✓✓✓✓✓
	✓✓✓	✓✓	✓✓✓	✓	✓✓✓✓✓✓✓✓✓

Figure 4.1   When prioritising problems with illiterate people, we can use pictures and symbols to signify problems, and rank priorities (see Table 4.2).

Selecting which problem to work on is always a very important decision. This may be the first time a community has come together to solve its own problems. Success is obviously important and may make all the difference to future co-operation and progress. Here are some criteria that will maximise the chances of success. Choose a problem that:

● will benefit many,

● has little or no opposition,

● has a good chance of success,

● can be solved quickly,

● will clearly show obvious visual change for the better.

Sometimes an obvious opportunity arises which has to be grasped quickly, as the example below shows.

Life in a slum

In one slum community, the major problem from the community's point of view was poor drainage, which made the only road into the slum almost impossible to walk on. People had to navigate through the water over a series of bricks, stones and boards. The government had recently finished building a community latrine complex, which was located on the edge of the community. Some senior government officials were coming the following day to inaugurate the complex. When the community heard about the up-coming inauguration, a community meeting was held to decide if the visit could be used to get something done about the waterlogged road. The community knew that they could never get such senior government officials to come again to see their plight. Therefore the community appointed some spokespersons who would speak to the visiting government officials and insist that they walk into the slum to see the road. The next morning, the government area engineer arrived early to see that the area was cleaned up for the inauguration and the visiting dignitaries. He had brought some workers to add some sand to the road to make it look better temporarily. The community refused to let them work on the road. When the dignitaries arrived, the community spokespersons told the dignitaries about the road and then accompanied them on a walk down the road. The senior government officials were aghast at the condition of the road and, impressed by the community unity and solidarity, ordered the same area engineer to see that a critical drain was built. Within a month, the drain was built and the road was no longer a river, but a road. (Kenya)

Step 2. Set objectives

Having decided with the community which problems to work on together, the next step is to set objectives. Here are some examples:

❶ To reduce the prevalence of moderate and severe malnutrition among children 1–3 years of age from 25% to 15% by the end of 2002.

❷ To install three tube wells in colony X within the next year.

❸ To provide home care for 30 people with AIDS in our community in the next year.

Why set objectives?

Setting objectives helps us to:

❶ **make specific and realistic plans**;

❷ **monitor our progress** in achieving those plans;

❸ **document and celebrate success.**

How do we construct a good objective?

An objective must be **SMART**:

A SMART Objective:	
S – Specific	Relates to a specific event, activity or impact.
M – Measurable	Has an indicator that is measurable.
A – Achievable	Can be accomplished bearing in mind strengths, weaknesses, opportunities and threats.
R – Relevant	Can reduce or solve a serious problem relevant to the community.
T – Time-bound	Can be accomplished in a specified period of time.

Practically speaking, it is better to construct objectives that represent relatively small steps to be accomplished over a short time period. We go through the steps shown in Table 4.3 to construct a good objective. We will use the third objective given above as the example.

Step 3. Construct the action plan

List the tasks required to accomplish each objective

These should be listed in order, with an estimate of how long each activity is likely to take. Remember that some activities can be carried out at the same time. For example, our objective is as follows: to ensure that 7 of our 10 deep wells function effectively during the next year, as reported weekly by community health volunteers to the women's CAG.

A list of activities to achieve this objective might be:

- Appoint a community health volunteer to be in charge of each well.
- Train the community health volunteers in monitoring and in simple pump repairs.
- Find out the problems affecting each pump/well and the estimated costs to fix them.
- Obtain funds to pay for parts and labour.
- Repair pumps/wells using community labour if possible.

Table 4.3 Steps to construct a good objective	
Step	**Example**
1. Restate the negative problem as a positive objective.	**Problem**: Some people with AIDS are not getting good home care.
	Objective: To provide home care for people with AIDS.
2. Make sure the objective is **SPECIFIC**.	**Objective**: To provide home care for people with AIDS *in our community*
3. Make sure there is a **MEASURABLE** indicator in the objective.	**Objective**: To provide home care for *30* people with AIDS.
4. Make sure the objective is **ACHIEVABLE**.	Consider:
	Do we have enough staff to provide care to 30 patients?
	Are there at least 30 people with AIDS who will require and request care from us?
5. Make sure the objective is **RELEVANT**.	Is AIDS a serious problem in the community and is the community concerned about it?
6. Make the objective **TIME–BOUND**.	**Objective**: To provide home care for 30 people with AIDS in our community *in the next year.*

- Monitor and make future repairs as necessary.
- Community health volunteers to report on progress and new problems weekly at the regular meeting of the CAG.

Plan each activity

For each task, answer the following questions:

1 **When should it start and when should it be finished?**

2 **Who does it?**

3 **Who is responsible for seeing it is actually carried out?**

4 **What materials are needed?**

When planning, think: WHO does WHAT WHEN and HOW.

More detailed planning about each area of activity is discussed in greater length in the relevant chapters.

Step 4. Monitor and evaluate the activity

What is monitoring?

Monitoring is the periodic checking of the progress being made towards meeting our objectives.

How can monitoring help us?

Monitoring helps us to:

- gauge our progress towards project objectives,
- identify problems,
- measure achievement of targets.

For example, take the objective above: providing home care for 30 people with AIDS in the next year. We can monitor our progress by keeping track of the number of households we start working with. If after 6 months we have been providing care to only eight people, as opposed to the ideal 15, we know there will be a lot of catching up to do. We must devote more time and resources in the second part of the year if we are going to meet this particular objective.

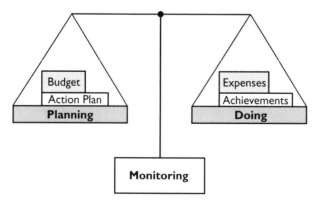

Figure 4.2   Monitoring helps us to keep track of and control project finances and activities.

What are indicators?

Monitoring, except of the simplest type, requires indicators. An **indicator** is a measurement that helps us to monitor our progress towards an objective (**process indicator**) or to assess the value of our activities (**impact indicator**).

- **Process indicators** are a way of measuring the **activities** we carry out to improve health. Examples are percentage of children 1–2 years of age who have received primary courses of immunisations, percentage of deliveries carried out by trained birth attendants, number of water points installed, etc. These are the commonest, and often the simplest, indicators used to monitor activities.

- **Impact indicators** measure the value or **effectiveness of the activities** we carry out. Examples, reflecting the same illustration used above are the numer of cases of immunisable illnesses which occur in the community, and the number of pregnancy related illnesses and deaths which occur. Impact indicators are ultimately more useful than process indicators, but usually more difficult to measure.

Indicators can also be classified as quantitave or numerical, or as qualitative or descriptive. Quantitative indicators are effective ways to help monitor improvements in health and environmental activities. But to monitor development activities or behavioural change, qualitative indicators can be more helpful. For example, compare the following qualitative and quantitative indicators for monitoring the empowerment of women.

- **Qualitative or descriptive indicators**: Women no longer cover their faces at public meetings, they are unafraid to express their point of view in front of community leaders, together they prohibited an illicit liquor shop from making and selling spirits.

- **Quantitative or numerical indicators**: The number of women's group meetings in a 12-month period, the average number attending per meeting.

Table 4.4 gives examples of process and impact indicators used to monitor objectives in health and environmental activities.

From the field: Using a simple indicator. Initial discussions with community members of a large East African slum suggested that a contaminated and inadequate water supply was a major problem. As part of the community diagnosis, the CHDP and community discovered the number of functioning water points in the community. They then used this number as an indicator. By resurveying every year they could see how this number changed as a way of monitoring whether progress was being made towards improving the water supply. (Kenya)

Source: Author visit.

It is important that we design our monitoring system wisely. It must provide us with information that we need to know but should not overburden the staff and community members. We should select a **few** indicators that are important to know about and **easy to find out about**, and which will be **useful** for planning. The specific indicators we choose must be sensitive to our chosen activities and their objectives.

Table 4.4 Some examples of indicators used in community health and development

Activity	Objective	Process indicator	Impact indicator
Health-related			
Giving at least 3 months' supply of iron tablets to all pregnant women	To ensure that as least 60% of women who deliver in the next 12 months will have received at least 3 months' supply of iron before delivery	% of women who have received 3 months' supply of iron prior to delivery	% of women who have delivered who are anaemic
Promoting breastfeeding from birth to 2 years of age and supplemental foods from age 6 months	To ensure that 75% of all infants 6–9 months of age during this year are still breastfeeding but also receiving supplementary foods	% of children 6–9 months of age who are still breastfeeding and also receiving supplemental foods	Nutritional status of children 1–2 years of age
Administration of measles vaccine	To ensure that 90% of children who are between 1 and 2 years of age at year end will have received measles vaccine	% of children 1–2 years of age who have received measles vaccine	Number of cases of measles
Environment-related			
Install tube wells	To install 3 tube wells in the community during the next year	Number of wells installed	Number of households per water point
Install community latrines	To construct 6 group latrines (8 latrines per unit) in the community during the next year	Number of latrines installed	Number of diarrhoea cases per child per year Number of households per latrine Number of cases of worm infestations per child per year
Encourage use of insecticide-treated mosquito nets	To arrange distribution of treated nets to 75% of children aged 0–5	% of households that use nets	Number of cases of malaria

The box below summarises this.

KISS!

Monitoring system: Keep It Short and Simple!

1. Select key indicators that will definitely be used.

2. Select indicators for which the data are easy to collect.

3. Do not overburden workers with collecting excessive data that will not be used.

4. Provide feedback to all participants and interested parties quickly.

5. Use the results.

6. Use a reporting format that makes analysis easy.

What is evaluation?

Evaluation is a more major assessment of the value or impact that a programme is having on the community. It will make use of information gathered through regular monitoring, especially through impact indicators, but also look beyond this to other sources, including team and community members. Cost effectiveness and sustainability are two issues that are often carefully looked at.

From the field: The women's groups organised by ASHA, a CHDP project in Delhi, monitor the health of their community at their weekly meeting when the community health worker presents the following:

1. All births that have occurred in the last week, whether they were conducted by a trained birth attendant, and any problems that arose.

2. All deaths that have occurred in the last week, the cause and circumstances of the death and whether it could have been prevented. They keep close track of the deaths of under-5 children and of women during pregnancy or delivery.

They maintain the data on a chart, which becomes part of the annual statistics that are presented at a community meeting when they make plans for the following year. (India)

Source: Authors

Evaluations usually take place every 3 to 5 years. Often outsiders with special expertise, who ideally also have some knowledge of the country and the project take part in this. They work together with members of the CHDP and the community. Quite frequently donor agencies request evaluations and pay for the costs. Sometimes they can be time-consuming which can add to the stress and overwork of project staff. However evaluations well carried out are useful to a variety of people:

- to **project staff and the participating community members**, who will use results and suggestions to reset objectives and plan for the future;

- to the **community-at-large**, which normally enjoys the participation and affirmation it brings;
- to **donors** who will know if their money is being spent responsibly and may wish to increase, decrease or target future support;
- to **government**, **agencies or other institutions** that have a vested interest in knowing whether the project is effective and achieving its objectives. This helps them to decide whether to continue partnership or support.

In summary an evaluation will help the programme to:

- see if its work is having an effect on the health of the community,
- plan future activities,
- determine reasons for success or failure,
- decide how to improve results.

Chapter summary

Following a community diagnosis the CHDP in partnership with the community constructs an action plan. This must fit in with the project's overall goals. The steps in drawing up an action plan include: prioritising problems, setting objectives, constructing the plan, and monitoring the outcome. This chapter includes, with the aid of charts and tables, a variety of practical ways to help in each of these four stages.

Resources

1. *Poverty and Health: Reaping a Richer Harvest.* M Feuerstein. Macmillan Education, 1997. Very good section on the use of indicators and participatory monitoring and evaluation. (Available from TALC.)

2. *The Use of Epidemiology in Local Health Planning.* A Kroeger *et al.* Zed Books, 1997. An excellent training tool for health workers to integrate basic epidemiology into: keeping records, calculating rates and percentages, making graphs, etc.

3. *Participatory Development Tool Kit: Training Materials for Agencies and Communities.* D Narayan, L Srinivasan. The World Bank, 1994. Good materials for participatory techniques.

4. *Participatory Evaluation: Tools for Managing Change in Water and Sanitation.* D Narayan. The World Bank, 1993. Has many practical examples.

5. *Partners in Evaluation: Evaluating Development and Community Programmes with Participants.* MT Feuerstein. Macmillan Education, 1986. Covers all aspects of evaluation of CHDP activities simply and with partnership in mind. (Available from TALC.)

6. *Planning Urban Community Health.* TALC, 1987. A set of slides about how to work with a slum community to develop a plan to deal with its problems.

7. *Facilitator's Guide to Participatory Decision-making.* S Kaner, L Lind, C Toldi, S Fisk, D Berger. New Society Publishers, 1996. Discusses the decision-making process, problems that can occur and how to deal with them.

5 Urban community health volunteers

Community health volunteers play an essential role in all CHDP activities. They show the community's interest in real participation and how committed they are to improve their health practices.

Who are community health volunteers?

Community health volunteers (CHVs) are people from the community, usually women, who receive extensive training in primary health care. They have two important roles: they **provide services** and they are **agents of change**. Worldwide a variety of names are used to describe CHVs, two common examples being community health workers (CHWs) or urban community volunteers (UCVs). Their rural equivalents are usually known as Village Health Workers (VHWs).

CHVs have a unique role in the community for several reasons:

1. They are **acceptable** to, and **respected** by, the community because the community selects them.
2. They **know** and **understand** the community because they live in the community. They can explain concepts using local language and ideas.
3. They are **available** to the community because they live in the community.
4. They are **cost-effective** because they are relatively inexpensive to train and they are paid relatively cheaply for their time and efforts.
5. They act as a **liaison** between the community and the CHDP.
6. They become **resources** for future activities, leading to empowerment of the community and sustainability of change.

> **Lesson from the field**: In the Yala Urban Health Programme in Patan, Nepal, the ward (smallest government unit) committee in the target area select women to serve as health promoters. Each promoter is responsible for 25–35 households in her immediate neighbourhood. The promoters visit each household at least once a month, identify health problems, give appropriate health teaching, and do referral and follow-up as needed. In one ward, the health promoter identified a severely handicapped child whose existence had been denied over the past 4 years of visits by the project Urban Health Worker.
>
> **Lessons learned**: Nobody knows a community better than the members themselves. And when sensitive issues arise, a friendly neighbour can lead the way.
>
> **Source**: C Preston, Yala Urban Health Programme, Patan, Nepal.

What are the functions and tasks of community health volunteers?

Community health volunteers have many functions. Different programmes will use them in different ways, and larger programmes may train CHVs to have more specialist roles. Here is a comprehensive list of possible functions and tasks:

They provide health care

- **Maternal/child health**: They educate and motivate; detect new pregnancies; provide antenatal care; recognise and refer women with complications of pregnancy and delivery; conduct deliveries; provide post-natal care; provide child care; detect malnourished children; give demonstrations on good nutrition and oral rehydration therapy, and assist in clinic.

- **Family planning**: They educate and motivate; provide contraceptives; and facilitate tubal ligations/vasectomies.

- **Illness and injury**: They educate and motivate; treat simple illnesses and accidents; and recognise and refer serious health problems. They have a particular role in the care and prevention of diarrhoea and acute respiratory infection.

- **Tuberculosis**: They educate and motivate; detect new cases; and act as observer and/or tracer for DOTS (Daily Observed Treatment, Short-course) programme. (See page 177.)

- **HIV/AIDS**: They educate and motivate; provide condoms; and provide, train and supervise home-based care. (See page 162.)

> Community health volunteers identify those who might be overlooked or excluded, such as the disabled or very poor. These are more likely to be sick or in need.

They work for a healthy environment

- **Safe water supply**: They educate and motivate; monitor wells, pumps and pipes; and chlorinate wells.

- **Safe sanitation**: They educate and motivate; and monitor drains, community latrines and walkways.

- **Housing**: They participate in the management and operation of the housing society.

They facilitate development

- **Mobilising the community**: They motivate, organise and facilitate community groups; encourage school-going and facilitate literacy activities, including community libraries.

- **Monitoring of community activities**: They educate and motivate; maintain records; and facilitate use of agreed indicators.
- **Advocacy in social issues**: They motivate and educate; monitor, counsel and refer in cases of domestic violence, alcoholism, and drug addiction.

> **From the field**: In some of the *favelas* (slums) of Rio De Janeiro, women from the community are chosen to be 'Sanitary Education Agents' (SEAs). Their selection is based, in part, on their communication skills. The selected women are trained in primary health care and urban environmental problems. Following the training the women are paid one and a half times the minimum wage by the municipality and work eight hours a day. Previous attempts using unpaid volunteers had failed. The job responsibilities of the SEAs include doing a baseline survey, house to house health promotion and sanitary education, and running street meetings as well as large community meetings to discuss environmental sanitation and health. These SEA's work in their *favela* for 2 years while the major environmental improvements are made and community members learn to take care of their environment. The programme then moves on to other *favelas*. (Brazil)
>
> **Source**: Author visit.

The training of community health volunteers

Where should the training take place?

Training should be held in the community, or as near to it as possible. This has many advantages:

- The community is available for practical parts of the training course.
- The site is convenient for the trainees and minimises dropouts and absenteeism.
- It is practical and economical to bring one trainer to the community rather than to take many trainees to another site.

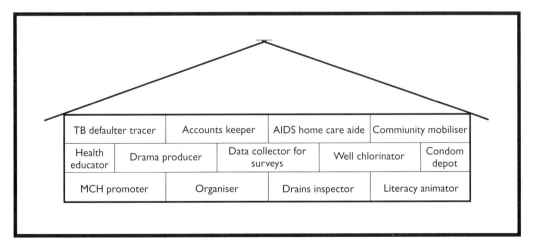

Figure 5.1   Some roles of Community Health Volunteers that help to build a healthy community.

One problem commonly arises: there is often limited space or no appropriate site within the slum. Sometimes a nearby community hall or room can be used, or space at the nearest health centre.

What should be the length of training?

The length and intensity of training will largely depend on what the role and functions of the CHV are planned to be. Ideally initial training should be daily, but CHVs may not have the time for a daily lesson. Adequate training in all components of primary health care takes 2–3 months if training is daily and proportionately longer if only done 2 or 3 times per week. Usually there is an intensive time of training for 1–4 weeks, and then regular (weekly to monthly) training sessions thereafter. Because of the wide range of skills needed and ever-changing situations in a slum, regular training and update must be built into the schedule of CHVs, during their entire term of service. Practical hands-on learning, and apprenticeship/mentoring from more experienced CHVs or staff workers should be part of this.

What should CHVs learn?

First of all CHVs must have the right attitude – even more crucial than knowledge and skills. Here are some key attitudes that need to be encouraged:

- willingness to share knowledge and skills with others;
- respect for **all** members and groups within the community;
- desire to serve the community;
- desire to learn.

> If the CHVs are literate and an appropriate book is available, organise the training around the book. Give each CHV her own copy to study from and to keep as a reference, and make sure she knows how to use the index.

Unhelpful attitudes that need to be discouraged include a strong wish for personal gain, promotion and financial reward.

The knowledge and skills of CHVs must cover the following areas:

- All aspects of **primary health care, environmental improvement** and **community development** as described earlier in this chapter. Chief among these will be:
    - care of mothers and children, including pregnancy care and nutrition
    - curative care
    - care and advocacy in social problems
    - improvement of water and sanitation services at community and household levels.

- **Communication** and **health education.**
- **Legal rights** of citizens, government policies, etc.

- **How to interact with government officials**, including effective letter-writing and competence in visiting offices.
- **How to present a need, case or viewpoint**.
- **Keeping records and simple accounts**.
- The **development process**: i.e. how to determine and prioritise needs, make and implement plans, and monitor progress.
- **Community participation** in all phases of the programme.
- **Motivating** people and **mobilising** community groups.

How training can lead to empowerment

- Focus learning sessions on community problems and how to solve them.

- Discover what CHVs already know and build on their knowledge and experience.

- Focus less on knowledge and more on problem-solving and communication skills and on changes in attitude.

- Promote interactive discussions through the use of role-playing, problem solving, puppet shows, pictures and videos.

It is inappropriate to have a highly trained person such as a doctor or nurse to train CHVs. More important is to train trainers to understand three key concepts: sustainable development, empowerment and the full roles which CHVs can play in the development process.

Many resources are available about the training and functions of health workers. Some are listed at the end of the chapter.

The selection of community health volunteers

Don't be in a hurry to select CHVs. First mobilise the formation of a Community Action Group and then help the CAG to choose the CHV with input from the Community Health and Development Programme.

Who chooses the CHVs: community or CHDP?

The community (often through the CAG) should select the community health volunteers. Often project staff with limited experience will be tempted to select, or suggest volunteers, with little community input into the decision. When this happens, a key chance for engaging the community in its own development is missed. In addition, other problems can occur:

- Since the community did not participate in the decision, it feels no obligation to recognise or co-operate with the volunteer.
- Both community and volunteer feel that the CHV is a part of the CHDP staff, and therefore should be a paid employee of the CHDP.
- The project may be unaware of circumstances that make a volunteer unsuitable – or unacceptable to certain segments of the community.

To avoid these problems, the community should select the CHVs themselves. Before they choose CHVs two things are essential: first helping the community to understand that the people themselves are responsible for making improvements to their own community. Second understanding the roles and functions of the CHV. Only then will the community choose CHVs with the right blend of caring attitudes and real determination to get things done.

Encourage the community to select volunteers from all segments of the community. Sometimes when free training is about to be offered powerful community members try to monopolise the selection process in order to get their relatives or friends elected. Help the community action group to resist these pressures.

From the field: ASHA, a community health and development project in New Delhi, India, first facilitates the organisation of a women's group in the community. The group then selects some of its members to undergo intensive training in primary health care. They select more women than they need for CHVs since some women drop out or are found to be unsuitable as CHVs. At the conclusion of the training, some of the women are then selected by the group to be CHVs. (India)

Lessons learned: Advantages of training many women and delaying the decision are:

① The knowledge and skills of many community members are improved.

② The community and the prospective volunteers have a better understanding of what is expected before final selection.

③ The community and the CHDP can get a better idea of who would make the most effective CHVs.

Source: Authors.

What qualities make effective CHVs?

Effective community health volunteers:

- are interested in the work,
- want to serve the community,
- are respected and acceptable to most members of the community,
- have good communication skills,

- have leadership potential,
- are intelligent though not necessarily highly educated,
- are supported and encouraged by their family. (This may not always be true initially and we should not be deterred by this. However, family support and encouragement help CHVs to be more effective.)

> It is especially important for volunteers to understand the community's responsibility in bringing about improvements, and their own role as agents of change.

How are the community volunteers supervised?

Accountability to the community action group

The CHV should be accountable to the community group, usually through the CAG, not to the project. This helps to reinforce the concept that the community is responsible for its own health care.

The CHV should report regularly to the CAG meeting. Here are some topics that can be covered:

- activities,
- vital health events in the community (births, deaths, serious illnesses) and concerns about the health of the community,

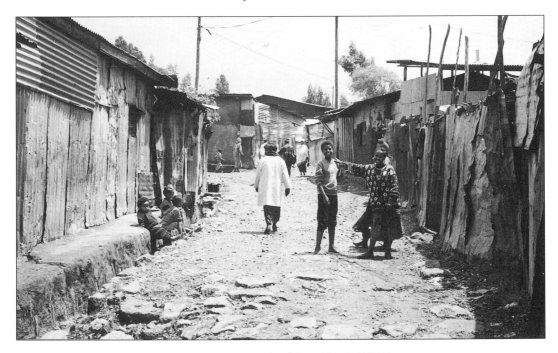

Figure 5.2   CHV talking to people in the community. (Kiran Martin/ASHA)

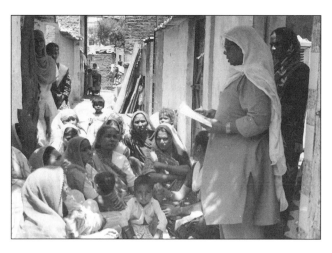

- environmental concerns (water supply and sanitation), and any improvements carried out,
- any other concerns or problems.

Figure 5.3   A CHV is giving her weekly report to the CAG, in this case a women's group. Regular weekly reporting encourages accountability of the CHV and involvement of the CAG. (Godfrey Martin/ASHA)

> The CAG should also protect the CHV who may be accused of not treating correctly a child or adult who dies.

Supervision by the CAG is important, especially when the CHV is new and inexperienced. Because the CHV is accountable to the CAG, that group, rather than the CHDP will usually be responsible for any correction or discipline that may prove necessary.

> The CAG will itself need to be trained in monitoring and supervisory skills so that it can work effectively with the community health volunteers.

Encouragement by CHDP staff

Although CHVs are largely accountable to the community, they will need encouragement and affirmation from the CHDP. Input by project staff will be needed:

- to encourage, motivate and support,
- to increase skills and knowledge through on-the-job training,
- to increase efficiency and effectiveness.

The support of CHVs is ideally co-ordinated by a trained supervisor who will provide regular training sessions, observe volunteers at work, talk with community members and guide the CAG in how best to encourage and support the CHV themselves.

Summary of the CHV's support systems

CHVs have major responsibilities, difficult jobs, and yet are members of the slum community who have had little experience in taking responsibility. They will only survive, and thrive, if strong and dependable support systems are in place for them. In summary this will come from:

- **CHDP staff**: It is not just the CHV who lacks experience in the beginning but also the community, which may have very limited understanding, belief or confidence in their recently elected CHV. Therefore, especially at the start, the CHDP will be a main provider of support. **CHDP staff should set the tone for the community by treating CHVs as colleagues and with respect**.

- **Other CHVs**: It is important to provide opportunities for CHVs to get together to generate a supportive peer group. Everyone can share his or her experiences – successes, failures or problems. Older, more experienced CHVs can provide newer CHVs with insights and suggestions on how to handle difficult situations. More formal mentoring can be set up where one or more inexperienced CHVs link up with a more experienced colleague.

> Experienced CHVs who have earned respect in their communities, should be involved with the training and support of newly appointed CHVs, both during the original phases of training and in developing their skills in community work.

- **Family**: Initially families, especially husbands of CHVs, may resent the time CHVs spend away from the home. With time, however, as the CHVs gain the respect of the community and as the community's health improves through their work, families become more supportive. Where families are unhelpful it is important to help them understand the role of the CHV at an early stage.

- **The Community Action Group**: In addition to its role in accountability, the CAG must also function as a friendly support group. Members of the CAG should assist the CHV by sharing tasks and responsibilities. For example, they can become 'lane volunteers' in which they are responsible for monitoring and improving the health of people living in a group of households.

Ways to keep CHVs motivated

At times the job of a CHV can be discouraging. Mobilising a community to become healthier is no easy task! Motivation becomes a key issue. Here are some of the ways this can be done:

- **Provide in-service training**: CHVs sometime forget skills and lose knowledge: they need to have refresher courses, and be part of a 'learning culture' in which the whole project encourages the idea of learning, and 'allows' members to show their ignorance and ask questions.

- **Train in new skills** associated with new activities and responsibilities, especially when work becomes monotonous and unrewarding.

- **Expose CHVs to successful work** being done in other communities.

- **Create opportunities for sharing with other CHVs**, especially those who are good role models.

- **Praise, encourage and support CHVs**, especially during difficult times both in their community work and personal or family life.

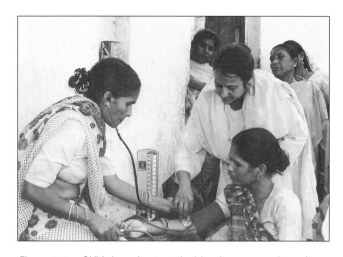

Figure 5.4   *CHVs learning to take blood pressures. Learning new skills helps to keep CHVs motivated. And when CHVs have special skills, the community respects and values them more. (Godfrey Martin/ASHA)*

- **Publicly affirm their work** during community events, or VIP visits.

- **Provide opportunities for socialising** with other CHVs and CHDP staff, such as birthday celebrations, outings and recreation.

- **Provide appropriate remuneration** for their work, in line with any agreement – and on time.

The payment of community health volunteers

Why should urban CHVs be paid?

Debates continue about whether or not CHVs should be paid for their time and effort. Valid arguments exist on both sides. Whether CHVs are paid or not, the idea of service to the community must be built on and encouraged. However there are strong reasons for paying CHVs who live and work in slums:

① They undergo extensive training and spend several hours each day working in the community.

② Some kind of paid work is generally available to slum-dwellers. Therefore it will be difficult to recruit people as CHVs if no payment is given. The cash economy of city life requires payment in order to survive.

③ It is cost-effective:
  - It reduces CHV turnover. When CHVs are not paid, many quickly become less motivated and interested and eventually stop working. Costly time and effort goes into training new CHVs to take their place.
  - Several CHVs can be hired for the same amount of money required to employ a single nurse. CHVs can perform many of the tasks of a nurse, and with their understanding of the community are often more effective.

④ It acknowledges the value of their work, and helps give status. Since CHVs are often women, non-payment for work reinforces the feeling that women's work has little value. This therefore becomes a gender and justice issue.

⑤ More can be reasonably expected of the CHV in terms of time and effort, making accountability more straightforward.

Life in a slum

Joella was a traditional birth attendant, who learnt her skills from her mother. She had lived in her slum community for the past 20 years, coming to the city with her husband in search of a better life. Her husband had died a number of years ago. She made some money on deliveries, but hardly enough to live on. Her two sons and a daughter were involved in their own struggles and couldn't help her much. When a new community health project came into her community a few years back, she was suspicious and fearful. They were caring for pregnant women and encouraging them to be delivered by someone who had received training they offered in what they called 'safe deliveries'. In fact, some people from the project had visited her and encouraged her to take the training. At first she refused but then one day a traditional birth attendant from another slum community came and talked to her and invited her to a one-day workshop. She attended the workshop and learned many things that she could do to make deliveries safer. Now she is the community health volunteer for her community. She is very proud of her certificate for completing a safe motherhood course which included spending a week in the local government hospital delivery room. Now, in addition to the fees she collects from people who have minor illnesses, she also has more deliveries since the women want to be delivered by a trained birth attendant. And now that she knows the hospital staff, she feels comfortable in referring women with complications of pregnancy or delivery to the hospital. She even goes with them to the hospital, which helps greatly since she is familiar with the hospital and staff. (Haiti)

How should CHVs be paid?

Paying CHVs can be done in a number of ways:

① **From the community at point of service**
   - The CHV can be paid a small sum when she treats someone from the community, or performs a service such as accompanying a patient to a health centre or hospital, or supervising a TB DOTS treatment.
   - She may have a kit of essential medicines to treat simple illnesses, which is supplied by the project at a subsidised rate or free of cost. She can earn by charging a proportion of the cost of the medicine, which she keeps herself. This means that the CHDP is actually paying for all or some of the drugs, but the community is paying towards the support of the CHV.

A key problem arises when the CHV is paid through the charges she makes for medicines. She is motivated to do ever more curative care, thus increasing overall project costs, and undermining her key role in promoting good health and preventing illness. One way to reduce this problem is for the CHV to charge for the consultation or home visit, rather than for the medicine she may or may not supply.

❷ Through the Community Action Group

Since the CHV is accountable to the CAG, it is appropriate for her to be paid by the CAG. Even if her allowance originates from the CHDP, or is subsidised by them, control and ownership are more likely to remain in the community than with the project, if the CAG is the actual body paying the allowance.

However it may be difficult to motivate the CAG to take responsibility for paying the CHV, especially at the beginning when her value to the community has not yet been demonstrated.

❸ Through an insurance scheme

Each community member or household pays a fixed monthly fee and receives medical services free of charge or at a reduced rate. The CHV is paid from these fees. For this to work various difficulties have to be overcome:

- Some people will refuse to pay, saying they don't need the services of the CHV.
- Some people may be eligible for government health care through their job.
- Wages for slum-dwellers may not be paid regularly, or may vary with the season of the year and availability of jobs. This makes it hard for householders to commit to a regular payment.
- Only when a CHV is known and respected are community members willing to pay in advance for services they might require.

> For insurance schemes to work, competent and honest local administration must be in place, CHVs must be well respected, and alternative health services should not be widely available to the majority of the community.

❹ Through government

Occasionally, some government scheme may be available to pay CHVs, or as a general grant to an NGO programme. When this occurs, we should definitely take advantage of such a scheme. However, we must remember that the scheme may be discontinued or the payments be slow in coming, meaning we should not be entirely dependent on it.

In practice it is usually difficult to persuade poor communities to pay CHVs full allowances, whatever method is used. Nevertheless we should keep encouraging the community to do this, making sure this issue is raised and understood from the very first meetings with the community. Because most CHDPs will need to subsidise the payment of CHVs, large annual expenses will be incurred, especially in larger scale and effective programmes. It will often take ingenuity to raise support, sponsorship or donations to cover this expense over a number of years.

❺ Through income generation projects

Sometimes the CHDP can provide matching funds or a loan so that the CHVs can start some small-scale business that generates income and also allows the women to continue to work as a CHV. This is often the most feasible way to provide CHVs with income.

From the field: The Undugu CHDP in Nairobi and the project CHVs contributed to a fund to start a tea kiosk. A problem was that it took a long time to collect the money.

Lesson learned: The poor do not have large sums of money. Therefore, extending loans with a long payback period is sometimes more practical than expecting community members to pay their share all at once.

Source: Harpham *et al.*, 1988.

Non-financial incentives: CHVs (and others) can be motivated with other incentives besides money. We can:

- Have a CHV of the month, with her picture displayed at project headquarters and in a prominent place in her community. Give pins for best immunisation coverage or least malnutrition.

- Issue a bi-monthly or monthly newsletter about what is going on in the different project areas.

- Display performance comparisons with graphs and pictures.

- Provide distinctive uniforms, pins, ID badges etc. that give a sense of identity and pride, and importance to the community.

What are some of the problems that can occur?

1 **Time to gain acceptance**. Credibility will develop more quickly if the project is already known and respected, if the CAG is active and representative, and if the CHV herself is known and approved before she is appointed. CHVs who provide curative care will face extra challenges when they don't give injections (for legal reasons and because most illnesses do not require them). Some projects will decide that their CHVs should not treat illnesses, though a medicine kit does provide a valuable entry point into the felt needs of the community, especially its poorest members.

2 **Early interest begins to fade**. This can be true of the community's attitude to the CHV and the CHV's own interest and motivation. This is most likely to occur when there is lack of supervision, support and encouragement. A good supervisor who can provide essential encouragement and support is the key to the solution.

3 **Rapid turnover**. Home and economic pressures may cause CHVs to drop out. If this does happen they will remain as informed community members, can still attend the Community Action Group, and may in time be considered for reselection as CHVs.

4 **CHVs recruited by other NGOs**. Other NGOs may follow unethical practices and lure CHVs to their projects through offering higher wages. More often CHVs will

come to hear of other opportunities for employment and apply where payments are highest. The solution is to know what other agencies are paying, work in co-operation with them as far as possible and try to harmonise levels of allowance.

⑤ CHVs recruited into government schemes. Sometimes NGOs will be working in close partnership with government, or government will 'contract out' primary slum health services to NGOs. However where governments are trying to run parallel community-based services alongside NGOs, CHVs are usually poorly supervised and lose motivation. Thus if CHVs switch to government service the community may in effect lose the services of a trained CHV.

From the field: In one community health project in an urban slum, the government began a programme that included community-based health workers. They were supposed to do the same type of work that CHVs were already doing in a programme run by an NGO. Although the government paid higher wages, their CHVs were poorly supervised and did little work. News of their higher pay from the government sector spread to the CHVs working with the NGO, who in turn started to demand higher wages. The project director met with the official in charge of the government scheme to explain what was happening. The government agreed to pull out of that community and go elsewhere. (India)

Lessons learned:

It may be difficult to retain workers in slums where other NGOs or government agencies are carrying out similar work. Frank discussion with the parties involved and facing issues together can often save the situation.

Source: Authors.

---

⑥ **CHV has incorrect motivation**. The CHV is working for personal advancement rather than the good of the community. If discussion and counselling fail to bring about change, it may be possible for the CAG to reach an agreement about asking the CHV to resign. It will usually be inappropriate for the CAG to dismiss their CHV unless there is clear evidence of bad conduct. Within the community she will have a group of supporters likely to take her side in any dispute.

⑦ **Legal and employment problems**. These usually hinge on the wish of the CHVs to be considered as employees of the CHDP. It is wise to draw up a contract that clearly states that the CHV is not an employee of the CHDP, and for the CHV to sign this at the time of her appointment.

To prevent union or legal problems:

- Generally avoid giving actual wages or salaries to CHVs, which sets the tone for an employer/employee relationship. Instead, provide them with an allowance or honorarium.

- Make sure that any payment method used and agreements entered into, abide by national employment laws.

- Set up a written agreement between the CHDP and the CHVs that defines the non-employer/employee relationship.

Chapter summary

Community Health Volunteers (CHVs) play an essential role in most urban health care programmes. They act both as provider of services and agents of change. The community as a whole or through the Community Action Group selects them. CHVs need extensive training in primary health care, environmental improvements and practical aspects of development. CHVs should be accountable to the community through the CAG and not primarily to the project. However project, CAG, fellow CHVs and the CHV's own family need to offer support and encouragement. This is especially needed when the CHV is first appointed or during subsequent periods of difficulty. In the urban setting CHVs should normally be paid for their services, ideally via the CAG, with money being raised either by item of service payments, insurance schemes or block grants from government, or from other donors. There are frequent challenges faced by CHV programmes, sometimes leading to failure. Whenever these threaten, issues need to be faced up to and robust action taken early.

Resources

1. *Jamkhed: A Comprehensive Rural Health Project*. M Arole, R Arole. Macmillan Education, 1994 A narrative of the experiences of Drs Mabelle and Raj Arole in developing a rural community health and development programme based on community health volunteers who were village women.

2. *A Guide for Training Teachers of Health Workers*. M Amri, P Ngatia, O Mwakilasa, (eds). The African Medical and Research Foundation, 1993. Good general reference for training teachers of any subject.

3. *Teaching Health-care Workers: A Practical Guide*. F Abbatt, R McMahon. Macmillan Education, 1993. Good resource for someone who is planning a community health training programme or teaching community health workers. It systematically covers deciding what should be learned, planning the course, teaching methods and evaluation.

4. *Where There is No Doctor: A Village Health Care Book*. D Werner, C Thuman, J Maxwell. The Hesperian Foundation, 1993 (revised English edition). This book is available in over 50 languages and is a simple but comprehensive resource for health care workers who are providing medical care. (Available from TALC.)

5. *Helping Health Workers Learn*. D Werner, B Bower. The Heperian Foundation, 1982 (now in 9th printing). Old, but excellent resource, especially if the health workers will be using *Where There is No Doctor*. (Available from TALC.)

6. *Health Care Together: Training Exercises for Health Workers in Community Based Programmes*. MP Johnston, SB Rifkin. Macmillan Education, 1987. Many exercises that help health workers to develop the essential skills of communication, leadership, team workmanship and community development skills. (Available from TALC.)

6 The programme team and the community

This chapter discusses the selection, training, tasks and motivation of the programme team. In this book the full name of the team is the Community Health and Development Programme (CHDP) team.

What is a programme team?

A CHDP team consists of all staff of the CHDP, including **health specialists** (e.g. nurses, doctors and lab technicians), **development specialists** (e.g. community organisers, trainers, water/sanitation specialists and social workers) and **support staff** (e.g. driver, clerks, secretary and cleaners). Community health volunteers are also members of the CHDP team but they are not CHDP staff.

The idea of working together as a team, with mutual support and flexibility, is of special importance in the work we are involved with. Here are some reasons:

- In community health and development, team members must be willing to be 'multi-purpose' workers, i.e. willing to carry out tasks when the need arises, which may not be included in their formal job description. This is especially important when a programme first begins and there may be only three or four staff members who between them must carry out all programme activities.

- It is important to 'practise what we preach'. We are encouraging our communities to put aside status, and work together towards a common goal. Our relationships with other staff must demonstrate that spirit.

- The success of the work the CHDP does depends upon the unique contributions that are made by each team member. But these contributions are only really effective when each member is working in harmony with others. The analogy which the Bible uses, that we are all individual parts of one body, is very apt in the context of how a team functions and relates together.

Community health volunteers, while members of the team, should NOT be considered to be CHDP staff for the following reasons:

It will seem to the community that the CHVs are CHDP employees, rather than community members who share the community's responsibility for the health and well-being of all.

It will seem to the Community Health Volunteer that she is an employee, entitled therefore to make demands for employee benefits. This will greatly increase the cost of the programme and could threaten its sustainability.

What qualities do we look for when choosing a programme team?

The success of the entire programme depends on the quality of its members. Therefore we must choose team members wisely, and without undue hurry. Attitude, manner and character are more important than qualifications, or even past experience.

1 **Commitment to the work**. People who work in community health and development must work long and irregular hours often in tough circumstances. Working in slum communities can be specially challenging:

- There may be no electricity, which means poor lighting – and no fans when the weather is extremely hot.
- There may be no safe water or sanitary latrines.
- Community members who are stressed by difficult circumstances may be rude or violent. There may be no telephone to call for help.
- Access may be difficult with a long commute to reach the slum; then within the slum, stinking, unsightly footpaths that may be waterlogged and cluttered with garbage, including human faeces.

Only team members with a strong sense of call, commitment or purpose will continue to work in these circumstances.

Life in a slum – the evolution of a CHDP staff member

Shakeela was not happy about her job in a beauty parlour. She had earned her bachelor's degree, but was not using any of those skills. Her sister-in-law suggested that she might join a community health programme in a slum. But she wasn't sure. She didn't know anything about community health and development work. And she didn't know if she really wanted to work in a slum. However she took courage and signed on as a multi-purpose worker. She received on-the-job training and was posted in a slum community. She had never been in a slum before. She shrank back from the stinking piles of garbage, and even from the people themselves. She even hesitated to eat or drink anything during her working hours, afraid she would catch some disease. Once she was accosted by a drunk slum dweller who had just lost his job; Shakeela almost resigned. But support from the health team, including the CHVs, gave her strength to continue. Slowly she began to see the people who lived in the slum as individuals, and her repulsion faded. Her hard work and leadership qualities led to her promotion as team leader. She led the team responsible for the health and development of a community of over 2000 people. Four years later, Shakeela was again promoted to the triple-role of supervisor, women's group co-ordinator and training co-ordinator for the health teams in eight slum communities.

2 **Willingness to learn from others**. Team members must be sufficiently humble to learn new attitudes, approaches and skills both from the team and from the community.

③ **Ability to work in a team**. Team members must be able to depend on each other, trust one another and help each other at times of stress, overwork or personal difficulty.

④ **Willingness to do whatever needs to be done**. The tasks in community health and development are many and varied. Drivers must be willing to weigh children and nurses must be willing to clean up the clinic.

⑤ **Patience**. The process of guiding a community through the steps required to sustainable development takes a very long time. There are bound to be setbacks and times of discouragement.

⑥ **Flexibility**. Working with communities is often unpredictable. Sometimes its members are fickle, changing course overnight. Team members will need to cope with last-minute changes in plans, or sudden problems that require urgent attention. This need to be flexible is especially difficult for people who have previously worked in government, institutions or other large organisations.

What orientation is needed for new staff members?

All new staff will require orientation. This is especially true for doctors and nurses who have received conventional medical training. These professionals must 'unlearn' much of what they have learned in medical school or from working in hospitals. Orientation, mostly on the job, should cover the following areas:

❶ **Realities of life as a slum dweller**: their joys and their difficulties.

❷ **Partnership with the community** and all that this means in practice.

❸ **Empowerment and capacity building**: the meaning of these concepts and how they actually come about.

❹ **Promotion of health and prevention of illness**: how these are greater priorities than curative care alone. How the 'tap of ill health' can be turned off.

❺ **Minimising the use of medicines**: how rational generic prescribing from an essential drugs list must be strictly followed – to reduce programme costs and prevent excessive use of medicines in the community.

❻ **The transfer of skills**: how knowledge and skills are not for guarding but for sharing – with other team members, with CHVs, with the community.

New staff should work along side experienced staff known to have appropriate attitudes. This learning by apprenticeship is more important than learning in the classroom. The most effective learning leaves dust on our shoes and the smell of the slum in our clothes.

It is worth highlighting the importance of a probationary period for all new employees. During this time both employee and CHDP can decide whether the person is right for the job. Work in slums is tough and many are not up to it.

A single unsatisfactory team member can cause a great deal of trouble, especially one with an uncontrollable temper or who expresses frustration publicly. The CHDP team is working in a community by invitation. If a team member offends a community member, years of patient work can be harmed in just a few minutes. Anti-programme rallies may be organised by the community, and the team may be locked out of the clinic or the premises vandalised. Just as serious, team and community morale may collapse. It is better to have the courage to fire an unsatisfactory employee than to bear the consequences of their action in the community.

In most developing countries, the low social status of women is a real barrier to progress. CHDP projects can expose the community to expanded roles for women. Therefore, project management needs to consider carefully the roles and responsibilities of female and male staff, and be aware of attitudes and interactions between male and female staff. Sometimes it is helpful to have 'gender workshops' for project staff that raise awareness and help people to work through gender issues.

What qualities does a programme leader need?

In community-based health care almost anyone in a programme can rise to positions of leadership. Therefore leadership qualities, while not essential, are useful aptitudes for all new members of the team. Many leadership skills can be taught or learnt through experience. An effective leader:

- **Leads by example**, empowering and affirming team members, who in turn will empower others.
- **Knows the vision and goals of the organisation** and is able to impart enthusiasm. A good leader is dynamic and enthusiastic about the work and can excite others.
- **Is a good listener**. Working in slums can be very stressful. A good leader listens to team members when they have a stressful experience or need to talk about personal problems.
- **Is fair and impartial**. A good leader assesses situations fairly. This is a strong reason for not hiring relatives.
- **Gives praise and credit where due**. The leader should create opportunities to commend the staff. Graphs and charts showing progress can be placed in a prominent place so that staff and guests can see them. When visitors come, the leader introduces staff and includes them in discussions.
- **Visits and encourages staff on the job.** Leaders willing to get their shoes dirty visiting staff have a better understanding of the work, share a sense of solidarity in the daily joys and challenges, and gain the respect of team members.
- **Supports and backs team members**. It is important for staff to know that their leader will support them in their actions and decisions. If this is not the case, team members will be reluctant to take initiatives and to make decisions on their own. This will slow down progress towards project objectives as well as limit staff development.
- **Disciplines staff in private**. At the inevitable times when corrective action is necessary, the leader faces the issues, offers counselling and where necessary exerts

discipline – but always in private. Some good rules are never to discipline staff or Community Health Volunteers in front of community members and to give praise at least ten times more often than to reprimand.

A good leader makes leaders

How can we motivate the programme team?

People who work in community health and development with slum communities have a difficult job. It is important to consider ways that the staff can be motivated to continue such challenging work.

What is motivation?

Motivation is an internal feeling that causes a person to act in a certain way. Motivation is strongest for the basic requirements for life: Food, water, shelter, clothes, and safety. Once these needs are satisfied, then comes need for love, respect, and satisfaction in our personal lives and in our jobs.

What can we do to motivate CHDP team members?

Here are some suggestions. We can:

- **Help them to achieve**: People like to succeed and accomplish something. We can enable this to happen in the team by giving members appropriate training, clear instructions, and the tools and materials needed for the job. We can establish short-

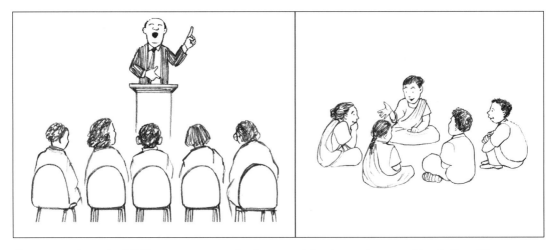

Figure 6.1   Does the CHDP encourage contributions, participation and partnership of all staff?

term objectives that can be achieved and observed, so that team members feel a sense of accomplishment when they see these being met.

- **Recognise good work and hard effort**: People like to be praised when they have done a job well. We can mention specific achievements or hard work carried out, at staff meetings, to outside visitors and in reports.

- **Make sure all team members understand the importance of the work they are doing**: People are motivated by doing something worthwhile. For example we can make sure that the person who cleans the clinic toilets knows the importance of this job because it reduces the likelihood of illness being spread in the clinic and demonstrates good practice to the community.

- **Enable team members to share in decision-making**: People thrive when they feel a sense of control over their work and can take part in decisions that affect their jobs.

- **Give team members responsibility**: When people have responsibility they are likely to do a better job. For example: we can give the clinic clerk the responsibility for collecting the monthly monitoring data. Delegation of responsibility must be clearly stated and understood: when responsibility is given, the power to carry out that responsibility must also be given, and understood by other team members. Written job descriptions can help to safeguard this.

- **Set up a fair complaints procedure**: Complaints are bound to occur – from team members or from members of the community. There need to be clear and agreed written guidelines, which everyone knows will be carefully followed.

From the field: Job Responsibilities and Work Assessment

The specific tasks of team members may vary over time, often because project activities change and there is continual staff turnover. Therefore job descriptions (JDs) must be flexible. Here is an example of how one project has ensured that JDs remain relevant, flexible and empowering, rather than outdated and restrictive. Each year in advance of their work appraisal, team members are encouraged to rewrite their own JDs to reflect the work they are actually doing. These are then discussed with their supervisor, ending up with a final product that both agree on. This document is used as part of the appraisal to discuss job performance. The main purpose of this appraisal is to help people discover their strengths and make the most of them, and to understand their weaknesses and learn how to overcome or minimise them. (Guatemala)

Source: Authors.

- **Reward good work with salary increases and promotion**: Pay rises and promotions are tangible recognition of work well done. Therefore it is helpful to have indicators on which performance can be judged by, as well as periodic reviews of performance with the supervisor. Salary increases and especially promotion should be based more on performance than on the number of years served.

- **Provide opportunities for self-improvement**: People need opportunities for personal and professional growth. We can provide educational opportunities and challenging tasks that require development of new skills or knowledge.
- **Promote team spirit**: People enjoy a sense of camaraderie and shared fun with their work mates. We can encourage these activities through setting up a social committee that organises parties, team sports and other activities that nurture fellowship and friendship. Combined acts of worship or voluntary times of prayer can also play their part.

> **From the field**: Several community health and development NGOs that work in one city come together twice a year for a sports competition and a time of fellowship. The function provides an opportunity for the staff of each NGO to have fun as a team, and for people from different NGOs to share experiences. (India)
>
> **Source**: Authors.

What demotivates team members?

Almost as important as setting up patterns to motivate the team, is the avoidance of actions that demotivate them. We should try to avoid going two steps forward, then one step backwards. Here are some practices that are known to undermine motivation:

- **Inefficient administration**: People do not like delayed payment of salaries, delayed transport, meetings that always start late or are cancelled without warning.
- **Poor supervision**: People lose enthusiasm for their work when no one takes notice, praises their efforts or helps them sort out problems.
- **Poor personal relations**: People resent favouritism. For example: it is essential that no one is given special treatment or privileges because they come from the same tribe, caste or geographical area as the programme director or supervisor, nor because they are distant (or close) relatives.
- **Poor leadership qualities**: Leaders who do not have honesty, fairness and competence lose the respect of their team.
- **Low pay**: Unfortunately, many NGOs pay fairly low salaries. Trained workers may leave the CHDP when other organisations attract them with higher pay or more perks. We must ensure that our salary structure is just, and that the rates we pay are fair and non-exploitative. We should pay pension or provident fund contributions, and abide by national employment laws, including minimum wage and maximum working hours.
- **Poor working conditions**: Staff members realise that working in slums is bound to be difficult. This needs to be acknowledged – and at times shared by the leadership. To help compensate for these hardships, real attempts should be made to make the general working conditions as pleasant and efficient as possible.

How should we supervise CHDP staff?

Fair and efficient supervision, or management, is one of the key factors determining the success of a project and the contentment of the programme team. There are three broad models:

① **Autocratic style**: Workers are told what to do. They are not allowed to influence what work should be done or how it should be done.

② **Anarchic style**: Workers are left to themselves without any supervision. They do what they like or think best.

③ **Democratic style**: Workers are encouraged to participate in all stages of the programme, from deciding what needs to be done, to planning the best way of carrying it out.

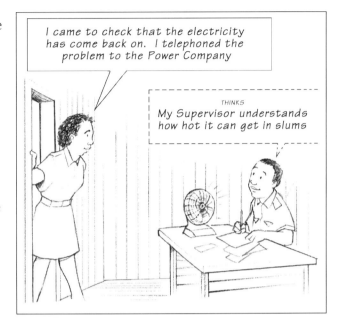

Figure 6.2   Support and understanding help staff bear difficult working conditions.

The democratic style usually works best in CHDPs. There are several reasons for this:

- **Participation and shared decision-making are core values and methods**. Team members trained in these methods are empowered to function effectively in scattered or isolated teams. When staff members are working in the community, circumstances will frequently arise that require immediate decisions and which health workers will need to make themselves. For example: a poor, sick community member comes to the clinic. The health workers must decide whether to refer the patient to hospital, and whether the project will help to pay the expenses.

- **Creativity is required**. When staff members come upon social or developmental problems in the community, they must be empowered to consider and share innovative solutions. The basis for success of a Community Action Group is for all members to consider a community problem and suggest ways of solving it.

A democratic style of supervision encourages brainstorming, where everyone is encouraged to put forward ideas and suggest solutions. The input is richer and the chance of success greater because all have contributed.

One word of caution: for a democratic style to work, staff members must be competent, experienced and reliable. This in turn will depend on regular training and empowerment.

There are a few occasions when a more authoritative approach is needed. Two examples might be:

- when workers are inexperienced or unreliable;
- in crisis situations requiring a rapid and co-ordinated response, such as when fire, flooding or rioting occurs in a slum colony.

What are the main tasks of supervisors?

When supervisors make the effort to visit workers in the field:

- Staff members perceive that the work they are doing is of value.
- Staff have confidence that the supervisor understands their situation and will provide help when needed.
- An opportunity for on-the-job training occurs.

When supervisors make field visits they should carry out the following tasks:

❶ **Monitor progress towards objectives**. For example, if a lady lane visitor programme is being implemented, the supervisor can check to see if they have been effectively chosen, and trained. The supervisor can talk with some of the lady lane visitors to see how well they understand their functions, and can provide on-the-job training during the visit.

❷ **Look and listen for any problems**. This is an opportunity for the staff member to discuss specific concerns and work-related problems. Some problems can be solved locally, others will require further action. For example, if garbage bins are not being regularly emptied by municipal garbage trucks, action may be needed by the CAG leaders to pressurise the Public Works Department. The supervisor can help to make this happen.

Supervisors are in an excellent position to cross-fertilise. They can apply solutions that they see at one site to similar problems that they come across at another.

❸ **Praise successes and encourage strengths**. In addition the supervisor can note how the particular knowledge and aptitudes of a staff member could be utilised in other ways.

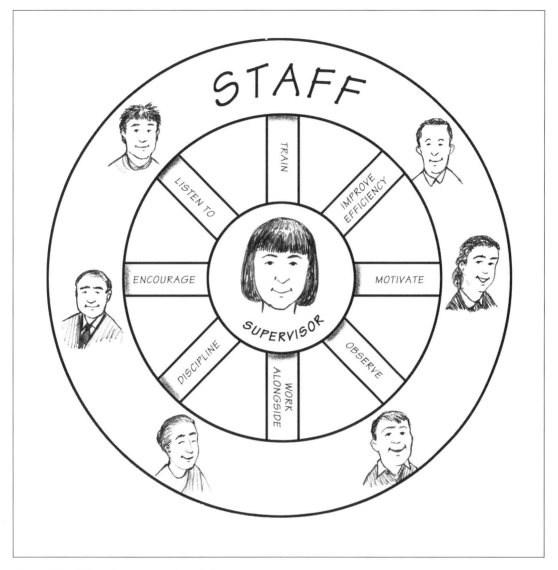

Figure 6.3   What does a supervisor do?

④ **Help the staff member to learn through failures and to recognise weaknesses.**
The supervisor can help the staff member to look for possible reasons why an
activity has failed, and to see if it might succeed if done in a different way.

Chapter summary

The Community Health and Development Team (CHDP) includes health and
development specialists, support staff and community health volunteers (CHVs,)
though CHVs are technically not members of staff as they are not paid by the project.
Working in slums requires exceptional qualities meaning that team members need to
be chosen with care. For most, commitment, attitudes and abilities are more
important than formal training or qualifications. All team members need careful

orientation, and leaders in particular need training in the appropriate styles and skills of leadership. Ways of motivating the team need to be thoughtfully planned and implemented: just ways of handling staff and good working conditions are key to maintaining staff morale. Supervisors have a key role in leading the programme forwards. They need to cultivate a democratic way of working and make regular field visits when they can train, trouble-shoot, and show a supportive approach to those working at the front line.

Resources

1. *Management Support for Primary Health Care: A Practical Guide to Management for Health Centres and Local Projects*. P Johnstone, J Ranken. FSG Publications/British Government Overseas Development Administration (now DFID), 1995. This book contains a wealth of useful information for those involved in managing community health programmes. (Available from TALC.)

2. *On Being in Charge: A Guide to Management in Primary Health Care*. R McMahon, E Barton, M Piot. WHO, 1992. A very comprehensive book for CHDP managers.

3. *Health Care Together: Training Exercises for Health Workers in Community Based Programmes*. MP Johnston and SB Rifkin. Macmillan Education, 1987. Many exercises that help health workers to develop the essential skills of communication, leadership, team workmanship and community development skills. (Available from TALC.)

4. *Managing to Empower: The Grameen Bank's Experience of Poverty Alleviation*. S Holcombe. Zed Books, 1995. Detailed case study of the very successful women's banking co-operative, with special emphasis on management of Grameen Bank staff.

5. *Training for Transformation: A Handbook for Community Workers: Book 1*. A Hope, S Timmel. Mambo Press, 1984 (and many reprints since). A practical handbook putting Paulo Freire's theory into practice. (Available from TALC.)

6. *Training for Transformation: A Handbook for Community Workers: Book 2*. A Hope, S Timmel. Mambo Press, 1984 (and many reprints since). Concentrates on participatory education. (Available from TALC.)

7. *Training for Transformation: A Handbook for Community Workers: Book 3*. A Hope, S Timmel. Mambo Press, 1984 (and many reprints since). Deals with the social analysis and management models. (Available from TALC.)

8. *Training for Transformation: A Handbook for Community Workers: Book 4*. A Hope, S Timmel. Intermediate Technology Press, 1999. Has practical modules on environment, gender, racism, multi-cultural understanding, and building participatory governance. (Available from TALC.)

Part 3

HEALTH CARE

7 Women's health

In this chapter, we shall consider:

What we need to know:

How does slum life affect women's health?

What are the health problems of women living in slums?

What are the special problems of adolescent girls living in slums?

What we need to do:

1. Promote safe pregnancy and delivery

2. Promote family planning

3. Detect domestic violence and help battered women

4. Prevent and detect sexually transmitted diseases

5. Promote the health of adolescent girls

What we need to know

Despite occasions for celebration, laughter and camaraderie, life for most women living in slums is a continual battle for survival.

How does slum life affect women's health?

In contrast to rural situations, women living in slums are more likely to be living in a nuclear family rather than a joint family

When a family is forced to move to the city, the youngest and ablest are the ones who go, leaving the old folk to protect and manage the little land they have. It is often a young couple who leaves when it is apparent that the family plot cannot sustain more mouths to feed. Although people who live in slums may have relatives in the city or even in the same community, most slum households are too small to hold extended family.

In practice this means:

- Relatives are less likely to be available to help care for children, and pass on practical skills and advice, such as on breastfeeding, weaning and how to bring up children.

- Unlike a village situation, neighbours may be from different areas, traditions and tribes. They may not even speak the same language. This often means they will be unwilling or unable to give support.

Women living in slums are likely to work as wage-earners for long hours outside the home

In practice this means:

- Their limited education, lack of job skills and time constraints confine them to the low-paid 'informal' sector with little pay, job security or benefits. Because they are vulnerable they are frequently exploited.
- Small children are deprived of care and protection.

Basic services such as water, sanitation and electricity are poorly developed

In practice this means:

- Women may have to spend precious time fetching water, disposing of household waste, and taking small children to an acceptable place for defecation.
- Women have no privacy for bathing, urination or defecation. Therefore they are prone to poor hygiene of the perineum, urinary tract infections and to harassment.

Women living in slums live in crowded and stressful conditions

Therefore:

- They or their partner may have multiple sex partners.
- Their partner or other family members may abuse them sexually, physically or emotionally, especially when unemployment, gambling losses, alcohol and drug abuse worsen the situation further.
- Neighbours or others may sexually abuse them.
- Women may be exposed to severe mental stress, including harassment and abuse when travelling or searching for work.

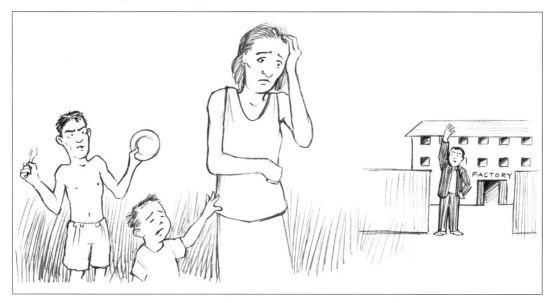

Figure 7.1   Women living in slums have conflicting responsibilities.

- Women are more likely to be abandoned, separated or divorced.
- Women may have to function as head of the household or as the only adult member, so carrying full responsibilities as parent and provider.
- Women themselves may smoke or be involved in substance abuse.

What are the health problems of women living in slums?

Many of the problems listed below are shared by all women living in poverty, but slum conditions can make them worse.

Health problems associated with pregnancy and delivery
During the antenatal period

- **Heavy physical labour**: Women often work on construction sites or in other jobs requiring hard physical work. They will often feel sick, or weak from exhaustion and anaemia. Even though needing to work less hard, they may lose their job if they complain or if their pregnancy becomes visible.

- **Poor antenatal care**: In practice women may have little or no access to antenatal care. They may be unable to take time off work; their husband or mother-in-law may consider an extra day's wages more important than a clinic visit whose purpose they don't understand. In the last few weeks of pregnancy women often return to their village so missing antenatal care at the most important time.

During delivery

- **Poor access to health care**: Women who live in slums theoretically have access to hospital care. However, they can't usually afford private health care so government facilities are the only choice, usually crowded, frightening and dirty. Only rarely can NGOs provide good quality alternatives.

- **Oxytocin abuse**: Many untrained practitioners, midwives or healers, whom slum dwellers often attend through desperation, use a drug called oxytocin when labour is not progressing quickly. Oxytocin increases the contraction of the uterus, and is dangerous to use outside a hospital. In most cities it is readily available and patients press for its use, often unaware of its dangers. Practitioners attract more patients if they use oxytocin or advertise its availability.

- **Traditional Birth Attendants (TBAs)**: Some slums have TBAs who are trained in antenatal care and how to conduct a safe and clean delivery. But more often, the training and hygiene of TBAs will be inadequate. There is often a high turnover of TBAs making it hard to monitor their effectiveness and safety.

- **Women often go to their home village for delivery**, where facilities and emergency care may be lacking.

Life in a slum

Banwari stood motionless, a hand covering his grief-stricken face. His four daughters sat motionless in a corner, not understanding the sight before them. The lifeless, frail body of their mother, Samwati, lay on the small string bed. Samwati had become pregnant soon after the birth of her fourth daughter. She and her husband had wanted a son. So many pregnancies, one following the other, had taken their toll on Samwati's health. She was severely anaemic, despite taking the iron–folate tablets given to her at the ASHA Health Centre. Although her previous four deliveries had all been conducted at home, the health team recommended she deliver in hospital. But her husband, balancing the cost of hospital with her success in four previous home deliveries wouldn't agree, even though during the later weeks of pregnancy, Samwati was too weak to get up. The health team pleaded unsuccessfully with Samwati's husband. He said it was Samwati's fault that they only had daughters so if she died, he might have better luck with another wife. The following morning, the family woke up to find Samwati had died, silently, during the night. (India)

During the post-partum period

- **Lack of knowledge**: Women living in slums are often poorly educated. They are cut off from traditional sources of family wisdom and support. They have no one to advise them about health care, and no access to books or the internet to help them. Their neighbours and friends may be too busy, or come from diverse ethnic groups with different patterns of child care.

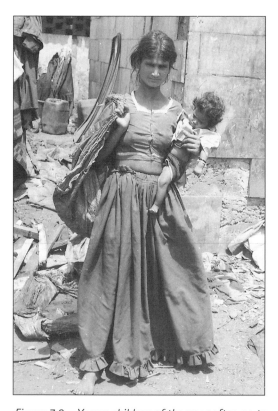

- **Early return to work**: The need for money may drive women back to work far too early leaving them exhausted and their baby at risk. Caretakers or older sisters may not give sufficient care, the work site may be dangerous or unwelcoming, and breastfeeding may be stopped, followed by inadequate replacement with other foods. Bottle feeding may compound dangers to the young infant.

Figure 7.2   Young children of the poor often go to work with their mothers. (Godfrey Martin/ASHA)

People living in slums often come from varied ethnic backgrounds with different traditional practices, some of which may be harmful. Health workers need to be aware of this diversity so they can provide appropriate care for each social group.

High fertility

Slums often appear to be teeming with small children. This is mainly because these communities contain a high proportion of young adults, many of whom have come to the city seeking work. These young adults are often recently married and beginning to have families. Add to this the many children born to mothers with no stable partner, or pregnant (again) against their choice. In addition there are few experienced adults to help care for the children, meaning many have to fend for themselves at a very young age.

High fertility creates extra health problems. With each additional child born, all children, especially girls, receive less time, space, food, security and care. This leads to increasing risks of:

- **illness**: especially diarrhoea, respiratory infections, measles and skin infections;
- **malnutrition** as children are weaned prematurely and insufficient food is available;
- **under-5 deaths** as malnutrition and illness added to other risks, reduce survival from infectious diseases and accidents;
- **maternal anaemia and exhaustion**.

These realities highlight the need for family spacing and effective birth control. A longer birth interval reduces infant mortality and improves the general health of children, and also improves school attendance.

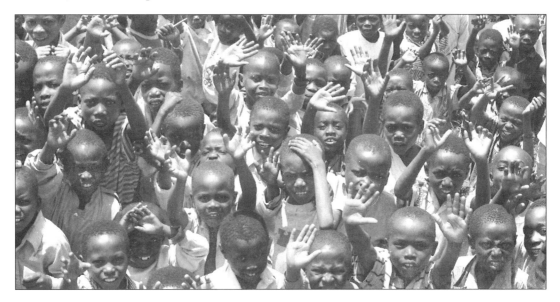

Figure 7.3   High fertility creates extra health problems. (Richard Hanson/Tearfund)

Domestic violence and sexual abuse

Domestic violence and sexual abuse, including rape are extremely common amongst those living in slums. Various factors contribute to this:

- **The pressures of living in poverty**, coupled with alcoholism, drug abuse, gambling and debt, are major problems.
- **Male unemployment** leads to increasing dependency on women as breadwinners resulting in humiliation and a need to demonstrate supremacy.
- **Social expectations**. In many cultures, it is accepted that women need to be disciplined and kept subservient. This in turn leads to mental, emotional, physical or sexual abuse, often all four together.
- **Overcrowded living conditions** make it difficult for women and girls to bathe and dress in privacy, so increasing the likelihood of sexual assault.
- **Respected older family members are not available** to provide counsel and a hand of restraint.
- **The low, dependent status of women**. In most poor communities, women have little recourse to help, advocacy or legal action, meaning they have no choice but to submit.
- **Women (and men or children) may have jobs as commercial sex workers** out of economic hardship.

A battered woman often has nowhere to go for help. In many cultures, wife-beating is an accepted and common practice – women need to be 'disciplined'. Her parents or siblings may not be willing to shelter her from an abusive husband if they cannot afford it or if it would be culturally inappropriate and would bring shame to the family. If an abused woman goes to the police, especially from an illegal settlement, further harassment and humiliation are likely.

Life in a slum

Rukhsana had been married off by her family to a man 30 years older than she. His first wife had died in childbirth leaving two young children still at home. They lived with her husband's brother and his wife in a city slum far away from Rukhsana's family. Rukhsana's husband was away a lot, and during his absence, her husband's brother often forced her to have sex with him. His wife knew what was going on and made Rukhsana's life miserable. Then one day when her husband had been away for many months, Rukhsana found herself pregnant. Fearing that her husband would suspect that he was not the father, she told her brother-in-law. He beat her, and then arranged for her to have an abortion. After the abortion she bled too much and her brother-in-law reluctantly allowed her to be taken to hospital. The abortion became common knowledge. When she returned home from hospital, her brother-in-law and his wife poured kerosene on her and set fire to her. She died of these 'accidental burns from a cooking stove'. When her husband returned the family told him that Rukhsana had been unfaithful and had to be killed to save the family honour. Her husband then went to find another wife. (Pakistan)

Sexually transmitted diseases (STDs)

Sexually transmitted diseases (STDs) such as gonorrhoea, syphilis, chlamydia and HIV infection are widespread in slums. Men and women are likely to have multiple sex partners for a number of reasons:

- **In many households one partner is absent**, such as the mother in her home village, or the husband working a long distance from home. Either or both may have other sexual relationships, sometimes with multiple partners.
- **Divorce and abandonment are more common, resulting in women-headed households**. Such women may seek a partner to give stability and protection to the household. These relationships often do not last long, resulting in a succession of sexual partners.
- **Women may be forced into prostitution to survive**.
- **Overcrowding and breakdown of traditional values lead to informal affairs**.

What are the special problems of adolescent girls living in slums?

Adolescent girls who live in urban slums are extremely vulnerable for several reasons:

1. **Crowded living conditions, with parents at work**, puts girls at risk of sexual abuse by neighbours or other family members.
2. **Girls may become sexually active at a younger age**, often before marriage. Often they will be ignorant of the risks of becoming pregnant or acquiring an STD.
3. **To prevent pregnancy, anal intercourse is common**, thereby increasing the risk of HIV infection.
4. **Families in severe poverty have easy opportunity to sell their daughters into prostitution or as domestic servants**. 'Sale' of a daughter brings in money, eliminates one more mouth to feed and postpones or eliminates the problem of providing a marriage dowry.
5. **Adolescent girls are relatively neglected by government and NGO health programmes**. Priority usually goes to younger children and to the care of pregnant women.
6. **Girls may not be able to attend school** because they are needed at home to mind younger siblings while parents are working, or to earn money. Parents will often given priority to educating boys rather than girls. Uneducated girls are less empowered to resist abuse.

> Girls may leave school when they start menstruating because there are no toilet facilities at school.

What we need to do

This section looks at women's health issues that are specifically related to cities. Resource materials on subjects such as maternal and family planning services, and on disease prevention and control are available elsewhere. Some are listed at the end of the chapter.

We will need action to:

Promote safe pregnancy and delivery

During the antenatal period

- **Train community women as lane health visitors**, responsible for 20 homes surrounding their own. Their tasks will include: detecting pregnancies early, providing advice during pregnancy and early motherhood, motivating women to attend antenatal clinics, and referring as needed. See also Chapter 6.
- **Consider holding antenatal clinics in the evening** for the convenience of women working outside the home. Also at sites as near to their home as possible.

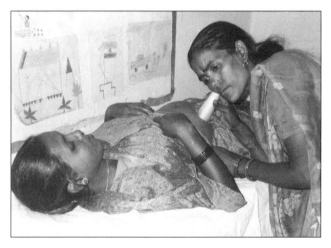

- **Provide tetanus toxoid coverage as early during pregnancy as possible** so that those women who return to their village later in pregnancy are fully covered.
- **Increase awareness amongst all family members about the importance of eating more and working less during pregnancy.**

Figure 7.4   Antenatal care is an essential component of safe motherhood. (ASHA)

During delivery

- **Ensure that there are sufficient trained traditional birth attendants (TBAs) or other trained midwives available in each community.** This will mean holding regular classes, or networking with government agencies or other NGOs that provide them.
- **Learn about the traditional practices of the various ethnic groups you are serving**: encourage useful practices, discourage harmful ones.
- **Arrange with the community a system whereby women delivering in hospital can be accompanied by a health worker, TBA or volunteer to act as friend,**

supporter and advocate. This is especially important if any medical complications have arisen, if there is no family member to accompany her or she feels especially vulnerable.

- **Advise women only to return to their village for the delivery if adequate maternal and child care is available**. This should include the presence of a trained TBA and adequate referral arrangements in case of complications.

- **Encourage models of co-operation between project members, TBAs and staff of the most frequently used referral hospitals and health facilities**. Building such professional links and friendships takes time because staff are continually changing and hospital staff may need to transform their attitudes to the poor. The rewards however are great. For example:
  - It helps develop more efficient and effective patient care with greater access.
  - Community midwives become more willing to refer and accompany their patients to hospital, in turn benefiting themselves by what they learn.
  - Hospital staff provide more friendly and appropriate care, especially for the poor.
  - It can help to encourage the 'Baby-friendly' and 'Mother-friendly' UNICEF/WHO programmes for maternity units.

During the post-partum period

- **Through trained volunteers ensure that breastfeeding for the first 2 years of life remains popular in the community and train mothers in its use**. Also instruct mothers unwilling or unable to breastfeed how to cup feed safely. Arrange parent-craft classes in the community, especially if slum families have few older people to give instruction.

- **Try to persuade the mother not to return to work for a period of 2–3 months after delivery**. This may involve explaining the benefits of this to other family members, especially the greater health and energy which the mother is likely to gain – to everyone's advantage. Be sensitive for times when mothers wish to return to work early because domestic situations are so stressful or threatening.

- **Encourage a work setting that permits breastfeeding**.

- **Ensure adequate post-partum care** including the speedy treatment of any infection and the ongoing **treatment** of anaemia.

Promote family planning

The promotion of family planning is made rather easier in urban areas. There are several reasons for this: family planning messages are frequently promoted in the media, on billboards and through mass campaigns; women working outside the home have a vested interest in avoiding pregnancy so as to hold down their jobs; there may be less opportunity for children to work as wage earners, as competition for jobs is tough.

However, early weaning because the mother must go to work each day, works against these factors as the contraceptive effects of lactation are lost prematurely, meaning that women can easily become pregnant again within a few months of the last child being born.

To encourage greater use of family planning services we need to:

- **Include family planning counselling** as a component of health education classes and of community services, including during the antenatal and post-partum period.

- **Ensure that condoms are always available from sources within the community.** Although useful as part of a family planning programme, the main value of condoms is to lower the risk of STDs and especially to reduce the spread of HIV infection. Community health volunteers or specially trained community 'depot-holders' such as local shopkeepers can provide this service. Condom supplies must be accompanied by pictorial instructions, easily understood by those unable to read.

- **Strongly encourage recently delivered women to adopt a child-spacing method**. A child whose mother does not have another child for at least 2 years has a significantly better chance of surviving and being well-nourished than a child whose mother becomes pregnant sooner. We need to explain the value of this to women and their partners, emphasising both the benefits to health of child and mother, and the money that the family can save.

- **Work as an advocate for on-site child-care facilities** (supervised creches, for example, staffed by members of a Community Action Group) that enable working mothers to continue to breast-feed and that provide a safe place for other pre-school children. This benefits everyone including older sisters, now able to attend school.

Prevent and detect sexually transmitted diseases

This has become a key issue in the past few years. Not only are STDs increasing worldwide, but the presence of an untreated STD greatly increases the risk of becoming infected with HIV during sexual intercourse. The most effective way to prevent STDs is to remain faithful in marriage and celibate outside of marriage. Failing that, the use of condoms greatly reduces the risk of becoming infected with an STD. In our programmes we can help reduce STDs in the following ways:

1 **Increase awareness about** how STDs can be caught, recognised and prevented:

By the beginning of adolescence and earlier in many societies, all young people need sex education. This should include how to recognise STDs and action to take if one is suspected. Even more important is knowing how STDs can be prevented, giving emphasis both on the value of stable long-term relationships as being the primary preventative measure, and always using condoms during sexual intercourse outside of such a relationship. Key groups to concentrate on include:

- all early adolescents to help establish good patterns of sexual health;
- commercial sex workers (ideally as part of a health and social programme);
- men working away from home, especially if employed as truck drivers – a known high-risk group responsible for the spread of HIV.

In areas where STDs and HIV infection are recognised as priorities, the programme should consider working in schools, either to teach the classes themselves or by giving in-service training to the school teachers. Linking with other NGOs working in education is also an effective strategy. Appropriate sex education needs to be built into the core curriculum of all slum-based schools.

② **Increase availability of condoms**. Condoms should always be available at the clinic, not just during family planning clinic times. Condoms should be also available in other places in the community where they can be obtained relatively inconspicuously and anonymously, and without embarrassment, e.g. from chemist shops or cigarette vendors.

③ **Detect and treat STDs early**. This is essential in stopping their spread. Health workers should know the signs and symptoms of STDs (in men, women and new-born). If diagnosis and treatment are not available they should know where to refer for convenient, compassionate treatment. WHO has developed a syndromic approach to the diagnosis and treatment of STDs (see resource section).

④ **Trace and refer STD contacts**: Health workers must encourage people with STDs to inform their sexual partners about seeking medical care. The health worker can also help to trace, counsel and organise referral/treatment for partners. Counselling needs to be done with sensitivity so as to maintain confidentiality and minimise the risk of causing anger or violence in the partner. Partners will often be poorly motivated or fatalistic about taking any action. Building relationships and explaining the value of treatment gives the best chance of success. See also Chapter on HIV, page 147.

The Five Cs of STD Control:

Compliance: ensure that patients complete their antibiotic course; use single dose therapy whenever possible.

Confidentiality: ensure that staff understand the importance of confidentiality.

Contract tracing: gain patient's trust and understanding; be sensitive, but persistent in tracking down contacts.

Counselling: educate about sexual health and transmission of STDs

Condoms: educate about usage and provide easy access.

Commercial sex workers

The health of commercial sex workers (CSWs) in and around a slum community can affect the health of slum residents:

● Women from the community – also teenage girls, older children and men, may themselves be commercial sex workers. For destitute families this provides good pay, and the pressures to enter the sex industry may be hard to resist.

● Some men from the community may be the partners of CSWs: others may use the services of CSWs. These men are at high risk of being infected with STDs including HIV disease, and will spread infections to others

If either or both of these practices are common, the CHDP should learn about the local commercial sex industry, and set objectives to reduce the degradation, abuse and disease it causes. Here are some strategies to help achieve those objectives:

1. Provide treatment of STDs. Clinics should:
   - be near the sex worker's workplace, have short waiting times and convenient hours;
   - have a welcoming and non-judgemental environment;
   - provide confidentiality;
   - provide other services (e.g. general medical care, contraception, maternal and child care).

2. Provide easy access to condoms.

3. Give education about safer sex.

   Education should include **these topics**:
   - safe and unsafe practices;
   - how and where to obtain good quality condoms and how to use them;
   - how to negotiate condom use;
   - how to discourage the use of alcohol and drugs to help reduce condom failure;
   - how to recognise STDs and where to seek immediate treatment.

   Education should be given to **these groups**:
   - the community at large which will include potential clients;
   - commercial sex workers;
   - brothel owners, pimps, etc., explaining how a healthy workforce will have financial and commercial benefits. (The underlying objective here is to reduce the spread of STDs/HIV.)

4. Provide support services to CSWs. These could include:
   - child support services to enable school attendance, with safe places for homework etc.;
   - welfare services, especially for those living with HIV/AIDS or the chronically ill;
   - legal advice and assistance;
   - advocacy with police, courts, brothel owners and pimps in cases of exploitation and cruelty;
   - counselling and support in cases of abuse;
   - training in self-defence.

In addition to these activities, the CDHP should think creatively about how to reduce the commercial sex-trade. We will have two objectives: the first is to reduce the pressures on community members to become CSWs in the first place. The second is to create alternative sources of employment for existing CSWs, especially those from households within the community.

We will need to call in expertise and resources from groups experienced in this work. In several cities including Mumbai (Bombay), and Bangkok, NGOs are setting up centres which empower women to find alternative sources of work through education and vocational training. Teenage girls from poor backgrounds in large cities are an important group to work with before they are drawn into the sex industry.

Detect domstic violence and help battered women

Detect domestic violence

Women who are abused often try to hide their injuries and protect the abuser. If they have a visible injury, they may make up a story to try and explain the injury. Abused women generally have very low self-esteem and tend to bear their burdens with resigned hopelessness. They see no way out of their problems and are too frightened for themselves and their children to accuse the abuser. Also they will rarely leave him, fearing he will soon discover them and become even more violent.

This means project staff must be aware of signs and symptoms suggestive of abuse (see Box on page 112). If domestic violence is suspected, staff should arrange to interview the woman alone or with a friend, in a safe place and without the abuser's knowledge.

> Empowerment of women to have control over their bodies, to learn assertiveness and to provide mutual and collective support can begin to break down the traditions that condone abuse of women.

Because many of the features of domestic violence are non-specific and have other causes we need to remain alert for the presence of abuse. Equally we must make sure we do not suggest abuse has happened without strong evidence indications.

Help battered women

Train project staff to work with victims of abuse

They must learn to:

- **Detect domestic violence and sexual abuse**.
- **Encourage and facilitate a setting that provides physical safety.** Domestic violence generally progresses, so delay is dangerous.
- **Give reassurance, advice and support, and where appropriate to arrange professional counselling.**
- **Record and preserve evidence of violence.**
- **Refer women to organisations that offer protection and advice in handling abuse situations.**
- **Seek specialist advice before attempting to counsel abusers.**

Seek out organisations that provide services for battered women

In practice these may be non-existent or very limited. If that is the case, and the community recognises abuse as a priority problem services can be set up. These could include care, advocacy or both:

- short stay homes to provide temporary refuge,
- counselling, including post-stress counselling,
- legal advice and assistance,

Signs and symptoms suggestive of Domestic Violence/Sexual Abuse

Signs

- Bruising, especially on face
- Unexplained missing teeth
- Recurrent nosebleeds
- Injuries produced by stabbing or blows
- Unexplained vaginal haemorrhage
- Deformities from previous injury (e.g. broken nose)

Symptoms

- Women who are anxious, fearful, and/or depressed
- Women who think that they are worthless or who refer to themselves as being stupid or incapable
- Women with frequent headaches, inability to sleep, or vague aches and pains
- Women who say things like:

  'He uses me'

  'He gets relief from me'

- child care facilities,
- long-term care for elderly, poor widows with nowhere to go.

The community itself can provide help to battered women especially through women's community action groups. The known existence of active groups will help to dissuade other abusers. In addition they can:

1. Apply community pressure to persuade men from causing abuse.
2. Encourage and assist women to seek help.
3. Give practical support to women in seeking solutions that will work in their own personal circumstances.
4. Approach the police, and insist that they take action.

Battered women usually have severe emotional problems, in particular low esteem and lack of confidence. They feel trapped with no options apart from self-survival. By providing such women with skills, it opens the way for employment and independence and helps to increase their self-worth. This can lead to the option of leaving the violent partner and setting up a new lifestyle.

Increase awareness and advocacy about domestic violence and sexual abuse

Individual efforts can only have a limited effect in reducing domestic violence which is prevalent almost everywhere, but especially where the status of women is low, and wife-beating is considered the norm. Real improvement will only come about if and when communities are transformed into believing that domestic violence and sexual abuse is an unacceptable, criminal offence.

If violence against women is a felt concern that the community wishes to address, then the CHDP can work with them, especially in terms of advocacy:

- **With police**: that they will acknowledge that violent acts against women are crimes, and that they have a moral and legal duty to protect women and arrest culprits. This will require police dealing with the situation in a sensitive manner, otherwise matters can be made worse.
- **With hospital staff**: that they will deal with the situation in a sensitive manner, preserve evidence and develop protocols for dealing with physical and sexual abuse.
- **With judicial authorities**: that they will recognise that violent acts against women are crimes and will enforce any protective laws in a just and sensitive way.
- **With the public**: that they will consider that violent acts against women are socially unacceptable criminal activities and that they will campaign for justice on gender-based issues and work to improve the status of women.

Promote the health of adolescent girls

Our purpose here is not simply to recognise and treat illness but to educate, and build the confidence of teenage girls so they can better survive in the slum environment. We will need to increase their self-esteem. This requires an approach involving adolescent girls, their families and the community.

Work with adolescent girls

The following should be our aims in any actions we take or programmes we set up:

- Increase awareness about how the body works, including the physical and emotional changes of puberty.
- Provide non-formal education at appropriate times of day such as evening classes.
- Discuss sexual activity and the risks of sexual promiscuity, including becoming infected with HIV. This needs a direct, interactive approach, appropriate to the age and cultural background of the participants.
- Increase awareness about options of safer sex using condoms and the value of long-term single-partner relationships.
- Ensure a source of condoms that is confidential, accessible and non-judgmental.
- Identify and treat anaemia and other chronic illnesses in young girls so that they enter their reproductive years in the best possible physical health.
- Seek out a legal assistance agency that can provide advocacy services for abused girls.

> **From the field**: An NGO implemented a sex and family education programme for low-income adolescent girls. They collected extensive amounts of preliminary data and then started weekly education sessions for adolescent girls. Attendance was very poor. Some community members thought that by teaching girls about sex, they would be more likely to want to experiment. The project then invited mothers and their daughters to the initial sessions. Later on, as trust developed, the girls wanted to have their own meetings and the mothers agreed. (Uganda)
>
> **Lessons learned**: From time to time programmes are likely to tackle subjects that are controversial to some segments of the community. If that is thought to be likely, build broad community acceptance before starting the programme.
>
> **Source**: Authors.

Work with families

- Increase awareness about the benefits of education for girls and alternatives to being sold into prostitution or domestic servitude.
- Increase awareness about the dangers that exist for young girls in a crowded community, especially if parents are working and there is no adult supervision.
- Encourage families to create a safe home environment.
- Encourage family members to seek help if the girl is being sexually or physically abused by a family member, neighbour or other person.

Work with the community

Two things we can do:

- Facilitate the setting-up of community-run day-care centres for young children so that older girls may go to school.
- Encourage or set up skills training for adolescent girls to improve employment prospects and reduce the need to enter prostitution.

> **From the field**: In the Puentes de Cristo CHDP, in Reynosa, Mexico, girls from 9 to 12 years meet each day before school for tutoring and help with their homework and to learn about new things, including child care, sex education, reproduction, and assertiveness. They are encouraged to bring younger siblings which allows those who are caring for younger siblings to come.
>
> **Source**: Gilberto and Maria Medina, Puentes de Cristo CHDP

Chapter summary

Living in slums seriously affects women's health. Services are poor and responsibilities are heavy – both to earn wages and care for the family. The environment is stressful and dangerous. Pregnancy and childbirth are especially vulnerable times. Women often face sexual and physical abuse and adolescent girls are exploited and sometimes sold into prostitution. Sexually transmitted diseases are an ever-present, but largely preventable threat. We need to facilitate imaginative and far-reaching programmes to empower women, provide care at vulnerable times, and mobilise a range of resources through a wide variety of networks. Empowerment through education and skills learning, temporary shelter, targeted health care, counselling and advocacy are key services that are always needed. The community needs full involvement and ownership of all programmes that are set up.

Resources

1. *Setting up Community Health Programmes: A practical manual for use in developing countries*, 2nd edition. T Lankester. Macmillan Education, 1999. Discusses maternal health issues in the context of a community health and development programme. (Available from TALC.)

2. *Men's Sexual Health Matters*. Healthlink, 1998. For health and community workers who work on sex and sexuality with men. Covers basic facts on reproduction, contraception, and safe sex for men, men's concerns about sexual and reproductive health and strategies for working with men in different settings. Free to readers in developing countries.

3. *Where Woman have no Doctor*. AA Burns, R Lovich, J Maxwell, K Shapiro. The Hesperian Foundation, 1997. A health guide for women/girls to help them identify common medical problems and treatment. Written clearly, simply and with lots of pictures. (Available from TALC.)

4. *The Family Planning Clinic in Africa*. 3rd edition. R Brown, J Brown. Macmillan Education, 1997. Very practical guide for health workers working in family planning. (Available from TALC.)

5. *Making Sex Work*. Network of Sex Work Projects/AHRTAG, 1997. An excellent review of the topic with systematic presentation of problems, needs assessment and interventions.

6. *Violence against Women: A Violation of Human Rights*. Institute for Development Training, 1995. A good resource guide for people who are working with battered women.

7. *Management of Patients with Sexually Transmitted Diseases*. Technical Support Series 810. WHO, 1991. Provides flowcharts for detection and treatment of sexually transmitted diseases that permit people with little medical training to treat sexually transmitted diseases with high likelihood of success.

8. *Training Manual for Traditional Birth Attendants*. G Gordon. Macmillan Education, 1990. Simple and has many simple pictures for training traditional birth attendants. (Available from TALC.)

9. *Women-Headed Households: Diversity and Dynamics in the Developing World*. S Chant. Macmillan Press, 1997. Explores the reasons for the formation and increase in women-headed households and their capacity for survival.

8 Children's health

In this chapter, we shall consider:

How does urban poverty affect the health of children?

Malnutrition

Diarrhoea

Acute respiratory infections

Vaccine-preventable diseases and vitamin A deficiency

HIV/AIDS

Other common illnesses

Injuries and accidents

Psychosocial problems: physical and sexual abuse

How does urban poverty put children to work?

What are the special problems of working children?

How can we help working children?

How can we work through children?

How do we form a children's group?

What does a children's group do?

Life in a slum

Ten-year-old Rashi came to the city with her family 8 years ago. The family was forced to move there during a drought as her father could not find enough fieldwork to keep them from starving. At first they had lived on the street. Each day her father sought work as a day labourer while her mother, carrying her baby sister and with her two younger brothers in hand, would beg on the streets. Eventually, Rashi's father was able to rent a cycle rickshaw, and then a few years later, he and his brother had saved up enough money to buy a second-hand rickshaw. By that time, Rashi's mother had found work cleaning people's houses. They now live in a one-room plywood house in a slum. Recently, Rashi's father has been diagnosed with tuberculosis, but the drugs were not available in the hospital pharmacy and he could only afford one week's treatment from the local chemist shop. Each day he gets weaker. To help the family, Rashi's 9-year-old brother stopped going to school and began to carry purchases for people from the store to their cars at one of the expensive shopping centres. Rashi continues to take care of her other younger brother and sister, as well as her father. Sometimes she and the youngest two children wander the streets going through rubbish in search of recycleable items. Rashi is proud of the money she has earns which helps to provide food for their family. Lately, though, her own health is deteriorating – she feels weak and has started to lose weight. ...
(Bangladesh)

As this story demonstrates, children of the urban poor in developing countries have a childhood completely different from that of middle or upper class children in their own country and in the same city. Commonly poor urban children will:

- **care for, or be cared by, other children**, often sisters or brothers;
- **not attend school**, either because their parents cannot pay school expenses or they want them to work instead;
- **work part or full-time**, sometimes while also attending school;
- **Live apart from their family**: e.g. alone, with their employer, with other children, or with a partner as they get older.

How does urban poverty affect the health of children?

The World Health Organization states that 7 out of 10 childhood deaths in developing countries are caused by malnutrition, diarrhoea, respiratory illnesses, measles and malaria, of which the first three are the most widespread. Severe urban poverty increases their danger. The factors linking this triad of illnesses are closely interwoven (see Figure 8.1). HIV/AIDS is also a major killer of young children in Africa, and is rapidly becoming so in Asia and other low-income countries. In addition children living in slums are at increased risk of injuries, accidents and abuse.

The sections below give the causes and background for these problems and suggest ways to reduce them. For more specific information on diagnosis and treatment, refer to primary health care/child health resources listed at the end of this chapter.

Malnutrition

In each family, the particular reasons and circumstances that lead to malnutrition will vary, but the root cause is poverty, which in turn creates conditions that result in:

1. **young children having inadequate food intake**, especially calories, but also protein, vitamins and minerals, and;
2. **young children having frequent bouts of other illnesses**, especially diarrhoea and acute respiratory illnesses (see Figure 8.1).

We will look at each of these in turn.

Reasons that children living in slums receive inadequate amounts of food

1. **Infants (children under 12 months of age) are less likely to be breastfed.**
   - Mothers are more likely to work outside the home.
   - Mothers are exposed to media, and gain the faulty idea that bottle-feeding is 'modern'.
   - Bottles and formula are relatively easy to obtain.
   - Mothers, separated from older relatives, learn little about breastfeeding and infant nutrition. Caretakers, often children themselves, may know even less.

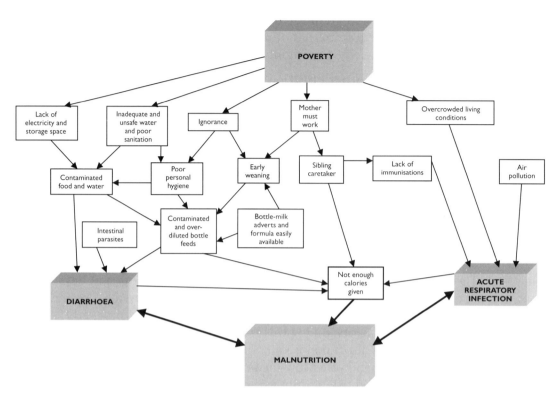

Figure 8.1 Factors that contribute to malnutrition in young children.

② **Infants are less likely to receive supplementary feeds**.
  ● The caretaker, often an older sibling, is unlikely to have the knowledge or the patience to provide the infant with appropriate kinds and amounts of food.
  ● Food must be purchased: often there is no money – meaning too little food – or no fuel for cooking.
  ● Earnings are often spent on cigarettes, alcohol or drugs.

> Families living in slums often only eat only twice per day, once in the early morning and again in the evening. Though adults and older children can survive on this, young children with their smaller stomachs will not get enough food, even if pacified by biscuits between meals. Children under 3 years of age need five meals per day to ensure adequate weight gain.

③ **Children living in slums have frequent bouts of illness**.

Diarrhoea and respiratory infections, including measles, are the main illnesses leading to weight loss. During acute infections children eat less, or nothing at all, leading to rapid weight loss. Illnesses increase the need for calories because fever and rapid breathing burn off more energy. In addition, diarrhoea prevents proper absorption of food. Children who are thin already soon start using body protein and fat reserves to provide energy, leading to loss of muscle mass.

There is also a widespread idea that sick children should not be fed. This is a dangerous belief and leads to further weight loss, just when food is desperately needed. Families seldom ensure that children receive extra food when they are recovering from an illness. Then just as the appetite is picking up another bout of illness strikes. Children can fail to gain weight for months on end, leading to a further life-long disadvantage – stunting of growth.

When children are recovering from an acute illness, they should receive an extra meal each day for the same number of days as their illness lasted. If they were sick for 3 days, they should be fed an extra meal for the next 3 days.

Diarrhoea and respiratory disease are discussed further later in this chapter.

Ways we can increase food intake in infants and young children

We will need to discover the main reasons underlying poor nutrition in the slums in which we work. The community diagnosis will give us ideas, especially if more detailed house-to-house surveys have been carried out looking at feeding practices, socio-economic patterns and the availability of food. Community Action Groups (CAGs) can also provide, or gather information, as well as being the main vehicle through which improvements are brought about. Our aim is to help bring about lasting changes in living patterns and behaviour, rather than looking at stopgap ways to improve nutrition for a limited period of time.

At a gathering of mothers and children, such as an under-5's clinic, identify well-nourished toddlers and then ask the mother their mothers how often they feed, what they feed, hand-washing habits, etc., to find out how they are able to produce healthy children. Let all the mothers there learn from these mothers.

Here are examples of actions the programme and CAG might take:

Encourage breastfeeding

- **Educate and motivate** mothers, daytime caretakers, pregnant women and adolescent girls about breastfeeding. This should include explaining its benefits and importance for the first year of life – why breast is best. Equally important is giving imaginative and practical ideas for successful breastfeeding – ideas likely to work for exhausted wage-earning mothers struggling with thin, cranky children in hot and crowded conditions.
- **Make postnatal visits** within 24 hours of delivery to assure breastfeeding is started and to help trouble-shoot any problems. This is best done by a female Community Health Volunteer or neighbour (trained lady lane visitor) who has herself breastfed children.

- **Organise day care centres** at the workplace so that working mothers may continue to breastfeed and have a safe place for their children to stay. This will involve explaining the benefits to employers, especially how healthier children means less absenteeism and a more contented female workforce, which will achieve greater productivity and increase company profits.

Help mothers and carers to feed children more nutritious food

- **Understand and follow the ABC of good nutrition**:
  A. Supplementary feeding from 6 months of age while continuing breastfeeding for at least the first year, and preferably through the second year.
  B. The correct balance of nutritious foods which are available, affordable and can be easily prepared in the context of slum life, including low-cost and simply made, nutritious snacks for use between main family meals.
  C. Feeding children under 3 years old, five times a day.

- **Motivate families to spend extra income on food** for the children, rather than **squandering** it on consumables for the adults such as alcohol and cigarettes.
- **Organise community alcoholic treatment groups**.
- **Increase household income** through development activities such as literacy, vocational training and locally based income generation.

> When planning income generation activities, concentrate on skills and programmes which will increase the earning power of women, and enable them to determine the way earnings are spent: women are more likely than men to spend their earnings on food and facilities for their children.

Diarrhoea

Factors that cause diarrhoea in slum children

Crowded slums, especially in hot, wet weather are breeding grounds for germs and infection. All the causes of childhood diarrhoea are increased in these settings. The combination of poor sanitation and inadequate, unsafe water supply are the underlying causes. In this context, water and food are almost bound to be contaminated with faeces, especially if young children (who often have highly infectious stools) defaecate in path-side drains or on the ground near their homes – the same areas in which they play.

Life in a slum

A small slum community clings to the side of a large drainage canal very near a road bridge that crosses the canal. Early in the morning, before light, the footpath at the side of the bridge is filled with women and girls defaecating, ignoring the occasional bus or taxi that passes by just a few feet away. An hour or so later, men and boys repeat the process. Before the main traffic rush starts a municipal cleaner with a wheelbarrow scoops up the faeces and by 7 am the footpath is seemingly clear. (India)

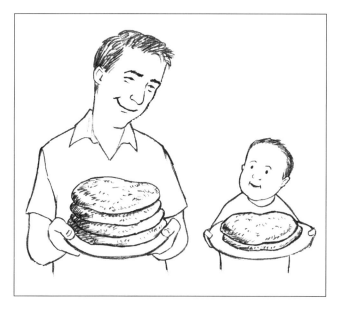

Figure 8.2   Each day a 2 year old should eat at least half the amount of food that her father eats.

Here is a summary of the reasons why slum children get such frequent diarrhoea:

The water supply is contaminated with human faeces
Local rivers, and ponds will be especially contaminated. Shallow wells are dangerous as germs can leech from the suface and contaminate groundwater supplies. Piped supplies may come from contaminated sources, or have leaks that suck in dirt and germs. This is especially true when water flow is intermittent, which may cause negative pressure within the water pipe. Water, once collected, may be stored in unclean containers or contaminated by dirty fingers or utensils. See Chapter 14, Improvements to the Water Supply.

There is not enough water
With little water available, especially in hot dry seasons, children (and those preparing food) are unlikely to wash their hands before eating, preparing meals, and after defaecation – or after cleaning a child who has defaecated. Germs also multiply in food left on unwashed dishes and utensils.

Bottle-feeding is more likely
Milk given by bottle is often diluted with contaminated water.

Ways we can prevent diarrhoea in infants and young children include
The most effective remedy is permanent improvement in the sanitation, water supply and total environment of the slum community. Chapters 14, 15 and 16 of this book describe how this can come about. If and until that happens we must do everything possible to reduce the faecal contamination of children's' food and drink. Our emphasis is on maximising personal hygiene in an unhygienic environment. Here are some priorities:

Prevent faecal contamination of water and food

We can do this by educating and motivating both children and their carers about the following:

- That mothers should exclusively breastfeed their infants for the first 6 months. This is the most useful thing we can do. See under malnutrition, page 119.
- That children should defaecate only in designated areas, separate from play spaces. They should avoid using open drains, and the centres or sides of paths.
- That children and all family members should wash hands before preparing food and eating, and after defecating or cleaning a child who has defecated. Advice needs to be relevant to the constraints of slum life and be relatively easy to carry out. (e.g. not involve large amounts of water which means even more queuing at the water tap).

In addition, we can make use of 'Child-to-Child' activities in which children are trained and empowered to understand the causes and prevention of illness. They use this knowledge to train and encourage their siblings, parents and friends in ways in which they can live more healthy lives. See an example later in this chapter.

Increase water supply

Individuals and families need a small amount of fully clean, uncontaminated water for drinking and larger amounts of water for washing which should be as clean as possible. There are ways that we can increase both the quality and quantity of water. Here are some examples of actions that can be taken:

- Organise the community to find out why there is not enough water and then to do something about it.

  For example, fix leaky pipes and broken pumps. Lobby appropriate government officials for more water points.
- Store water in clean containers and prevent contamination within the home.
- Encourage collection of rainwater where appropriate.

Ways we can treat diarrhoea and dehydration in slum children

Ensure that all mothers and community members know how to recognise dehydration and use Oral Rehydration Solution (ORS)

Specifically they will need to know:

- where to buy ORS packets and how to make home based supplies or food-based substitutes (e.g. rice water), if packets are unavailable or too expensive;
- how to feed the correct amount of ORS to dehydrated children and those with diarrhoea;
- that breastfed children with diarrhoea should continue to receive breast-milk;
- the signs of dehydration;
- when a child needs referral to a health centre, e.g. if he is too sick to swallow ORS;
- that children with diarrhoea should be fed nutritious food as soon as they are willing to eat.

Monitor the use of ORS in the community

Make sure that family members do actually use ORS in cases of diarrhoea. Members of a children's group could do this or it could be a 'Child-to-Child Activity'.

Ensure that a local, affordable supply of ORS packets is always available

The Community Action Group could be responsible for this.

Discourage families from taking children with simple diarrhoea to health centres for unnecessary medicines or injections

Mothers and carers should be taught how to use ORS.

Acute respiratory infections

Life in a slum

Johri lives in a hut made of plywood with a tin roof. Seven people live in the 2 metres by 2 metres hut. Johri's father smokes and his mother cooks their meals on an open fire. Johri coughs most of the time, but especially during the cooler, rainy season. When he gets fever, his mother gives him medicine that she buys out of her meagre earnings from the chemist shop. (Uganda)

Causes of respiratory infections in slum children

The World Health Organization states: 'Acute Respiratory Infection (ARI) is the leading cause of death in children under 5, killing over 2 million children each year. Up to 40% of children seen in health clinics are suffering from ARI, and many deaths attributable to other causes are in fact "hidden" ARI deaths.'

People living in poor urban communities, as in crowded refugee camps, are more prone to respiratory infections than others. Here are some reasons:

Exposure to disease-causing organisms

Reason for exposure to disease-causing organisms are:

- Overcrowding and poor ventilation lead to poor air quality.
- People constantly arriving from outside communities bring in new strains of organisms, for which existing members of the slum have little immunity.
- Malnutrition and chronic anaemia. These lower resistance, making children more likely to become ill and to remain infectious to others for a longer period.
- HIV/AIDS is worsening the situation in many communities.
- Tuberculosis, a disease of poverty, is more common.

The small, overcrowded houses, which often have no windows because of lack of space and security concerns, encourage respiratory infections, which are transmitted through coughing and sneezing. In addition to colds and flu, measles and TB are transmitted in this way.

Exposure to respiratory irritants and toxins

Causes of exposure to respiratory irritants and toxins are:

- cooking indoors with smoky fuel (wood, cow dung, etc.),
- indoor tobacco smoking,
- traffic pollution,
- air pollution from nearby factories or industries.

Air pollution irritates the respiratory tract, making respiratory infection more likely and more serious.

Ways we can help to prevent respiratory infections in slum children

As with preventing diarrhoea, major changes in the slum environment are the key to reducing respiratory illness. This depends on improving the quality of housing, increasing ventilation, and reducing overcrowding (see Chapter 13). In the meantime there are useful activities which the community can carry out:

Reduce exposure to diseases-causing organisms

- Take action to improve nutrition. Well-nourished children are less likely to die from ARI and measles.
- Ensure infants receive BCG and measles vaccine.
- Facilitate an effective TB control programme based on passive casefinding, careful caseholding and aiming for 85% cure rates (see Chapter 10).

Reduce exposure to respiratory irritants and toxins

- Educate the community about dangers of:
  - smoking tobacco, including the hidden danger of passive smoking – non-smokers especially children, breathing in the smoke of others;
  - using smoky fuels indoors;
  - windowless houses which concentrate germs and pollutants.

- Demonstrate and encourage use of smokeless fuel or smokeless stove, or cooking outside.
- Organise employees to protest against industrial pollution, especially the effects of any factory in the immediate area, or up-wind from the slum.
- Press for the enforcement of existing anti-pollution laws and the passing of stronger ones. With pollution becoming a worldwide concern, opportunities exist to network with environmental agencies.

Arrange prompt treatment for acute respiratory infection

Respiratory illnesses can kill quickly especially if pneumonia develops. Most cases of ARI do not need treatment with antibiotics, but for some they are essential and must be started urgently.

- Train CHVs in the diagnosis and treatment of children with respiratory infections according to the guidelines developed by WHO. Treatment depends upon the age of the child, respiratory rate and other easily recognised clinical signs. References for these guidelines are included in the resources at the end of this chapter.

- Always have supplies of antibiotics readily available. If CHVs have medicine kits, ensure they **always** have a supply of antibiotics (within legal constraints) and know how and when to use them.

Vaccine-preventable diseases and vitamin A deficiency

At the time of writing, seven illnesses are targeted by the World Health Organization for universal immunisation:

- diphtheria, pertussis and tetanus, the 'D', 'P', and 'T' of the DPT immunisation;
- polio, which is on the verge of eradication;
- measles, which can cause respiratory illness;
- tuberculosis, for which BCG is given (this is most useful in preventing tuberculous meningitis rather than respiratoy TB);
- hepatitis B which causes severe liver infection and greatly increases the risk of liver cancer in later life.

Vaccines are also widely available against other diseases including two forms of meningitis (meningococcal, prevalant in large parts of Africa and elsewhere), and haemophilus B, which is prevalent in most countries of the world). Vaccine is also available against pneumococcal infection, which can cause pneumonia and meningitis. Urban yellow fever is an increasing risk in cities of South America and West Africa, e.g. in Santa Cruz, Bolivia.

Blindness due to advanced vitamin A deficiency is becoming less common, but it has recently been recognised that in children who have milder forms of vitamin A deficiency, acute respiratory infections, measles and diarrhoea are more severe. Vitamin A can be given as a regular supplement along with childhood immunisations. It reduces the death rate from ARI and measles, as well as having other benefits. All countries will have national guidelines on immunisations, and most on vitamin A. Information is also available from the World Health Organization, (see resources at end of chapter).

Reasons slum children do not receive the WHO-recommended primary series of immunisations

Although urban children usually live near clinics and should be easily reached, there are also reasons why uptake is lower than it should be:

- Families are frequently on the move, meaning children can easily miss their immunisations.
- Mothers are at work during clinic hours.
- Government services, including immunisations, may not be available to those living in illegal settlements.
- Families pick and choose health care, often using untrained or private practitioners who may not provide immunisations.
- Health-care providers are not trained to immunise children at all opportunities, not just at formal immunisation clinics.

Ways we can help to ensure that slum children are immunised

Educate all community members and families
Community members and families should know:

- which illnesses can be prevented by immunisation;
- the age when children should start immunisations;
- details of nation-wide immunisation programmes and National Immunisation Days (NIDs);
- the locations and opening times of health centres that provide immunisations.

> We will also need to correct misperceptions about the danger or purpose of vaccines and help to answer widespread concerns. Incorrect rumours may need confronting.

Ensure access to immunisation services, including vitamin A supplements

- Follow national immunisation guidelines.
- Make certain that the cold chain is carefully maintained: check refrigerators regularly and have an alternative fuel supply if there are frequent electricity cuts.
- Keep records of immunisations via clinic registers, project computers or CHV lists, and send reminders through CHVs or lane health visitors. These follow-up activities of defaulters and non-attenders are known as 'mopping up operations'. They help to raise immunisation coverage to the level that reduces the dangers of community-wide epidemics – especially important with measles.
- Organise services at times of day community members can attend without having to miss a day's work, e.g. early morning and evening.
- Offer immunisations through project health centres to all eligible children, whatever their reason for attendance (not just at 'immunisation' clinic).

> Most acute illnesses in children are NOT a contraindication to immunisation!

HIV/AIDS

Life in a slum

Kim is 3 years old. She contracted AIDS from her mother at birth. Her father was a truck driver and died of AIDS before she was born. Since her father died, Kim's mother has earned a living by running a food stall near their house. Kim would spend the day at the food stall with her mother. But in the past few weeks Kim's mother has been sick with diarrhoea and weight loss and hasn't been able to run the food stall. Kim's older sister has come to help but she doesn't have much time to take care of Kim. (Thailand)

AIDS is more common in urban areas because of the high prevalence of sexual promiscuity and injected substance abuse. AIDS may affect children living in slums in a number of ways:

- **Children may themselves have HIV-AIDS**. Children can become infected from their mother during pregnancy, at birth or when breastfeeding, or from sexual abuse or from receiving a contaminated blood transfusion.

- **Children may be orphaned**. Children whose parents die may not have other relatives nearby to take them in. Their extended family may not be aware that the parents have died or may not be able to cope with the added burden.

- **Children may become more prone to poverty and neglect** if a household member has AIDS. The loss of income and the cost of medical care mean less food and other necessities for the family.

- **Children may have an increased risk of contracting tuberculosis**, which unless treated with the correct drug combination can develop resistance. In overcrowded slums the danger of spreading TB, often multi-resistant, to other members of the household and community is high.

For more on HIV/AIDS, see Chapter 9, and page 148.

Other common illnesses

Skin infections and **conjunctivitis** are common in slums because of inadequate amounts of water, which combined with ignorance, prevents adequate hand washing, bathing and washing clothes. In addition to personal hygiene issues which were discussed earlier in this chapter and in Chapters 14 and 15, we should motivate children's' families to ensure they receive prompt treatment from CHVs or neighbourhood clinics. It is ideal if CHVs, who use medicine kits, have a supply of antibiotic/antiseptic cream, antibiotic eye drops, and oral antibiotics (within legal constraints), with clear instructions how and when to use each.

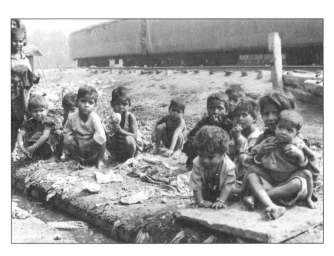

Figure 8.3   With children, defecation and play are often done in the same place. (Godfrey Martin/ASHA)

Worm infestations (e.g. round, pin, whip, hook and tapeworm) are common in children living in slums. In the case of roundworms especially, this is because children play in areas where humans, often other small children, have defecated. In some East African cities almost the entire child population has one or more types of intestinal worm. Heavy or prolonged infestations can cause stunting of growth and reduced alertness and intelligence. If worm loads are known to be heavy consider regular deworming every 4–6 months.

Urban malaria is common in some Asian cities and **dengue fever** is a rapidly growing threat to children's health in Asia, Latin America and parts of Africa. Both are spread by mosquito, but the *Aedes* mosquito which spreads dengue can breed rapidly in small amounts of water, such as air conditioner vents and water-filled hoof prints. It also tends to bite during the day. Where either of these illnesses or other insect-borne diseases are common, e.g. filariasis, arrange community distribution of permethrin-impregnated bed-nets which as well as preventing bites, kill insects that land on them if resoaked every 6–12 months. Also work with the Community Action Group to minimise breeding sites. Government spraying teams and community-wide prevention measures will be needed, especially to deal with dengue, and we may need to advocate for them to visit regularly. In the case of malaria, make sure drug treatment is quickly available.

Schistosomiasis (bilharzia) is invading urban areas in many parts of Africa, and some in South-east Asia. This blood fluke breeds in water which contains certain species of snail and which is contaminated by human faeces or urine. It causes blood, not always visible, in the urine or faeces, which can lead to anaemia and often to serious long-term complications. Where this illness is common train the community not to allow children (or adults), to bathe, play, urinate or defecate in open water sources. Consider yearly distribution of praziquantel tablets if infection rates are high.

Injuries and accidents

Children who live in slums are exposed to hazards in the home, the workplace and the community. Accidents are common. They have been described as the great unseen epidemic.

Factors that cause accidents and injuries in slum children

Children are poorly supervised

In rural areas most households include grandparents, parents and children. In urban slums, families are usually nuclear, containing only one or two generations. If both parents work outside the home, children may be left to fend for themselves or are left in the care of a sister or brother not much older than themselves. This multiplies the dangers of accidents and injuries.

Hazards in the home

- Homes are so small and crowded that there is no place in the house to store toxic household chemicals, such as kerosene.
- Open fires are often used for cooking or heating.
- Homes may be used as a workplace and work tools, toxic substances or other dangerous materials left or stored in easy reach of children.

Hazards in the community

- overloaded, exposed electrical wiring,
- dense housing made of, or containing, highly flammable substances, leading to the danger of flash fires,

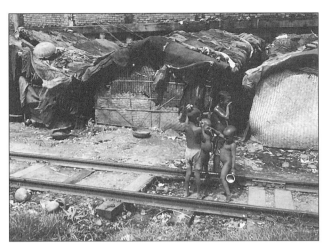

- nearby roads without walls or fencing,
- open drains,
- flooding,
- toxic waste from factories and industries,
- poor access for emergency vehicles.

Figure 8.4   Slums are located in hazardous places, especially for young children. (Richard Hanson/Tearfund)

Life in a slum

James and his family were scavengers. Piles of materials that would be sold later surrounded their house. One night a fire broke out while the family slept. A leak in an illegally tapped natural gas line was the cause and kept feeding the fire, which spread with terrifying speed. The footpaths were so narrow and the houses so packed together that people could not escape. James and his father were just able to get away but his mother and two younger sisters died. Over 1000 huts were burnt that night before firemen controlled the blaze. They were unable to bring in fire-fighting vehicles because the paths between huts were too narrow. (Kenya)

Ways we can prevent accidents and injuries in children

Before we take any action it is important to know the common causes of injuries or accidents in our particular community We may need to arrange a sample survey, or questionnaire. The CAG can organise this or might gather information through other means. They could draw a map locating main hazards in the community. Then they can target solutions for the common and serious problems in the community. Here are some examples of useful activities:

1. Encourage the women's group to organise a day-care centre for children of working mothers.
2. Encourage the community to designate an open area for recreation where children can play safely.
3. Start a child-to-child programme to make homes safe. Teach children about hazards and how to reduce or eliminate them. Then let them check their houses and the houses of neighbours for hazards and look for ways to reduce them.
4. Encourage children's or women's groups to approach the government for a key community improvement with maximum benefit, e.g. covering a dangerous drain or removing a large pile of garbage.

⑤ Help the community to approach the electricity or natural gas authority for legal connections. The Community Action Group and project could work on this together.

⑥ Help the community to develop a disaster plan for times of flooding or fire, etc.

Psychosocial problems: physical and sexual abuse

Factors that contribute to abuse of slum children

Children are often the main victims of the intense social problems that are present in slums, made worse by extreme poverty and the breakdown of traditional values. Commonly this leads to child abuse – physical, sexual or both. Specific factors include:

- **Extreme poverty** with seemingly insoluble problems faced by adult members of the household.
- **Severe overcrowding** and lack of privacy.
- **Absence of an older adult** to provide security, though sometimes older men, including fathers or uncles are abusers.
- **Male unemployment**. Men who are idle and demoralised, more quickly become violent or unreliable in their behaviour.
- **Alcoholism, and drug abuse** are the precipitating factors in many communities.
- The **high divorce/abandonment rate** so that children are more likely to be living with their mother's new husband or partner, who is not the child's father. The children become unwanted reminders of times gone by.
- **Pornographic and violent material** on video may increase the likelihood of abuse.

Life in a slum

Issa's mother earns money cleaning houses. His father is a day labourer. When he doesn't have work, he frequently beats Issa's mother if she won't give him money to buy liquor. One time Issa tried to stop his father from beating his mother, but his father just beat Issa. So now when they fight, Issa leaves the house and sleeps at a friend's house. (Tanzania)

Sexually abused children and those forced into commercial sex work are at increased risk for becoming infected with HIV:

- They often do not know how HIV is transmitted or how to protect themselves.

- Even if they knew, they would find it difficult or too expensive to buy condoms.

- Even if they obtained condoms, they would find it hard or impossible to insist that their clients should use them.

- When children have sex with an adult, genital injury often occurs, allowing easier transmission of HIV. Anal sex, usually more traumatic and therefore a higher HIV risk, is relatively common in order to avoid pregnancy when men have sex with young girls.

Adapted from: *Street and Working Children*, p. 24.

Ways we can help to detect and prevent abuse in children

Many aspects of abuse require specialised areas of help. We should try and discover any sources of specialist care, advice or information that we can use when cases of abuse come to our notice. We should ensure that programme staff and Community Health Volunteers have a broad understanding of these issues and know what procedures to follow if they suspect a child is being abused.

1. Train staff and Community Health Volunteers to detect child abuse (see box below).

2. Help families to become aware about issues surrounding abuse.

3. Provide a centre for recreation (a temporary safe haven) where children know they will be out of danger.

4. If children are in danger, help find a safe place for the them to live (family, friends or institution).

5. Provide counselling and support services for families in which abuse is occurring. This requires a highly sensitive approach and careful professional training. Until project staff acquire these skills we should make use of other service providers.

6. Encourage the Community Action Group to apply pressure on the abuser, but only to inform the police if essential. Often their insensitive approach can make the problems worse.

7. Raise the status of women. (See Chapter 7 on Women's health in slums.)

Suspect child abuse if one or more of these features is present:

1. The child's injuries seem to be greater than might be expected for the reason given.

2. The child has injuries of varying ages, such as old fractures or scars, when presenting with fresh injury.

3. The child has burns in unexpected places such as stomach and back rather than hands or feet.

4. The child is fearful or won't talk when a certain relative/person is in the room.

5. The child volunteers that they have vaginal or anal bleeding or injury.

6. The child gives a story suggestive of abuse.

We must never start taking action against abuse unless we have firm evidence. Through training and experience we must avoid the twin dangers of failing to recognise abuse, and incorrectly assuming it to be present.

How does urban poverty put children to work?

Life in a slum

Eight-year-old Juan and his family moved to Cebu 4 years ago when his father couldn't find work in their small fishing village. His father makes deliveries for a store that sells stoves and refrigerators. Juan's mother died a few years ago in childbirth, and his father married again, though rarely comes home. His stepmother and older sister run a stall in the market. Juan spends his day scavenging. He and two friends rent a cart and then at the end of the day sell their findings to the cart owner, making a profit of just $0.50 (US) for the day. He uses his money to buy food for his younger brother and himself. In the evening Juan comes home in time to cook dinner for the two of them. Then he goes to a night school where he is finishing his primary education. He gets home about 10 pm, the time his sister and step mother usually arrive back from their stall. Recently Juan cut his hand on a sharp lid in some garbage he was sorting. He wrapped it in a piece of cloth, which stopped the bleeding, but his hand has become swollen, red and painful. Finding money to pay for treatment has proved difficult. (Philippines)

Many children who live in slums must work in order to help to provide food for their family. They may work in a family enterprise, such as delivering tea or washing dishes at a family food stall. They may not be paid for such work, but their labour does produce income for the family. Children may beg, scavenge, shine shoes or sell small objects. Often they must pay someone for the 'right' to work on a particular street corner or in a particular garbage dump. That person protects their spot and bribes police to leave them alone. Children may work in people's homes, cleaning the house and minding the children. Children, especially girls, often take care of younger siblings and the house. They are not paid, but they do free up adults who can then work outside the home.

What are the special problems of working children

Unfortunately, it is unrealistic to try to prevent children from working. A family's survival often depends upon child labour. It is important, however, to understand what the problems are so we can take action to improve working conditions and ban forms of labour that are dangerous or abusive.

1. **Working children are exploited**. They usually work in the informal, unregulated sector, leading to long hours and low pay. They will usually have no protection from injustice or unsafe practices. Underage working children are powerless and therefore open to all forms of danger and exploitation.

2. **Working children may have been sold or kidnapped into bondage**. This means that worldwide there are millions of child slaves. For a particular family this process often starts as they slip deeper into poverty and debt, until those to whom they owe money gain full control over the family and their labour. Children can be severely exploited in these circumstances. Being inexperienced and often lacking skills they may perform badly or break equipment adding further to the family's debt and hardship.

③ **Working children may perform tasks that are dangerous or harmful to their health**. Common jobs performed by slum children include scavenging on rubbish dumps where accidents can easily occur from sharp objects, begging or selling at traffic lights with dangers from accidents and toxic fumes, and in many cities, child prostitution.

④ **Working children often are not able to attend school**.

How can we help working children?

It is important for us to see working children as self-reliant, resourceful young people. They are helping both themselves and their family to survive. Often any alternative to child labour is worse both for the child and their family. This idea may seem unacceptable to those from wealthier backgrounds but it is a fact of life for millions of children worldwide. Our interventions must help to empower and protect families and not deny them the very means of survival. In practice we have two options:

- The first is to help ban those forms of child labour, which are by nature dangerous and exploitative. An example of this is child prostitution. But as we take action against one form of labour **we must ensure that other forms of employment are available**.
- The second is to help make existing working conditions, safer, healthier and with shorter working hours.

In both cases we must ensure children have access to education whether at school or through informal arrangements. Here are some suggestions:

① **Advocate banning child labour**, especially if the work is dangerous with unacceptable or illegal hours and working practices. Seek out any NGOs, or other organisation that has expertise in this area and work with them, or through them.

② **Provide training in appropriate basic skills in literacy and numeracy** to protect children from being taken advantage of in the streets or in the workplace.

③ **Provide schooling opportunities** in the evening or early morning hours.

④ **Provide vocational training** to provide young people with safer and better-paid alternatives. Involve the trainees in planning content and timings so they feel empowered by their involvement.

⑤ **Help child workers organise to work for better working conditions, and for savings programmes**. This will mean understanding labour laws and may mean seeking legal advice.

⑥ **Provide training in basic job-seeking skills**, such as personal presentation, time-keeping and letter-writing, and, where appropriate, in basic business skills such as simple accounting, and computer skills.

From the field: The Columbian College of Olongapo, Philippines started a programme (Reach-Up) to help children of the urban poor. Among other activities, the programme has encouraged working children to form associations, so now there are a bus washers' association, a scavengers' association, a pushcart boys' association, etc. Now, uniforms identify them to the clients and the public, savings programmes have been organised, and contracts negotiated.

Lesson learned: Organisation and advocacy activities can make a very big difference in the lives of slum children.

Source: Black, 1991.

Street children

The majority of 'street children' who are seen working or living on the streets in low-income countries are children from slum households. But not all. There are several types of street children, and each has a different set of characteristics and problems.

1. **Children who live on the street with their family**. These children live on pavements or other open spaces with their families, often with little or no shelter. The family is often new to the city and is still looking for employment and a permanent place to live. Some families live on pavements for extended periods, having found a nearby water point, local jobs and police willing to be paid bribes to let them stay on. Children living in such circumstances have little chance of receiving any form of health care, immunisations or schooling.

2. **Children who live on the street without their family**. These children live on the streets having left their family. Younger children are more likely to have been orphaned or abandoned, and older children more likely to have been abused. Street children without families often live in groups which provide informal protection and support. Sometimes a group of such children live in a slum hut, but more commonly they sleep on the streets, at railway or bus stations or in shop doorways. They are often unable to bathe and have no safe place to keep their very few possessions. They frequently turn to glue sniffing or other addictions, then need to steal to feed their habit.

3. **Children who live at home with their family but spend most of their time on the street**. It is this type of street child who usually lives in slums. In most cities this group makes up the majority of street children. They may spend much of their day working on the streets, shining shoes, begging, scavenging, or washing car windscreens, but come home at night to sleep.

How can we work through children

In Chapter 2 on Working with the community we saw the importance of the community needing to own the project and also the need for there to be a 'vehicle' such as a Community Action Group to take programme activities foward. Similarly when working with children, we can encourage them to set up their own programme and carry out activities through a children's group or club. Children should decide themselves which problems they wish to tackle and how they want to go about it. Even with younger children, we can encourage them to express their ideas and point of view, and to take an active role in the life of the community. The Child-to-Child programme (see resources at the end of this chapter) gives many ideas of how this can be done.

> Children who grow up in slums take on adult responsibilities early. Therefore we must resist the temptation to treat them like children and work for them. Instead, we should take advantage of their abilities and work with them to solve their problems and those of the community that affect them.

Sometimes children who live in slums have time on their hands. Their parents and older siblings are usually working. They have no place to play and have energy, which if not guided, can lead to destructive behaviour. They also crave attention. Formation of children's club helps to turn their energy into positive actions for the community. The objectives of a children's club will include:

1. To discover obstacles which prevent children and the wider community from being healthy.
2. To take action to address the problems they find.
3. To pass on their knowledge and experience to younger children.

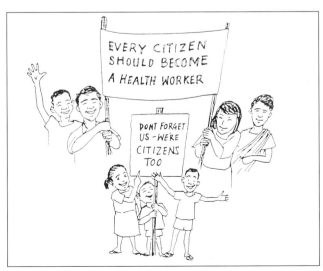

Figure 8.5   All children are health workers.

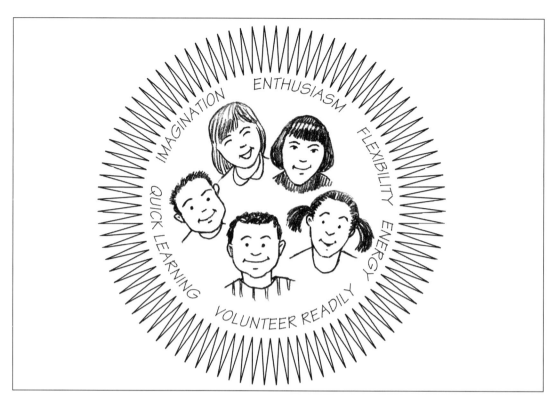

Figure 8.6   Children have many characteristic that make them excellent agents of change.

How do we form a children's group?

❶ **Mix informally with the children**. Play games with them, get to know them and gain their trust and confidence. In some communities we will need to take care that others do not misunderstand our actions.

❷ **Organise meetings**. The best time is usually in the late afternoon after school hours. We bring the conversation around to discuss problems the children experience in the community. Common examples are: no place to play, frequent attacks of diarrhoea, no place for defecation, nothing fun to do and bullying.

❸ **Organise the group**. Older children become the group leaders and take a lead in planning activities.

> Each meeting will need to include at least one fun activity that will hold the children's interest and increase future attendance by making them look forward to the next meeting of the club.

❹ **Provide training, especially for group leaders**. Just as with adults, children leading the club will need special training in communication, how to organise meetings, write letters and talk to officials

From the field: In one slum community, children who were members of a children's club decided to make their community a more pleasant and a safer place by trying to reduce the number of young children who defecated in the pathside drains. The caretakers, usually mothers or older sisters, didn't want to walk all the distance to the community latrine complex. The children decided on two activities:

1. They made an effort to take their younger brothers and sisters to the latrine complex when possible, so saving their mother or older sister the time, and showing their commitment in helping to help solve the problem.

2. They took responsibility for educating neighbouring families assigned to them about the dangers of open defecation and the benefits of having cleaner drains and paths.

They did this by patrolling their designated area each afternoon after school and keeping track of how many times they saw a child defecating, or noticed faeces in the drain or on the paths. If they knew which family was at fault they would visit and remind them. The children plotted the number of violations on a chart and were very excited to note that after a few weeks, the numbers fell substantially. (India)

Lesson learned: Children with their energy and enthusiasm can be effective agents of change.

Source: Authors.

The Child-to-Child Approach

A Child-to-Child Programme was developed at the University of London, Institutes of Child Health and Education, with the input from colleagues all over the world. It is based on the belief that children need good health but also are very able to give health to others. Child-to-Child activities give children new knowledge, skills and understanding about health issues, especially those that concern their own health. The activities are designed to make learning fun and interesting. Child-to-Child programmes can be school- or community-based. The Child-to-Child Trust has published books and other materials that describe in detail how to set up a Child-to-Child Programme. Some of the publications are listed in Resources at the end of the chapter; a full list can be obtained from Child-to-Child Trust, whose address is listed in Appendix 2.

What does a children's group do?

Here are some working examples from different slum communities:

1   They can help make a **community diagnosis**.
    - **Make a community map**. Children can either join in when the adults are making their map, or better, make their own map, then compare it with the one made by adults. It will help to show what children see as priorities, and begin to give them a sense of ownership of community life and what they can do about it.

- **Do a survey**. Each child is assigned 5–10 houses to investigate a subject which the group has identified to be interesting or important to them. For example each child can keep track of the number of children who have diarrhoea and the number who have been treated with oral rehydration solution. They can see which groups of houses use ORS most regularly, and then point this out in an appropriate way.

➋ They can carry out **specific actions or tasks** each of which has value in itself.

Here are some examples:
- **They can educate other children, child caretakers or other segments of the community**:
  – by writing and performing songs, dramas or puppet shows,
  – by drawing posters or arranging a poster-drawing competition.
- **They can help make their community to become a better place to live**:
  – by cleaning drains around their house,
  – by planting trees,
  – by holding a general clean-up day.

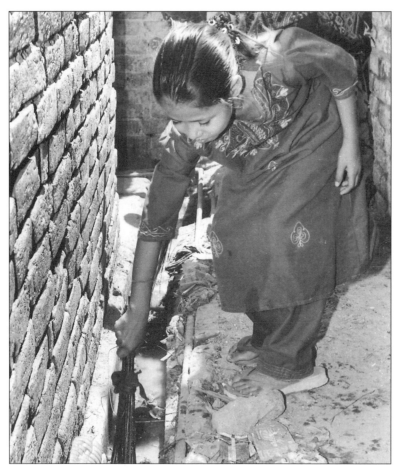

Figure 8.7   Children can participate in making their community cleaner and healthier.
(Godfrey Martin/ASHA)

- **They can track the health of babies or pregnant women**:
  - Each club member can 'adopt' a newborn baby who lives nearby. The child reminds the mother when immunisations are due, helps with regular weighing, encourages the use of ORS when the baby gets diarrhoea, and where appropriate give a hand with childminding as the baby gets older.
  - They can compare the health and weights of children being 'adopted' with that of a similar (control) group not being adopted by children's club members. Learning to plot weights on a growth chart can improve students' graphing skills learned in school.

Chapter summary

Children living in slums are vulnerable to a whole range of illnesses, accidents and abuse. Poverty coupled with a poor water supply and sanitation underlie most illnesses, including malnutrition, diarrhoea and acute respiratory infections. Each can be greatly reduced by education and specific interventions. Injuries and accidents through open drains, unguarded chemicals, vehicles and faulty wiring can be largely prevented by community-wide precautions. HIV/AIDS is an increasing problem in slums, caused through infected mothers, child abuse and prostitution. One of the most effective ways to promote children's health is to form children's clubs which empower children to recognise problems of importance to them and take action to deal with them. This helps childen to grow up to be responsible citizens. Children are an important and overlooked resource for improving their own health and that of the slum environment.

Resources

1. *Setting up Community Health Programmes: A Practical Manual for Use in Developing Countries*, 2nd edition. T Lankester. Macmillan Education, 1999. Discusses specific child diseases, including diagnosis and treatment, in the context of a community health and development programme. (Available from TALC.)

2. *Stepping Forward: Children and Young People's Participation in Development Process.* V Johnson, E Ivan-Smith, G Gorden, P Pridmore, P Scott-Villiers. Intermediate Technology Publications, 1997. Discusses the key issues and challenges on involving children and youth in the development process.

3. *Malaria: A Manual for Community Health Volunteers.* WHO, 1996. Simply written, comprehensive review for community health workers.

4. *The Management of Acute Respiratory Infections in Children.* WHO, 1995. WHO guidelines for diagnosing and treating acute respiratory infections in infants and young children.

5. WHO is responsible along with UNICEF for the *Expanded Programme on Immunisation: Information, Resources and Newsletter. (Available from WHO.)*

6. *Street and Working Children: A Guide to Planning.* J Ennew. Save the Children Publications, 1994. Very practical and extensive discussion on how to work with street children.

7. *Where There is No Doctor: A Village Health Care Book*. D Werner, C Thuman, J Maxwell. The Hesperian Foundation, 1993 (revised English edition). This book is available in over 50 languages. It covers the diagnosis and treatment of most of the common health problems of children. (Available from TALC.)

8. *Facts for Life: A Communication Challenge*. UNICEF, WHO, UNESCO, UNFPA, 1993. A booklet that communicates the essential messages for child health in critical areas such as breastfeeding, birth spacing, immunizations, diarrhoea and respiratory infections. (Available from TALC.)

9. *Children for Health: Children as Communicators of the Facts of Life*. H Hawes, C Scotchmer. The Child-to-Child Trust, 1993. Provides practical ways that children can convey the important health issues from the Facts for Life book. (Available from TALC.)

10. *Child-to-Child: A Resource Book Part 1: Implementing the Child-to-Child Approach*. H Hawes, D Bailey, G Bonati (eds). The Child-to-Child Trust, 1992. A comprehensive resource book containing sections on the Child-to-Child concept, methodology, evaluation and running workshops. (Available from TALC.)

11. *Child-to-Child: A Resource Book Part 2: Child-to-Child Activity Sheets*. D Bailey, H Hawes, G Bonati (eds). The Child-to-Child Trust, 1992. Activity sheets on a wide variety of health topics. (Available from TALC.)

12. *Child-to-Child and Children Living in Camps*. C Hanbury (ed.) The Child-to-Child Trust, 1999. Although directed at children living in refugee camps, their situation is in many ways the same as slum children, especially the environment. This book has many practical ways to include children in making their situation healthier. (Available from TALC.)

13. *Philippines: Children of the Runaway Cities* (part of Innocenti Studies on the Urban Child in Difficult Circumstances). M Black. UNICEF International Child Development Centre, 1991. In depth study of children of the urban poor in the Philippines, giving good insights and many case studies of successful projects.

14. *Urbanization and its Implications for Child Health: Potential for Action*. WHO, 1988. A good review of health problems of children of the urban poor.

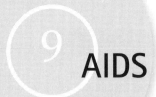

AIDS

At the time of writing the World Health Organization estimates that there are approximately 35 million people living with HIV/AIDS. This number is increasing by between 15 and 20% per year. In many major cities of sub-Saharan Africa, 20–40% of adults in the 20–45-year-old age-group are HIV-positive, and AIDS is the major killer in that age-group. In the major cities of Asia, including India, Thailand and Cambodia, the epidemic is growing at a rapid pace. HIV infection spreads especially fast in cities, where injected drug abuse and prostitution are more common.

There is no cure for HIV infection yet, although combination therapy with expensive drugs is available for the tiny minority who can afford them. Combination drug therapy can greatly increase the length of survival, but it is beyond the reach of the urban poor in developing countries.

In addition to causing misery and death, HIV/AIDS further increases poverty, as it consumes scarce resources that could be used for other pressing needs. It also tends to kill adults of reproductive age, in other words the main wage earners and care providers, thus causing a double impact on children, many of whom are eventually orphaned.

What we need to know

What is AIDS?

AIDS (Acquired Immune Deficiency Syndrome) is a disease caused by the Human Immuno-deficiency Virus (HIV). HIV attacks the immune system so that an infected person is unable to resist infections, and eventually dies.

Table 9.1	An HIV Glossary.
AIDS	Acquired Immune Deficiency Syndrome; a group of signs and symptoms caused by the Human Immuno-deficiency Virus (HIV)
ELISA	The most common test to detect antibodies against Human Immuno-deficiency Virus (HIV)
HIV	Human Immuno-deficiency Virus; the virus that causes AIDS
HIV–positive	HIV antibodies are present in the blood. Usually, this means that the person is infected with HIV
HIV–negative	HIV antibodies are not present in the blood. Usually, but not always, this means that the person is not infected with HIV. It takes up to 3 months from the time of exposure to the time when the ELISA and Western Blot HIV tests becomes positive. During this 'window period' people are still infectious even though they test HIV-negative
Immune deficiency	The body's immune system is weakened making it less able to fight off infections
Immune system	The body's system that defends against infections caused by bacteria, viruses and other infectious agents
PLWHA	A common term to describe those infected with or affected by HIV/AIDS. It stands for People Living With HIV/AIDS
Transmission	The way in which an infection is spread from one person to another
Western blot	A test to detect HIV antibodies which is more accurate (and more expensive) than the ELISA test

How do people become infected with HIV?

HIV is present in the blood, semen and vaginal secretions of an infected person. To become infected, the virus present in the affected person's semen or blood must come into contact with the uninfected person's bloodstream. In practice there are three main ways a person can become infected with HIV:

Through sexual activity with an infected person

This is the most common way of becoming infected. When having sex, the virus passes from the semen of an infected man, or from the vaginal secretions of an infected woman, into the bloodstream of the uninfected partner. The virus does this by passing through the lining of the vagina, or penis.

Several factors increase the risk of infection:

- **Women** are more likely to be infected than men.
- **Uncircumcised** men are more likely to become infected than circumcised men.

- **Sexually transmitted diseases**, especially those that cause ulcers such as syphilis, herpes and chancroid, greatly increase the risk of infection by making it easier for the virus to pass into the bloodstream.
- **Anal intercourse** has a high risk of infection for the receptive partner because injury to the rectal mucosa easily allows the virus to enter the bloodstream.

Through exposure to blood from an infected person

Uninfected people can be exposed to the blood of an infected person in several ways:

- when receiving a **blood transfusion** from an infected donor, or less commonly through inadequately prepared blood products such as immunoglobulins;
- through **intravenous drug abuse** where drug abusers share unclean needles and syringes;
- through **needles and syringes recently used** on a person infected with HIV, then being used to inject others;
- through **tattooing**, **ear and nose piercing**, **shaving** etc. when needles or blades have recently been used on a person infected with HIV;
- in the case of health workers, from **needle-stick injuries** and other instruments which accidentally pierce the skin during operations on those infected with HIV. Blood spills on damaged skin can occasionally spread infection.

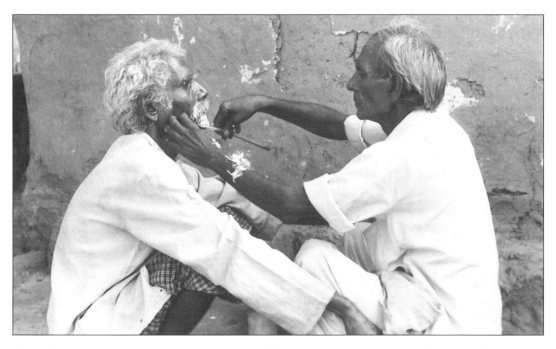

Figure 9.1   Any object that comes into contact with blood is a potential source of HIV infection. (Godfrey Martin/ASHA)

From mother to child

A woman who is infected with HIV can pass the virus on to her fetus or infant. In developing countries, about one-third of infants born to HIV-positive women become infected, either during pregnancy, during delivery or through breastfeeding.

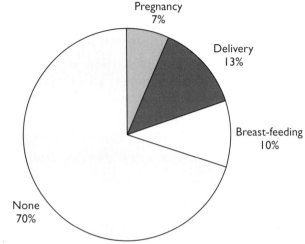

Figure 9.2   Ways in which mother-to-infant transmission of HIV occurs from HIV-positive mothers in developing countries.

HIV infection cannot be spread by close social contact, including touch. This means that those caring for people with HIV/AIDS are at minimal risk providing they take care to avoid the causes of spread mentioned above.

What happens when a person becomes infected with HIV?

After infection, the virus targets certain cells in the immune system, which respond by trying to kill the virus. The immune system is able to fight off HIV infection for months or usually years. Therefore, people who are infected with HIV have no symptoms of infection, i.e. do not suffer from AIDS, until the immune system begins to break down.

This means there is a long period when no symptoms are present, but when people are nevertheless highly infectious, usually without realising it. During this time they can spread the infection to large numbers of partners.

Months to years of being without symptoms means that one person can infect many others before it becomes obvious that he or she is infected.

After months or years, as the immune system breaks down, the person becomes less able to fight off other kinds of infection, including tuberculosis. At first the patient may respond to treatment, but soon becomes so weakened that antibiotics no longer have an effect. Death soon follows.

In industrialised countries, the common interval between exposure to infection and the onset of clinical symptoms of AIDS is over 5 years, usually between 8 and 10 years. Anti-retroviral drugs given in combination prolong this disease-free interval. Being so expensive they presently have little use outside developed countries except amongst the richest minority.

In developing countries, the disease progresses much faster. Although good data is lacking, the average time between exposure and death from AIDS is about 5–7 years, and often much less. There are several reasons for this more rapid progression of the disease:

- poor general health and nutritional status;
- greater exposure to infectious diseases such as pneumonia, tuberculosis and other infections of the respiratory tract, bowel and skin;
- lack of access to medical care when other infections occur;
- lack of access to medical therapy against HIV infection.

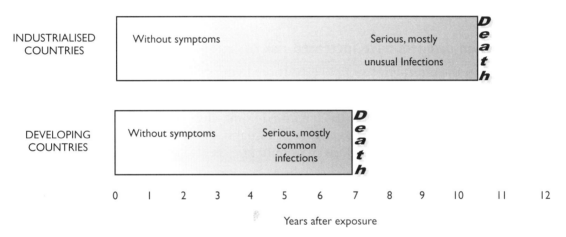

Figure 9.3   The clinical course of HIV/AIDS: Industrialised vs. developing countries.

How does HIV/AIDS impact on people living in slums?

Life in a slum

Kai is a 3-year-old girl who is dying from AIDS and tuberculosis. Kai's father became HIV-positive several years before Kai was born. He was a drug addict who shared needles with others. He died when Kai was just a few months old. Kai became ill with chronic diarrhoea and frequent infections and was found to be HIV-positive when she was 18 months old. She was probably infected through her mother, though her mother has no symptoms and has not been tested for HIV. When Kai was 2 years old, her mother moved in with her new boyfriend, and Kai was left in the care of her elderly grandmother. Kai's mother has just given birth to a son. It is not known if he is infected with HIV.

Kai and her grandmother live in the corner of a relative's shack. The grandmother is not able to work because of her age and because Kai is so sick. They receive no support or help from Kai's mother. A local NGO recently helped to set up a community response committee which now provides assistance to people with AIDS and their families. Since that time neighbours have regularly provided Kai and her grandmother with food, and look after Kai when her grandmother has to be away. They also accompany Kai and her grandmother to the hospital clinic and help to explain the instructions given by health workers. (Thailand)

The poor are disproportionately affected by HIV/AIDS. They are more likely to become infected with HIV and they have less access to medical care.

How does poverty contribute to the spread of AIDS?

- The poor and illiterate have less access to information about prevention.
- The poor have less access to condoms and the treatment of sexually transmitted diseases.
- Women who are poor and uneducated find it harder to insist that their partner uses a condom and avoids sex with other partners.
- Women who are poor and uneducated have few job opportunities outside the home and may have to resort to commercial sex work.

Why do slum dwellers have increased risk of being infected with HIV

In addition to the direct effects of poverty, those living in slums are more likely to become infected with HIV because of the unique features of slum life:

- Men from slums are less likely to be married or may live apart from their wives. This makes them more likely to engage in casual sex with more than one partner, especially if they live and work away from home.
- Women in slums are more likely to be widowed, divorced or abandoned and/or live in women-headed households. These women are more likely to have casual sex with multiple partners.
- Poverty, lack of education and social tradition often make it hard for women and young girls to find jobs, meaning they may be forced into prostitution to earn enough money to survive.
- Families are more likely to be nuclear rather than joint, resulting in a breakdown of family values. Poverty and slum life further contribute to this breakdown.

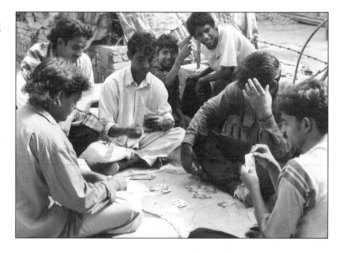

Figure 9.4   Men forced to come to the city to find work often leave their family behind in the village. They can become infected with HIV from commercial sex workers and infect their wives on return to the village. (Godfrey Martin/ASHA)

- The unsafe water supply and high cost of infant formula usually means that HIV-positive women must continue breastfeeding. (Here risks must be balanced: even though there is a 10% chance of the infant being infected with HIV, there may be an equal or higher risk of death from artificial feeding, see page 161).

> People with HIV have a greatly increased risk of developing active TB, and spreading their infection to others. Poorly ventilated and overcrowded houses typical of slums increase this risk further.

Slum dwellers are less able to cope with HIV infection

There are several reasons for this:

- Many People Living With HIV/AIDS (PLWHA) do not have the economic and caring support of extended families.
- PLWHA may not qualify for government medical or other benefits because the government does not recognise the slum. They may not be able to obtain a voting card or other identification that qualifies them for services.
- Other treatment and care facilities may be non-existent or completely inaccessible to PLWHA.

What are the problems affecting women, youth and children?

Women

- **Women have little or no power to implement HIV preventive measures such as negotiating condom use, abstinence or mutual faithfulness.** They fear displeasing their partner in case he abandons her, thus leaving her with no means of economic support.
- **Women living in slums are subject to the pressure of entering prostitution in order to survive,** especially when they are the major wage-earner for the household, as in women-headed households. Prostitution is often the only alternative for women who are uneducated and unskilled.
- **Women and girls carry the major burden of caring for people with AIDS.** In some cases this means pulling a girl out of school to care for her sick father. The lack of extended families compounds this problem.

Life in a slum

Rui is 23 years old. When her husband died of AIDS, her in-laws threw her and her 2-year-old daughter onto the streets. They wanted their other son to inherit their small piece of land. Rui and her daughter are now living with another woman. Rui cleans houses to earn some money, and takes her daughter with her. She does not know whether she is HIV-positive and refuses to be tested, as she knows she can't afford treatment and fears suffering even more sadness, rejection and shame. She has met a man and has regular, unprotected sex. She is thinking of moving in with him. (India)

Youth

Over half of all new HIV infections occur in young people between the ages of 15 and 24 years. About 90% of these young people live in developing countries.

Adolescent boys and girls are sexually active at an early age, often by their mid-teens. Many, especially boys, will have had sex with more than one partner before they are 18. The age of first sexual experience is falling and the age of marriage is rising. Therefore, more young people are engaging in pre-marital sex, so further increasing their risk of HIV infection and other sexually transmitted diseases. We have seen how nuclear families, less parental supervision and the erosion of family values, add to the social problems of slum communities. These factors also make pre- and extra-marital sex more likely and increase the average number of sexual partners. In addition young girls (and boys) may enter or be sold into prostitution.

Apart from these factors, living in cities brings exposure to films, satellite and cable television, web-sites and magazines that glamorise sex and suggest that 'everybody is doing it'.

Children

HIV/AIDS can affect children in a number of ways:

1. **Children in affected households suffer a greater degree of poverty**. People with AIDS cannot work and inevitably drain household resources. In addition children are surrounded by the emotional turmoil of someone seriously ill or dying in the household. Girls in particular will often become the primary carers, so that unaffected adults can continue to work. The caretaker role prevents girls from attending school, so perpetuating poverty.

2. **Children suffer from the rejection and social stigma of being a member of a family with HIV/AIDS**.

3. **Children in affected households may contract tuberculosis** from a household member with HIV/AIDS who has developed pulmonary tuberculosis.

Sick children of HIV-positive women are sometimes not brought for health care as it is commonly assumed they have AIDS and are likely to die anyway. Many people believe falsely that all children born to HIV-positive mothers are themselves affected. In fact two-thirds of such children are normal and unaffected.

4. **Children can become infected**. Infants can become infected from mothers through breastfeeding. Children can also become infected through sexual abuse.

They may outlive their parents, be cared for by grandparents or neighbours, or be abandoned or taken to an orphanage.

⑤ **Children may be orphaned or abandoned when parents or carers die**. Most AIDS orphans are cared for by extended family members, often grandparents. A single set of grandparents may be caring for several of their own orphaned grandchildren. The burden of caring for extra children, some of whom are HIV-positive, often overwhelms their ability to cope.

For children living in slums, the death of both parents can be life-threatening for the surviving children. Any relatives in their original village may not be aware of the deaths. The stigma of HIV/AIDS, which often carries the perception of illicit sex, may prevent the child's parents from telling other family members. Under these circumstances, the future care of their children is often the greatest concern of a dying parent.

Neighbours may adopt them, but sometimes believe wrongly that they or their children might 'catch' HIV. Sometimes the most helpful people are others who are HIV-positive, but still relatively well.

In developing countries, half of the children who are infected before birth, at delivery or during infancy will survive beyond their fifth birthday. This means that they often outlive their parents who die of AIDS.

What we need to do

The rest of this chapter looks first at ways in which HIV can be prevented, and then outlines practical steps in setting up an HIV/AIDS programme.

Understand how HIV/AIDS can be prevented

HIV/AIDS is largely a preventable illness! For each of the three main ways that HIV is spread, very specific measures, if implemented, can greatly reduce its transmission. The difficulty, and our challenge, lies in persuading people to practise the safest behaviours.

Prevention of HIV infection caused through sexual activity with an infected person

The practice of having multiple sex partners is the main reason for the spread of AIDS in Africa, Asia and most developing countries. In order to halt the AIDS pandemic, the basic values and attitudes of society and individuals must undergo a fundamental change that results in safer sexual behaviour.

BEST OPTIONS

- Remain faithful to a faithful partner **OR**
- Abstain from sexual intercourse

GOOD OPTION

- Use condom **AND**
- Treat other sexually transmitted diseases

Prevention of HIV infection caused through exposure to blood from an infected person

BEST OPTIONS

For drug abuse:
- Stop abusing any drugs **OR**
- Switch to non-injectable drugs

For injections:
- Avoid unnecessary injections for minor illnesses

For tattooing, body piercing, shaving by barbers:
- Avoid

For blood transfusions:
- Only receive blood when strongly indicated **AND**
- Test blood for HIV before transfusing **AND**
- Use known unpaid volunteers

GOOD OPTIONS

- Use disposable sterile needles and syringes, then destroy them after single use **OR**
- Use a carefully monitored needle/syringe-exchange programme **OR**
- Sterilise needles and syringes after each use

- Seek care only at reputable health care facilities that use disposable needles and syringes

- Ensure that new sterile needles/blades are used

- For transfusions, any alternatives are too risky

Prevention of HIV infection transmitted from infected mother to child

BEST OPTIONS

- If known to be HIV-positive, have no further children and undergo tubal ligation

GOOD OPTIONS

- Take a specific anti-HIV drug such as zidovudine (AZT) during the latter stages of pregnancy, delivery and during first weeks postpartum **AND**

- Consider avoiding breastfeeding (weigh against likelihood of infant dying from diarrhoea and/or malnutrition)

Decide whether to start an HIV/AIDS programme

Learn about sexual beliefs, knowledge, attitudes and practices in the community

Each of these four aspects is important to learn about. The first stage is to discover what **high-risk practices** are going on in the community. We will need to answer questions such as:

- **Sexual practices**: To what extent do people use commercial sex workers? At what age do young people start sexual activity? How many men are living apart from their families? How many widowed, divorced and abandoned women live in the community? How many commercial sex workers are there in the community?

- **Injecting drug users**: What are the most commonly used drugs? How many people between 15 and 25 inject drugs? What are common practices about reuse and sharing of needles and syringes?

- **Injections from health workers**: What is the average number of injections received in the past year from health-care workers? Are needles and/or syringes reused and if so how are they sterilised? How common is injection of medicines by unqualified practitioners?

- **Breastfeeding**: How common is breastfeeding and what is the average length of time? What is the cost and availability of infant formula, along with access to clean water?

We will need to be sensitive when enquiring about sexual practices:

- Hold focus group discussions with people of the same gender and approximately the same age.

- People are often more willing to discuss the sexual practices and experiences of 'friends' rather than their own. By decreasing hesitancy and embarrassment, this method can lead to frank and open discussion.

In most communities direct questioning and surveying will not be possible. Through focus groups, and discussion we will gain data that is usually sufficient to guide us on the future direction of the programme.

We also need to understand more about the 'sexual culture' within the community. This is a slightly less sensitive area than discussing actual practices, and sometimes we can ask more direct questions once we have established sufficient trust with the community. Focus groups will also be a useful way of discovering this information. We will need to know the about the **beliefs**, **customs** and **attitudes** concerning topics such as:

- premarital and extramarital sex,
- prostitution,
- sex education,
- use of condoms,
- beliefs about HIV/AIDS: how people believe it is spread, how it can be avoided and what will bring a cure.

For example in parts of east and southern Africa there is a widespread belief that an HIV-positive male can improve his health by having sexual intercourse with a virgin. Or that when a man's wife dies he should have sex with her sister.

Find out how widespread HIV/AIDS is in the community

We will already have formed an idea of the type and extent of high-risk behaviours. It is also helpful for us to know just how prevalent HIV/AIDS actually is.

We will need to estimate the prevalence of HIV, i.e. the percentage of people who are HIV-positive in the groups tested. In this way we can estimate the problem in our city and compare it with that of others.

There are two main 'indicator groups' which are commonly monitored, (because HIV testing is easier to carry out in these groups). The first group represents groups known to practise high-risk behaviour: commercial sex workers and those attending STD clinics. The second group represents groups that are assumed to reflect the situation in the general population: women attending antenatal clinics and volunteer (as opposed to paid) blood donors.

The HIV/AIDS epidemic can be classified into three phases. If effective preventive activities are not in place, then the epidemic will progress from the nascent phase, through the concentrated phase and on to the generalised phase (see Figure 9.5).

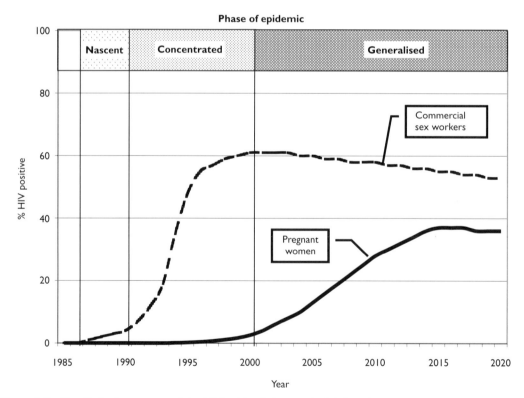

Figure 9.5   The likely time course of the HIV epidemic in a typical Asian city.

1. **Nascent** (The epidemic is limited to high-risk groups and is of fairly low intensity): HIV prevalence rates in high-risk groups (e.g. commercial sex workers, STD clinics, etc.) are less than 5%.

2. **Concentrated** (The epidemic is still limited to high-risk groups, but is increasing in intensity): HIV prevalence rates in at least one high-risk group is more than 5%, but prevalence among women attending urban antenatal clinics is less than 5%.

3. **Generalised** (The epidemic has spread to a serious degree to the general population): Prevalence among women attending urban antenatal clinics is greater than 5%.

Prevalence data can usually be obtained from the city health department, from STD clinics and hospitals and from state or federal HIV/AIDS offices. UNAIDS, which is the UN office for HIV/AIDS, has excellent data, and offices are usually located in country capital cities. WHO is another good source of data. There may be NGOs specialising in HIV/AIDS that we could contact.

Discover if the community is interested in tackling the HIV/AIDS problem

Trying to prevent an HIV epidemic always raises a dilemma. Intervention at the earliest stage possible is the best way to prevent HIV infection. But the epidemic develops unseen for many years, and strong taboos about discussing sexual behaviour and HIV add to this secrecy. **Communities only appreciate the danger and want to take action when they can see the effects of AIDS**, such as knowing friends or relatives who have died from it. By this stage the epidemic is beyond the nascent stage and only massive and expensive interventions can prevent the epidemic from turning into a crisis.

This problem is made more challenging because the only way to control the epidemic is to help bring about behavioural change. This in itself takes time and often meets with frank opposition.

This therefore leaves the CHDP responsible for creating awareness and to link with others in the community, city or nation who understand the issues and are prepared to take public initiatives.

In many cities of Africa, the AIDS epidemic is already in the generalised phase. In Asia, the onset of the epidemic has occurred 10 or more years later than the onset of the African epidemic. Hence many Asian cities are still in the nascent phase; others are in the concentrated phase. Intensive and effective efforts NOW could significantly reduce the magnitude of the epidemic in Asia. In Thailand, the annual number of new cases of HIV-positives is going down, presumably the result of intense efforts to increase the use of condoms.

Plan and implement prevention activities

Three conditions will need to be present before we start a programme for HIV/AIDS:

1. High-risk practices are going on in the community.
2. There are at least some community members motivated to join with us
3. We have the time, personnel and finance to start and maintain a programme, without detracting from other equally important priorities. (If we don't have resources ourselves we could link with another NGO that does, preferably one with experience in setting up effective programmes.)

If we do plan to go ahead we can work through an existing community organisation such as a women's group or a youth group. Or we can facilitate the development of a new group which can concentrate on issues to do with HIV/AIDS. This 'HIV Action Group' will need to work closely with other groups in the community, help to inform them about the issues and make sure that everyone is giving a similar message. A disadvantage of a separate HIV Action Group is that people may hesitate to join, afraid that others will think that they are HIV-positive. On the other hand, sometimes people who are HIV-positive feel more welcomed to a group that has a specific concern for PLWHAs.

> It is essential that all members of the team, including CHVs, have an open and accepting attitude so that people with HIV/AIDS or known high risk behaviour, will feel safe in coming forward with their cares and concerns. *Stepping Stones* (published by ACTIONAID, available through TALC), is an excellent training resource for groups working in the area of HIV/AIDS.

Community Health and Development Programmes (CHDPs) can help communities in two broad areas:

1. **HIV/AIDS prevention**
2. **Care and support of People Living With HIV/AIDS** (PLWHA) – these are people who are infected with or affected by HIV/AIDS, in practice largely those with HIV/AIDS along with members of their families and loved ones.

HIV/AIDS Prevention

Our prevention activities will need to tackle the three main ways HIV infection is spread: (1) through sex; (2) through blood transfusions and dirty needles; (3) from mother to infant. We will look at each in turn.

Reduce transmission of HIV by modifying sexual behaviour

1. **Raise awareness about how sexual transmission can be prevented.** People will need to know about the following:
   - How HIV is spread.
   - How likely they are to become infected.
   - What behaviour puts them at risk.

- How risky behaviour can be avoided. This will include the knowledge and skills to negotiate safer sexual practices with partners, e.g. the use of condoms (see next section), and how to resist peer pressure to have multiple sex partners or to drink excessive alcohol, etc.

The most effective workers in AIDS prevention and support programmes are often community members who are HIV-positive.

- They can be especially helpful in reaching members of high-risk groups. For example, HIV-positive ex-drug abusers have credibility among current drug addicts.

- As peer educators, taking action helps to boost their self-esteem, and can make it easier for them to cope with their illness.

- They can evaluate educational material to help modify behaviour in their own high-risk group.

- They can be powerful advocates to raise public awareness and to impact on policy making.

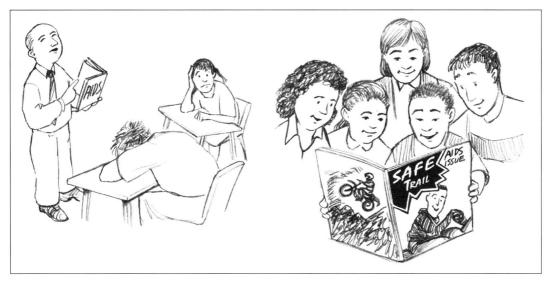

Figure 9.6   Authority figures are usually ineffective in bringing about behavioural change. Use instead dramas, stories or comics written by people with AIDS or by sports or folk heros.

Concentrate on high-risk groups, especially youth.

- Teach the basics: they have heard about AIDS but they are misinformed about risks and how HIV is spread.

- Support and encourage questioning of norms that encourage high-risk behaviour, including pre- and extra-marital sex and frequent change of partners.

- Train peer educators.

❷ Increase the use of condoms during casual sex and ideally during any sexual act, except within long-term stable relationships.

- **Train family planning workers and CHVs** (and others who distribute condoms) to teach women how to negotiate condom use by their partners.
- **Ensure sensitive promotion and distribution of condoms to all women**, including those who are not served by the family planning or maternal/child health clinic, such as unmarried adolescent girls.
- **Include men in promotion and sensitive distribution activities.** It is difficult for a single young man to walk into a regular clinic and ask for condoms. Street hawkers make good providers. They are usually young men and the transaction can occur quickly.

Condoms should be accessible. The supply should be:

- easy to access day or night,
- from a source unlikely to cause embarrassment,
- easily affordable,

Some barriers to condom use are:

- high cost,
- difficulty to obtain them when needed,
- embarrassment, or fear that your partner will mistrust you,
- the worry that others will think you have AIDS, or may be a prostitute,
- the unfounded fear that if the condom breaks inside the vagina it will lead to infection or infertility,
- the notion that using a condom interferes with pleasure,
- other beliefs and ideas specific to each area or community.

Cost of condoms can be a significant barrier to use. For the urban poor, a condom can cost 10–20% of the cost of having sex.

From the field: In Lesotho, southern Africa, footballers have been organised by CARE into Footballers against AIDS. Footballer volunteers speak to youth groups, fans and the general community about AIDS. Some of the matches are designated as HIV/AIDS awareness matches, and an educational, football theme comic has been developed. As well as encouraging youth to practise safer behaviour, some of the footballers have changed their own sexual behaviours as a result of their participation.

Source: UNAIDS, 1998.

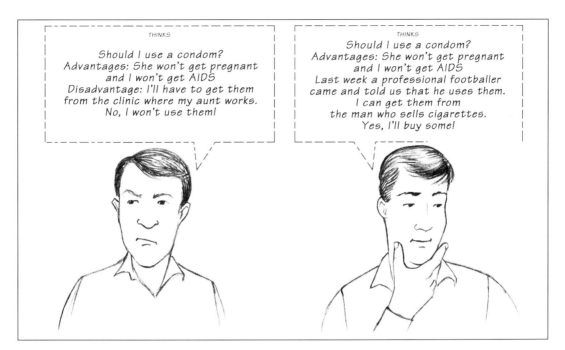

Figure 9.7   People look at the advantages and disadvantages and then decide.

❸ **Reduce the prevalence of STDs in the community**. We have seen that untreated STDs increase the likelihood of becoming infected with HIV. The community treatment of STDs is essential, especially when an epidemic is in its early phases. In our programmes we need to ensure:

- **STDs are treated in ordinary clinics**. Many people, especially women and girls are unwilling to attend STD clinics. We should include treatment in general, family planning and Maternal and Child Health clinics.
- **Ensure that staff and CHVs are trained to recognise and treat STDs**. This depends on understanding the syndromic approach – how clusters of symptoms suggesting different forms of STD are treated by specific treatments.
- **Ensure privacy** in examining all patients, and especially women and girls
- **Trace and treat contacts**. We need to make a sure a sensitive and confidential system is set up for doing this.

STDs are common in young adults, especially women. Women are more easily infected than men, often have no symptoms and are more likely to have serious complications, including persistent infection, which can cause infertility.

④ Advocate for women and girls

> The low status of women contributes greatly to the spread of HIV infection. Women who are socially and economically dependent on men, with few alternatives because of illiteracy, lack of skills and social pressures, lack the power to refuse unprotected sex.

We can help to empower women in the following way:

- Ensure that girls attend school, and women become literate.
- Ensure that girls understand about their own bodies, reproduction, and sexuality, as well as how HIV is prevented and spread.
- Promote female-controlled prevention methods as they become available, such as female condoms and vaginal microbicides – medical foams or creams that can be inserted into the vagina and will kill HIV.
- Support activities that strengthen the economic independence of women such as credit and savings schemes, income generation projects and vocational training.
- Support policies that strengthen the human rights of women: issues include marital rape, property rights, widow inheritance and divorce laws.
- Ensure that men and boys are also targeted for education and awareness activities.

Reduce transmission of HIV through blood transfusions and dirty needles
There are various actions we can take:

① **Raise awareness about the risk of blood transfusions** especially from unknown or untested sources. Those accompanying severely ill patients to hospital should be aware of these risks and be assertive in monitoring hospital treatment. The CHV is sometimes able to do this.

② **Assist addicts to quit abusing drugs or decrease the risk of HIV transmission** through:
- **Referral to treatment programmes.**
- **Minimising the attraction of drug abuse** by: developing youth recreation programmes, as alternatives to idle time spent on the streets and encouraging youth training schemes. We can network with agencies who offer these services.
- **Encouraging the use of needle and syringe-exchange programmes** – where under careful supervision and without intimidation, addicts are able to exchange their used needles and syringes for a supply of clean ones. The CHDP will need to be aware of programmes being run by other agencies.

③ **Minimise injections from health care workers**

This is a matter of continuing education both of community members and of health care workers. We will be fighting against pressure from drug companies, and the wrong perception that injections are always better than pills. We must teach, and demonstrate, the following in our clinics:

- **That injections are seldom needed for common illnesses**. Oral medicines are as effective as injections, and sometimes no medicine is needed at all.
- **That injections carry with them the risk of HIV as well as hepatitis B and** C. The World Health Organization estimates that 12 million cases of hepatitis B are caused each year through the use of unclean needles. Hepatitis B, spread in a similar way to HIV, is 100 times more infectious.
- **That a disposable needle and syringe should be used for all injections, including immunisations**. If that is not economically possible rigorous re-sterilisation must be carried out.

> **From the field**: In an immunisation clinic, the health worker was asked how she disposed of used disposable needles and syringes. She said that she used to just throw them away outside the clinic, but the community complained because children would find them and play with them. So now she just throws them out on the street on the way home. (India)
>
> **Lesson learned**: We must train health workers to dispose of needles and syringes properly.
>
> **Source**: Authors.

Reduce transmission of HIV from mother to infant

① **Raise awareness about how HIV transmission from mother to child can be reduced**.

This is our first task. Our next action will depend on the HIV status of the mother, see below.

② **Action for women who know they are HIV-positive:**
- If women are not pregnant, offer family planning advice with the option of having tubal ligation.
- If women are pregnant or very keen to have a child, provide counselling about the pros and cons of breastfeeding. For most children of HIV-positive women living in urban slums, the risk of dying from AIDS acquired through breastfeeding (about 10% risk) is usually less than the risk of dying from diarrhoea and malnutrition caused by artificial feeds. One alternative, if acceptable, is wet-nursing by women known to be HIV-negative (who must practise safe sex during the period she is breastfeeding). Women with AIDS or those infected during pregnancy or while breastfeeding of the infant are at greater risk of transmitting HIV infection. They should consider using infant formula instead. (See Resources, HIV and Infant Feeding: A guide for health care managers and supervisors, and updates for current guidelines.)

> The likelihood of an infant becoming infected through breast-milk is proportional to the length of time the infant is breastfed. The risk from diarrhoeal infections is greatest in the first 2 months. For mothers who decide to breastfeed, 2 months is is a good time to change over to bottle-feeding.

③ Action for women who do not know their HIV status:

Encourage and arrange voluntary and confidential counselling and HIV testing. Mothers found to be HIV-positive can then make informed decisions about contraception and infant feeding most appropriate in their circumstances.

From the field: In Abidjan, Ivory Coast the HIV counselling and testing centre run by the Sisters of Dorothy also provides treatment for minor health problems and sells photocopies. Through this strategy, if people attend for HIV counselling or testing and meet someone they know, they are able to say that they are there for some small medical problem or to have something photocopied.

Lesson learned: The stigma of AIDS forces people to keep their illness secret, sometimes preventing them from seeking help. In addition to helping change attitudes in the community, we need to think of creative ways to support individuals.

Source: Williams *et al.*, 1995.

④ Consider specific treatment that decreases transmission rates.

Much research is being done in the area of preventing HIV transmission from mother to child. Keep up-to-date with the latest research and any medicines or other aids that reduce transmission risks.

AIDS Action is a newsletter that can help us to keep current about AIDS prevention, education and care. It is available from Healthlink (free to developing countries).

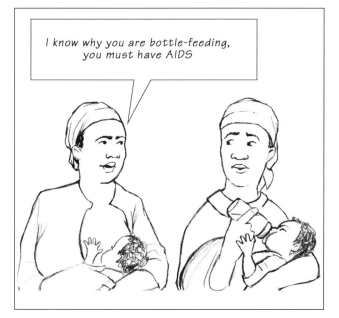

Specific therapy with anti-HIV drugs

Recent studies have shown that treatment of HIV-positive mothers with zidovudine (AZT) during the final weeks of pregnancy and through delivery greatly reduces the risk of transmitting infection to the baby. Treatment is expensive, but prices are coming down and treatment regimes becoming shorter. GlaxoWellcome, which manufactures AZT under the trade name Retrovir, is making subsidised supplies available to public health programmes.

Figure 9.8   When bottle-feeding is not the usual practice, HIV-positive women who decide to bottle feed need sensitive advice and support.

When low-cost treatment becomes widely available, it will be important for pregnant women to discover if they are HIV-positive so that treatment can be started to reduce their chance of giving birth to an infected child. We will then need to ensure:

- That access is easy for voluntary and confidential counselling and HIV testing, with encouragement, but not pressure to agree.

- That efforts are intensified to detect all pregnant women to tell them about voluntary counselling and HIV testing.

- That HIV-positive women who become pregnant are monitored carefully and started on treatment where this is appropriate.

- That a programme is set up to treat HIV-positive women before, at the time of delivery and during breastfeeding to prevent mother-to-child transmission.

Breast-milk substitutes

UNICEF, UNAIDS and WHO have recommended that breast-milk substitutes be made available to HIV-positive women with young infants. As and when these become freely available or easily affordable, we should help mothers to obtain them, and teach them how to use them hygienically. **However, we must strongly discourage their use amongst women who are not HIV-positive**.

Low-cost interventions thought to reduce transmission

1. **Give vitamin A to the mother**. Vitamin A deficiency is known to increase the risk of transmission from mother to child. Vitamin A is cheap and available. A recommended dose is 25,000 IU each week in the last month of pregnancy.
2. **Cleanse the birth canal during labour and delivery**. This is now under study and may decrease transmission.

Care and support of People Living with HIV/AIDS

Home-based care of people with AIDS has evolved over the last 10–15 years from the experience in many African countries. Here the AIDS epidemic has overwhelmed the capacities of hospitals and health centres to cope. In addition many people can be cared for more comfortably in the home provided that family members are trained and supported by health workers. In countries with very high rates of HIV, e.g. 20–40% of the adult population, home-based programmes can only succeed when the community is strongly involved. The role of the CHDP is to help the community to recognise and use its own resources and to link up with support services outside the community.

Advantages of Community-based Home Care of People with AIDS
For people with AIDS

- They are usually happier staying among family and friends.

- They can be as active as they like.
- Knowing that AIDS is incurable, many prefer to die at home.

For the family

- Home care is cheaper than hospitalisation, which requires travel, providing food and paying fees.
- It keeps the family together, and members can participate in care.
- It disturbs household routines less since caretakers can also perform other tasks.
- It provides an opportunity for CHDP staff to know and support the family.

For the community

- It helps to reduce the fear and stigma of HIV/AIDS, as CHDP staff and community members take part in providing care.
- Home care is a felt need and gives the programme an entry point both for care, educating the family and community how to prevent HIV infection, and for tracing contacts.
- It relieves hospitals so they have more time and resources to treat other patients.

Activities of a community home-care programme
These can include:

❶ **Medical care**: The programme has access to a physician or nurse who supports the community volunteer. The volunteer, after appropriate training, can diagnose

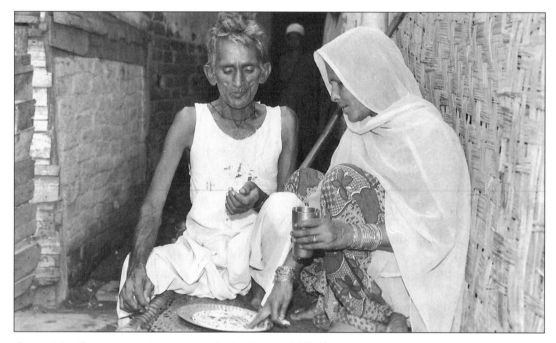

Figure 9.9 Community volunteers are the backbone of AIDS home-care programmes. (Godfrey Martin/ASHA)

and treat simple illnesses. The volunteer can also ease pain and discomfort and help to avoid pressure sores.

It is important to remember that most people with HIV/AIDS in developing countries die prematurely of treatable diseases such as pneumonia, typhoid fever and tuberculosis. Explain to People Living With HIV/AIDS, the symptoms of tuberculosis so that they can be started on treatment as early as possible. Treat other illnesses early and aggressively since in the earlier stages of HIV infection patients respond well to treatment.

② **Nursing care**: The volunteer can teach family members how to give medicines, bathe, change dressings and feed the sick person.

③ **Emotional and spiritual support**: Community volunteers provide comfort and solace. They hold hands or pray with the sick person and the family.

④ **Practical support for the patient and the family**: Volunteers learn to look for what needs to be done. They may sweep out the house, give a back rub, sit quietly, buy some vegetables. They can teach family members how to avoid contact with blood and other body fluids and to wash hands immediately after handling soiled articles.

⑤ **Counselling and awareness raising about HIV/AIDS**: Initially sick patients may not want others to know that they have AIDS, even though they often suspect it. We must respect their desire for confidentiality. However, counselling and the development of trust often breaks down this barrier.

⑥ **Contact tracing**: After trust is developed it is important to track down possible contacts.

In the early stages of a programme community members may not welcome home visits, as they will not want others to know that they are HIV-positive. A programme that cares for people with a range of chronic illnesses may be more acceptable.

Training needed by home-care volunteers
CHVs or Home-care Volunteers should receive training in:

- recognition and treatment of common, simple illnesses in people with AIDS;
- recognition of serious illness, which require a visit from a nurse, or more specialized care;
- counselling techniques, including how to be a good listener.

(See Resources for more discussion on clinical care)

CHDP staff and community volunteers must never betray a trust. They must keep the confidence of the sick person and family members. Betrayed trust can adversely affect the whole programme. When word gets around that confidentiality has not been kept, others will be very hesitant to come forward and share sensitive issues such as their HIV status and the names of their contacts.

From the field: The Chishilano Centre is a base for community HIV/AIDS activities in Nkwazi, Zambia. Although foreign donors built the Centre, people elected from the community manage it. Activities of the Centre include support groups, income-generation activities and HIV prevention activities. Peer educators carry out street theatre about STDs, sexual behaviour and HIV/AIDS. The Centre also organises healthy recreational activities for out-of-school children.

The Centre is also a base for the home-care programme. Fifty-two community volunteers visit the chronically ill, many of whom have AIDS. Two nurses make home visits 3 days a week. They meet ahead of time with the volunteers to decide which homes should be visited. The volunteer goes with the nurse to the home. The centre also runs a weekly clinic for chronically ill people who are able to walk. Volunteers accompany patients when they must be seen by a physician.

The impact of AIDS on the community: In Zambia, AIDS is taking a severe toll. One out of five adults is HIV-positive. Nkwazi is a slum with a population of 30–40 thousand people. In 1998, 440 patients were registered for the home-care programme (about 1% of the population). About 50 patients, most of them with AIDS, are seen at the weekly clinic. It is estimated that one out of three households is looking after one or more orphans.

Source: Blinkhoff *et al.*, 1999.

Chapter summary

AIDS (Acquired Immune Deficiency Syndrome) is caused by the Human Immuno-Deficiency Virus (HIV). HIV attacks the immune system so that people with AIDS are progressively less able to fight off infection. HIV is spread in one of three main ways: by sexual contact, through infected blood and dirty needles, and from mother to child. People living in slums are especially vulnerable to infection by HIV and to its adverse impact on their lives. Specific measures can be taken to prevent HIV infection. Setting up a programme can be done in various stages. First estimating whether the problem is severe enough and resources are sufficient to start. Second planning activities to try and prevent each of the main methods of transmission. Raising awareness, facilitating behavioural change and empowering women are key strategies in this: new treatments are also being developed. Third setting up a community-based home-care programme for the huge numbers of people now affected by the AIDS pandemic.

Resources

1. *HIV and Infant Feeding: A Guide for Health Care Managers and Supervisors.* WHO/UNAIDS, 1998. Current guidelines on this important topic, which are likely to be revised frequently.

2. *Prevention: International Case Studies of Effective Health Promotion Practice in HIV/AIDS.* UNAIDS, 1998. Many case studies to learn from.

3. *Positive Development.* Global Network of People Living with HIV/AIDS (GNP+), 1998. A very practical manual for people living with HIV/AIDS on how to set up groups and advocating for change. (Available through Healthlink.) Free to readers in developing countries and organisations of people living with HIV/AIDS.

4. *Men's Sexual Health Matters.* Healthlink, 1998. For health and community workers who work on sex and sexuality with men. Covers basic facts on reproduction, contraception, and safe sex for men, men's concerns about sexual and reproductive health and strategies for working with men in different settings. Free to readers in developing countries.

5. *Confronting AIDS: Public Priorities in a Global Epidemic.* World Bank/Oxford University Press, 1997. Very good overview of the HIV/AIDS epidemic, but not written in simple language.

6. *Caring with Confidence.* Healthlink Worldwide, 1997 Practical information for health workers on preventing and treating HIV infection in young children. Single copies free to developing countries.

7. *Stepping Stones: A Training Package on HIV/AIDS, Communication and Relationship Skills.* A Welbourn. ACTIONAID, 1995. Very good resource of training exercises in skills needed in HIV/AIDS projects, such as communication, dealing with prejudice, negotiating skills, etc. (Available from TALC).

8. *Helpers for a Healing Community.* K Dortzbach, N Kiiti (eds.) MAP International, 1995. A very practical manual for HIV/AIDS counselling written in very simple English.

9. *Under the Mupundu Tree: Volunteers in home care for people with HIV/AIDS TB in Zambia's Copperbelt.* P Blinkhoff, E Bukanga, B Syamalevwe, G. Williams. Action Aid, 1999. Part of a series on HIV/AIDS, Strategies for Hope, which presents many case studies about how communities have dealt with the AIDS epidemic. Very practical and informative for groups wanting to become involved in HIV/AIDS to see how others have done it. (Available from TALC.)

10. *AIDS Management: An Integrated Approach.* ID Campbell, G Williams. Actionaid, 1990. Describes an integrated approach to the clinical care of people with HIV/AIDS, specifically outlining care that can be given in the home.

11. *The Caring Community: Coping with AIDS in Urban Uganda.* G Williams, N Tamale. Action Aid, 1991. Good review of the problems associated with HIV/AIDS in cities and gives guidelines for home visiting.

12. *AIDS Orphans: A Community Perspective from Tanzania.* MC Mukoyogo and G Williams. Action Aid, 1991. A very good discussion of the problems and needs of AIDS orphans. (Available from TALC.)

13. *AIDS: A Guide for Community Work*. G Gordon, T Klouda. Macmillan Education, 1988. Very good guide for people working in AIDS prevention and counselling with many case studies. (Available from TALC.)

14. *AIDS Home Care Handbook, UNAIDS*. A practical handbook for families and communities to provide safe and compassionate AIDS care at home.

10 Tuberculosis

In this chapter, we shall consider:

What we need to know:

What is tuberculosis?

How do people become infected with TB?

What happens when someone becomes infected with TB?

Why are slum dwellers at high risk for TB?

What we need to do:

Decide whether to start a TB programme

Decide what our aims and objectives should be

Plan and implement activities

Life in a slum

Eighteen-year-old Rebekkah lived with her parents and three brothers and sisters in a small 2 by 3 metre hut. For several months Rebekkah had felt very weak and had frequent fevers and coughing bouts which allowed her little sleep. Soon, she was bed-ridden. Her mother never told Miriam, her community health volunteer, about Rebekkah. But she did take Rebekkah to several private practitioners. Although the medicines prescribed were expensive, they didn't improve her health. Miriam, a health worker who lived in the community, found out from concerned neighbours that Rebekkah was ill. She visited Rebekkah and her mother, and told Rebekkah's mother that her symptoms were probably due to tuberculosis, which could be cured by medicines. Miriam went with Rebekkah and her mother to the local government hospital for a sputum test, which confirmed the diagnosis of tuberculosis. The doctor started Rebekkah on DOTS anti-TB treatment. For the first month of therapy, Rebekkah was too weak to go out, so Miriam visited her each evening to make sure she took her medicine. When Rebekkah felt better, she started to come each morning to Miriam's house. Within 2 months, Rebekkah felt so much better that she was able to care for her younger brothers and sisters, cook and keep house again while her mother was away at work. (Kenya)

What we need to know

What is tuberculosis?

Tuberculosis (TB) is a serious illness caused by *Mycobacterium tuberculosis*, a bacterium that is sometimes called AFB (acid-fast bacteria) for short. It most commonly affects the lungs. In developing countries, TB is the major killer of adults in the working age group. Overall, one-third of the world's population is infected with TB, and about 10% of these people become ill or infectious at some time in their life. Someone in the world is newly infected with TB every second.

TB is spreading rapidly in all developing countries, and also in the former Soviet States and Eastern Europe. There are several reasons for this:

- neglect (in case-finding and in treatment);
- lack of political (government) will;
- increasing HIV infection;
- increasing urbanisation with people living in over-crowded houses in densely populated communities;
- increasing prison populations with absent or inadequate TB treatment;
- corruption in the government health system causing shortage of drugs;
- increasing poverty with malnutrition;
- increasing air pollution;
- the spread of multi-resistant TB which is more difficult and expensive to treat;
- poorly managed programmes which, through having low cure rates, spread resistance.

Nearly 75% of the world's TB cases live in just 13 countries: Bangladesh, Brazil, China, Ethiopia, India, Indonesia, Mexico, Pakistan, Philippines, Russia, South Africa, Thailand, and the Central African Republic.

How do people become infected with TB?

When those with TB of the lungs cough or spit, they release droplets into the air that contain infectious particles. Others become infected when they breathe in the air that contains those droplets. The spread of TB usually occurs indoors where droplets are concentrated and persist in the air for longer. Direct sunlight quickly kills the TB bacteria, but in the dark inside of a house, they can live for several hours. Good ventilation quickly disperses infectious droplets.

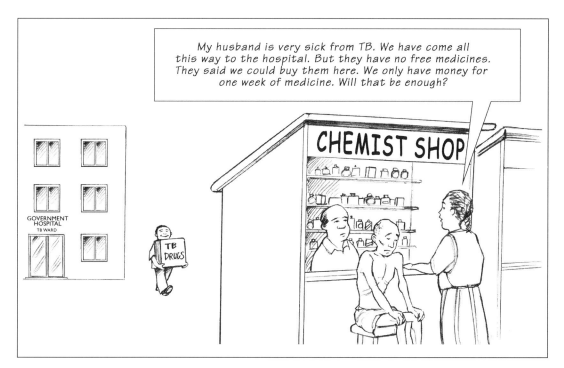

Figure 10.1   Non-availability of medicines is a common problem in government TB programmes.

One cough by someone with TB can produce 3000 infectious droplets.

Source: Harries *et al.*, 1997.

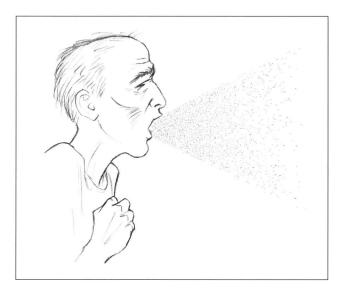

Figure 10.2   TB is spread through coughing. On average each infectious patient will spread TB to about 10 to 15 other people each year.

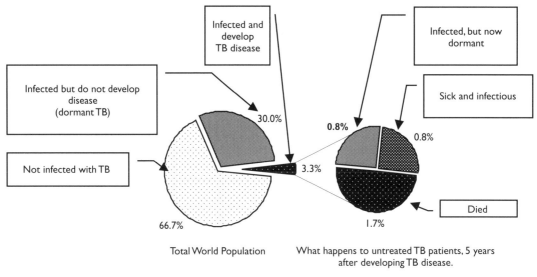

Infected and develop TB disease

Infected but do not develop disease (dormant TB)

Not infected with TB

Infected, but now dormant

Sick and infectious

30.0%

0.8%

0.8%

3.3%

Died

66.7%

1.7%

Total World Population

What happens to untreated TB patients, 5 years after developing TB disease.

Source: Adapted from: TB: A Clinical; Manual for South East Asia. WHO. 1997

Figure 10.3   Tuberculosis infection in the world.

What happens when someone becomes infected with TB?

About nine out of ten people who become infected with the TB bacteria, do not go on to develop active disease (see Figure 10.3). This is because their immune system is strong enough to prevent it. The bacteria remain, however, and have the potential of causing active TB if the immune system weakens. Malnutrition, HIV infection and other illnesses can cause the weakening of the immune system. HIV infection is a major reason for the rapid increase in TB especially in Africa and Asia.

When a person develops active TB, the most common site of infection is the lungs and the disease is known as pulmonary tuberculosis. People with untreated pulmonary TB often have TB bacteria in their sputum, which can be detected when a glass slide containing a smear of sputum is specially stained and viewed under a microscope. People who have TB bacteria in their sputum have 'sputum-positive' TB. They are the most likely to spread the infection to others. When sputum-positive cases are treated effectively, nearly all become sputum-negative within 2–4 weeks of starting therapy and become relatively non-infectious.

Active TB can also occur in other places in the body (called extra-pulmonary tuberculosis). This is more common in people with HIV/AIDS. In extrapulmonary TB, the risk of spread to others is very low: common sites are the kidneys, bowels, bones, skin, and lymph glands in the neck.

Common symptoms of pulmonary TB in adults and older children are cough for more than 3 weeks, (often with sputum, sometimes with blood); weight loss, tiredness and fever especially in the evening and night. Young children often have non-specific symptoms. They sometimes cough and are usually losing weight for no obvious reason. Often there is a household member with infectious TB.

When people with active TB are not treated, about half will die within 5 years, one-quarter will remain chronically ill, and one-quarter will get better on their own. When people are effectively treated for TB and complete a full course of therapy, up to 95% of them are cured.

Why are slum dwellers at high risk for TB?

TB spreads easily in slums because:

- **Houses** are small, overcrowded, poorly ventilated and dark.
- The **community** is densely populated.

If the household contains someone with infectious TB, these factors will increase the concentration of infectious droplets in the air, making spread to others more likely.

Slum residents are more likely to develop tuberculosis for a number of other reasons:

- Because **TB is so common** their risk of becoming infected is proportionally higher.
- Poverty means that many patients will be **untreated or partially treated**.
- **People dying of TB, who are highly infectious** in the last weeks of life, may remain in the slum because they have no alternative.
- **Multi-drug resistant TB** spreads fast because of incomplete treatment.
- **Malnutrition** weakens the immune system.
- **Cigarette smoking** and **air pollution** weaken the lungs.
- **Many are migrants**, meaning they are exposed to greater numbers of people and are less likely to complete courses of treatment.
- **Crowded public transport** is the main way in which slum residents travel.

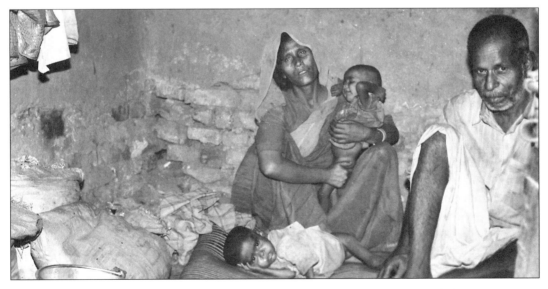

Figure 10.4 The crowded conditions of slum housing are ideal for spreading tuberculosis. (Godfrey Martin/ASHA)

What we need to do

Decide whether to start a TB programme

Tuberculosis is both difficult and expensive to treat. Poorly managed treatment programmes actually make the problem worse by spreading resistant germs. Before we start a programme we must carefully consider several issues.

❶ Is TB common in the community?

We should only consider a TB programme if the level of proven or suspected TB cases is greater than 1%. For example, if the population of the slum community is 5000, are there 50 or more known or suspected cases of tuberculosis? In practice most slums will have higher rates than this if investigated thoroughly.

❷ Is the community concerned about TB?

Does the community want to have a TB programme? Will community members help to run it? An effective TB programme needs motivated community health volunteers, and community members with sufficient interest to take action and ensure that those with persistent cough in their own households come forward for testing.

> Awareness raising is often needed for a period of time before the community is ready for full participation.

❸ Is TB already being adequately detected and treated in the community?

Is there an effective and well run TB programme, carried out by the government or by another NGO? For example in many states of China very successful programmes have been set up by the government in association with the World Bank. In most cities, however, government programmes seldom function well, and treatment, supposed to be free, is usually only available at a high price from private doctors.

❹ Do we have the necessary resources to run a TB programme?

- A **doctor** to advise and provide clinical care?
- A **laboratory and lab technician** who can make and read sputum smears?
- People to serve as **community supply-holders of antituberculous drugs, and as observers and tracers for DOTS regimes** (see below)? The Community Health Volunteer is an ideal person for this, if well trained and trustworthy.
- **A reliable supply of the correct drugs which will never run out.** Sometimes the government is willing to provide a CHDP with medicines. If so, is the government supply reliable, will the agreement be affected by changes in government personnel or policies, and are back-up supplies available?

- **Money** to run the programme for at least 5, and preferably 10 years? The programme is expensive, especially if medicines must be purchased rather than donated.
- Effective **management** to run the programme?

To answer these questions we may have to gather further information:

1. Do a quick sample survey of the community to determine:
   - the percentage of community members currently on treatment (and ask where they are being treated);
   - the percentage of people with suspected symptoms: cough for 3 weeks or more is the prime indicator for adults and teenagers: others include pain in the chest or unexplained fever for 3 weeks or more, and coughing up blood.

2. Discuss knowledge, attitudes and commitment to a programme with members of the community, in particular the Community Action Group

3. Visit government health centres and hospitals in the area. Could they provide an informed and committed doctor and a reliable laboratory for sputum testing?

4. Talk with donors.

Decide what our goals and objectives should be

For a comprehensive TB programme, the overall **goals** should be:

1. To reduce death, illness and the rate of transmission.

2. To prevent the spread of multi-drug resistant TB.

Our **objectives** should be:

1. To cure at least 85% of new sputum-positive cases: this automatically leads to control of TB.

2. To detect at least 70% of existing cases of sputum-positive TB.

3. To ensure a high uptake (e.g. 85%) of BCG to infants, as soon after birth as possible.

When we achieve an 85% cure rate, we can pursue more active case-finding in the community

It will take a long time to achieve these **objectives**. We should set realistic objectives in our 1, and 3 year, action plans. We may discover that some activities are already being done by the government and we can actively co-operate with them. For example they may have an effective BCG programme and be able to provide laboratory facilities.

It is essential that we work with the National TB Programme (NTP), which usually follows the WHO guidelines for national programmes, and follow their procedures, guidelines and treatment regimes.

Tuberculosis can be controlled if we detect and cure 85% of new sputum-positive cases.

Plan and implement activities

We will need to carry out the following steps, not necessarily in the order given below. Several steps will also be going on at the same time.

Step 1. Set up an effective management structure

Many programmes fail because of poor management, inadequate supervision,and lack of forward planning. We therefore need to ensure that:

- **A programme leader is appointed**, empowered and trained to give effective leadership.
- **All CHDP members are given basic training** in the aims of the programme and how it will be implemented.
- **The Community Action Group and Community Health Volunteers are involved and trained.**
- **Defined links are made with the NTP**, and any government agencies, hospitals or NGOs who will be working with us.
- **Drug regimes are followed according to NTP guidelines**, supplies are obtained and back-up sources identified.
- **Good quality laboratory back-up is ensured**, and methods of sputum collection, delivery and reporting are set up.
- **Hospital back-up is identified** for severely ill patients.
- **A community network of DOTS observers and tracers is arranged.** This will involve identifying, training and supervising this team (see Step 6 below).
- **Funding is available**, for at least 5 years.
- **Reporting and monitoring systems are in place** (see Step 7 below).

Step 2. Educate the community

We will need to educate the community about how TB can be **prevented**, and that TB can normally be **treated** successfully.

Within a slum community there will be a variety of beliefs about TB. Is it a curse? Can it be cured? We will need to start where people are, understand their beliefs and then gently correct their wrong ideas. The key facts we must help the community understand are these:

1 Prevention:
- how TB is caused and spread, especially the dangers of coughing without covering the mouth with hands, and spitting;
- how poor ventilation and overcrowding speeds the spread of TB;
- the common symptoms of TB.

2 Treatment:
- that TB can be treated;
- that the earlier treatment is started, the quicker and cheaper the cure;
- that courses of treatment must be finished;
- the locations and opening times of the nearest treatment centres.

At the same time we must make sure that any clinics we set up have convenient opening times, short waiting times and friendly and welcoming staff.

Step 3. Detect cases of infectious TB using passive case-finding

Initially we should concentrate on carrying out sputum tests on those referred or self-referred to the clinic with symptoms suggestive of TB. Often when word gets around about a new TB programme, patients are referred from private doctors and clinics, and even from government centres, especially if the medicines are free of charge. This type of TB case detection is known as **passive case-finding** because at this stage we do not actively search for cases in the community, we just wait for people to come forwards. Usually those who do come to the clinic are the more seriously ill and therefore the most infectious to others.

Most patients we start on treatment will be sputum-positive adults or older children. Sometimes patients will be sputum-negative but we may strongly suspect they have infectious TB because of their symptoms. An X-ray can help us decide in these cases, **but should not be routinely carried out on TB patients: it is a waste of time and resources**. Sputum tests are much more reliable than X-ray.

Young children tend to swallow sputum and will often have non-specific symptoms such as failure to gain weight for no obvious reasons.

Whenever we start a patient on TB treatment we should categorise them according to which of four case definitions they come into (see definitions under Step 7 below, Recording Information).

Only when we achieve cure rates of 85% or more should we consider the option of **active case-finding**, when we try and discover untreated cases in the community (see Step 9 below).

Step 4. Treat sputum-positive TB cases

We should follow these guidelines:

- Use drug regimes and guidelines as recommended by the National TB Programme (NTP). This will involve ensuring a good quality supply, careful storage and distribution, and a thorough understanding of how the drugs should be used and their possible side effects. Also treating patients with their full understanding and co-operation.
- Monitor patients at recommended intervals. Guidelines are also laid down for this and depend on the drug regime being used.
- Follow the DOTS approach of supervised treatment (see Step 6 below)

Details on all these guidelines and definitions, including recommended drug regimes, can be obtained from the National TB Programme and from books listed at the end of this chapter.

Step 5. Encourage TB patients to complete treatment ('case-holding')

In the past, people with TB needed to take medicines for 12–18 months in order to be cured. Even with the shorter 6 or 8 month courses now used, patients begin to feel better after a few weeks and then stop taking their medicine. A **defaulter** is a person who stops taking anti-TB medicines before completing the full course of treatment. When a person stops taking anti-TB medicines before finishing the course, three serious things can happen:

1. They will probably not be cured.

2. They may continue to spread the disease through living longer as a result of having partial treatment.

3. The tuberculosis may become Multi-Drug Resistant (MDR), i.e. at least two of the commonly used drugs become ineffective. MDR-TB is much more difficult, and hugely more expensive to treat. Those with MDR strains easily pass these on to others.

It is not surprising that defaulting is such a major problem (see Figure 10.5). It is very difficult for low-income patients to afford a full course of treatment. Often patients are seen once per month, and given a further month's prescription. To receive free medicines (the only ones within reach of almost all slum residents), patients have to be seen at a regional government centre, often some distance away. Often these hospitals have run out of medicines and so the patient ends up paying for them (or going home disappointed without any medicines).

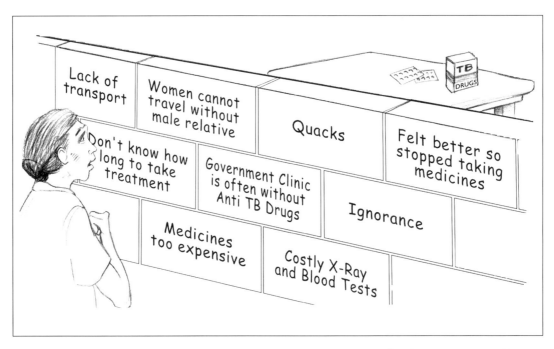

Figure 10.5   Many obstacles prevent the poor from completing a course of anti-TB drug therapy. How can we help build a door in this brick wall?

Step 6. Set up a DOTS programme (Directly Observed Treatment, Short-course)

DOTS is one key strategy for building a door in the brick wall in Figure 10.5.

What is DOTS?

DOTS is a new strategy in the treatment of TB that has been used increasingly since the early 1990s. It is proving an effective way of controlling TB and reducing the default rate. As part of the DOTS strategy, a powerful combination of anti-TB drugs is given, which permits a shorter course of therapy (6–8 months). To ensure that patients take their medicines, an observer watches each patient take each dose, at least for the first 2 months of therapy. DOTS stands for:

- **Directly**: We **Direct** resources to detecting and treating people with sputum-positive TB, because these are the main sources for spreading TB to others.
- **Observed**: A health worker or trained community volunteer must **Observe** the patient swallowing each dose of medicine.
- **Treatment**: TB patients must be given a complete course of **Treatment** and be regularly monitored to ensure they are being cured.
- **Short-course**: The correct combination of anti-TB drugs must be given in the **right combination for the right (shorter) period of time**.

Before setting up a DOTS programme, we must make sure a management structure is in place as described in Step 1. Three key features of this will be:

- **Trained volunteers**. We must set up a network of community volunteers willing to observe treatment and trace defaulters (CHVs are often ideal people for this).
- **Laboratory facilities** to make and read sputum smears. Ideally the CHDP should have its own competent, motivated and trustworthy lab technicians so that sputum smears can be looked at on site, and treatment started on the same visit. If that is not possible, we can search out a nearby government hospital or clinic and enter into a collaborative arrangement.
- A **reliable supply of anti-TB drugs**. Increasingly governments and NGOs are working together to tackle TB. The government may be willing to supply the CHDP with anti-TB medicines.

> TB is most likely to be controlled if national and city governments along with local NGOs, work in active partnership, following National TB Programme guidelines, and implementing a well managed DOTS programme with the active involvement of the community.

Setting up an urban DOTS programme: initial tasks

1 Work out the tasks and responsibilities of each agency involved in the programme (community, government, private, other NGO, etc.). The main tasks will include:
  - education/awareness activities,
  - BCG immunisations of infants,
  - clinical care including diagnosis,
  - clinical follow-up and patient monitoring,
  - setting up laboratory testing of sputum,

- provision of anti-TB and other drugs,
- observing treatment,
- tracing defaulters,
- training staff and volunteers, including observers and tracers.

From the field: In Patan, Nepal, a collaborative effort between government, the private sector and NGOs is carrying out an intensive tuberculosis programme using the DOTS strategy. Diagnosis and therapeutic decisions are made at a 'treatment centre' which is based in a government or private hospital. The patient can then choose to come to the treatment centre for medicines, or go to a sub-centre (run by the NGOs) near home or workplace. No new staff members have been added. Several existing staff members rotate the observer duties. Community Health Volunteers take a 2-day Late Patient Tracer Course. If a patient fails to come for a dose, the tracer is contacted and generally brings the patient the same or the following day.

Lesson learned: Collaborative efforts are effective when government and NGO make their own unique contributions within a well managed programme.

Source: C. Preston, Yala Urban Health Programme, Patan, Nepal.

Tuberculosis and HIV

TB and HIV/AIDS cause a lethal combination. Those who are HIV-positive are 30 times more likely to become sick with TB than those who are HIV-negative. TB is the cause of death in about one-third of all people with AIDS. At the time of writing, 2000 AD, HIV is causing about 1.5 million cases of TB which would otherwise not have occurred.

In practice:

- HIV infection reactivates TB, meaning that many TB patients will be HIV-positive.

- Patients with HIV often respond well to anti-TB treatment and should be managed in a similar way and with the same drugs as those who are HIV-negative (though thioacetazone must not be used).

- Community volunteers who are providing home care for people with HIV/AIDS can also serve as observers for the DOTS programme.

❷ Develop written guidelines on the responsibilities of each collaborating agency and plan to meet regularly to assess progress and clarify any misunderstandings.

❸ Train all members of the CHDP in the tasks they are responsible for as well as understanding the structure of the programme and the roles of others involved in it.

Setting up an urban DOTS programme: treatment and observation

Treatment of TB: This is divided into two phases, the initial phase and the continuation phase. The **initial** or intensive phase involves the rapid killing of TB bacteria with the aim of making the TB patient non-infectious within the first 2–4 weeks, with a marked improvement in health. Directly **Observed** Therapy is especially important during this phase when drug resistance easily occurs if treatment is missed. The initial phase usually lasts 2 months, depending on the exact drugs used.

The **continuation** phase is longer, usually lasting 4 or 6 months, but is less intensive and fewer drugs have to be given. Ideally, Directly **Observed** Therapy should be continued during this phase. Follow NTP guidelines about which drugs to use during the intensive and continuation phases.

Observation of treatment: When a patient is first registered, the CHV or other person appointed as observer, should make a home visit to build relationships with the patient and his family, and to confirm the location of the house. Later, if the patient misses a dose, the tracer can then find the house more easily.

The patient and the health team determine the specific arrangements for the observed treatment. Patients can come to the observer's home or to the health centre at a set time to take their medicines. It must be at a time and place convenient for the patient (otherwise they are likely to default) but also acceptable for the observer (otherwise they will lose motivation). If patients fail to attend, the tracers needs to find them and discover why, and then ensure they take their medicines.

Sometimes at the beginning of a course of therapy, the observer must go to the patient's house each day as the patient may be too sick to leave the house.

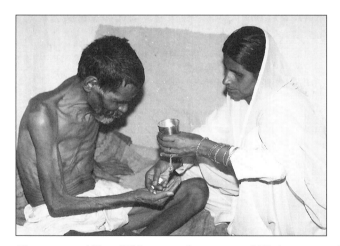

Figure 10.6   When CHVs act as observers, anti-TB therapy can be given close to home. (Godfrey Martin/ASHA)

Step 7. Monitor the effectiveness of the programme

We will need to choose indicators as laid down by the World Health Organization and adopted by the National TB Programme. By using these indicators we can both

Women and TB

Women with TB are usually less likely than men to be diagnosed and treated:

- Women have less time to attend clinics.

- Families are less likely to spend money for medical care on females.

- In some countries, women need to be accompanied by a male relative.

- In some countries where women cannot be examined by male health workers, there are few female health workers to care for them.

- Women are more likely to be illiterate and uninformed about the issues.

In our programme it is important to recognise this imbalance and make sure that women have equal access to the TB programme.

monitor our own programme and compare our results with other programmes anywhere in the world.

WHO sets the objective that at least 85% of patients with newly diagnosed sputum-positive TB should be cured. If we fall below that rate we are in danger of causing MDR-TB to develop, see page 176.

The main indicator to monitor each year is the cure rate:

$$\textbf{Cure rate } (\%) = \frac{\text{Number of newly diagnosed sputum-positive patients who were cured}}{\text{Total number of sputum-positive patients that were treated}} \times 100$$

We can only use patients that have been treated for 8 months (or longer for defaulters). Therefore it is practical to take patients who were diagnosed in the previous year. For example if it is currently July, 2001, then look at the records of patients who entered the programme from July, 1999 through June, 2000 and look at their outcome. To calculate the cure rate, the total number of newly diagnosed sputum-positive patients registered during that period will be the denominator (goes below the line in the above equation), and of those patients, the number of them who were cured will be the numerator (goes above the line in the above equation).

Step 8. Organise an effective, simple recording system

This will be needed both for annual monitoring and for more detailed evaluations. We need to categorise all TB patients started on treatment, according to both a **case definition** and a **treatment outcome**. These categories have both been internationally defined.

There are four categories of **case definition**.

1. **New case**: A patient has never had treatment for TB or has taken anti-TB treatment for a total of less than 4 weeks.

2. **Relapse**: A patient has been declared cured of any form of TB in the past after one full course of treatment, and has become sputum-positive since.

3. **Treatment failure**: A patient, who while on treatment remains or again becomes sputum smear-positive 5 months or later after starting treatment, OR a patient initially smear-negative before treatment but became positive after the 2nd month of treatment (see also definition of Treatment Outcome below).

4. **Default** (also known as 'Treatment after interruption'): A patient who interrupts treatment for 2 consecutive months or more and returns for treatment with smear-positive TB or is judged clinically to still have active TB.

There are six categories **treatment outcome** for patients started on treatment.

1. **Cure**: A patient is sputum-negative at or within 1 month of completion of treatment and on at least one other occasion.

2. **Treatment completed**: A patient has completed treatment but without proof of cure (for example smear results are not available for at least two occasions before completion of treatment).

3. **Treatment failure**: A patient who remains or again becomes smear-positive 5 months or later, after starting treatment.

4. **Died**: A patient dies for any reason during anti-TB drug therapy.

5. **Defaulted**: A patient whose treatment has been interrupted for more than 2 consecutive months before the end of the anti-TB therapy

6. **Transferred out**: A patient who has been transferred to another treatment centre and whose treatment results are not known.

The NTP will probably have reporting forms that we can use. In addition or instead, we can create a TB Patient Register that records data according to the above categories. The register in Table 10.1 would provide the information we need. When the patient is enrolled, we would enter the data for the first four columns. When the patient completes anti-TB drug therapy, we complete the last two columns.

Table 10.1	TB patient register				
Serial number	Name	Date therapy started	Case definition category	Date completed therapy	Treatment outcome category

A recording system for a community DOTS programme usually includes the following:

- patient TB card (kept by patient),
- patient TB card (kept in health centre),
- TB patient register,
- sputum register,
- observer patient register if treatment site is not at the health centre.

If the project keeps computerised records all except the first can be maintained in the database.

Step 9. Consider active case-finding

If and when our treatment programme is successful with a cure rate of greater than 85% we should consider active case finding. Here, we actively search for people in the community who have sputum-positive TB. It is the equivalent of the mopping up operations in childhood immunisation. We concentrate on this group of people because they are the ones infecting others.

> If our cure rates are less than 85% then we are harming rather than helping the situation. A higher priority is to achieve high cure rates (thus reducing multi-drug resistance) rather than increasing the case detection rate.

Here are some suggestions for active case-finding:

1. **Examine all patients coming to the health centre** if they have suspicious symptoms and signs. This includes those who have come for other medical reasons, and any attending relatives.
2. **Follow up the household contacts**, especially children under 5, of newly diagnosed sputum-positive patients. This can be undertaken by the CHV.
3. **Encourage the CHV to refer any patients with features suggestive of TB**, who they know themselves or have heard about through lane health visitors or members of the CAG.
4. **During community surveys encourage any household members with suggestive symptoms** not already under treatment, to attend the clinic.

Step 10. Arrange BCG immunisation of new-borns

BCG is probably already being given as part of the government's Expanded Programme on Immunisation (EPI). BCG should be given as soon after birth as possible. Those born in hospital may receive BCG there, but this needs to be confirmed for each child. Those born in the community should ideally receive BCG on the first post-natal visit.

WHO recommends that in high TB prevalence countries, all children should receive BCG except those with signs and symptoms of HIV/AIDS. In low prevalence countries, BCG should not be given to HIV-infected children.

Chapter summary

Tuberculosis (TB) kills more people than any other infectious illness and is increasing worldwide among most poor communities. It is spread through the cough of a person with infectious TB. Those living in crowded, unventilated slum houses, are most at risk especially if malnourished or HIV-positive. We need to decide if the community is ready to start a programme and whether our CHDP has the necessary resources. All programme activities need to be done in close collaboration with the national TB programme following its guidelines for treatment and monitoring. We should aim for cure rates of 85% or more, through passive case finding. A key strategy is DOTS standing for Directly Observed Treatment, Short Course. Here treatment is carefully supervised in the community, with each dose of medicine swallowed, being observed by a community volunteer. Accurate recording systems need to be set up according to standard case and treatment category definitions. We must ensure that our programme gives equal access to women, that we develop an integrated strategy for those with HIV infection who are at high risk of developing TB and that infants are immunised with BCG.

Resources

1. *Clinical Tuberculosis (second edition).* J Crofton, N Horne, F Miller. Macmillan, 1999. An extremely helpful book covering all aspects of TB in clear language. (Available from TALC).

2. *TB: A Clinical Manual for South East Asia.* A Harries, D Maher, M Uplekar. WHO, 1997. A very comprehensive review of all aspects of the clinical management of people with tuberculosis.

3. *Treatment of Tuberculosis: Guidelines for National Programmes.* D Maher, P Chaulet, S Spinaci, A Harries. WHO, 1997.

11 Vulnerable households: households that cannot cope with misfortune

In this chapter, we shall consider:

What we need to know:

Why people are unable to cope when misfortune occurs

Types of households that are vulnerable for destitution

What we need to do:

Phase 1. Choose high-risk factors for our community

Phase 2. Discover which households are at high risk

Phase 3. Carry out specific interventions for high risk groups

This chapter gives ideas about how to care for the poorest of the poor. In practice many of these will be those with special needs, and will therefore require specialist help. Community Health and Development Programmes can help to identify and empower those in greatest need and link groups with special needs to people and programmes able to help them.

Many slum dwellers live on the margins of survival. They can just manage to live and work as long as no misfortune strikes them. If it does, they may no longer be able to provide themselves with food, water and shelter. The misfortune may be something that happens to a family member, such as serious illness or the loss of a job; or it may be a community crisis such as fire or flood.

What we need to know

Why people are unable to cope when misfortune occurs

Like the poor anywhere, people who live in slums are poorly equipped to cope with misfortune or deal with unexpected events. Their income is barely able to pay for food and shelter. They have little or no savings, and are usually in debt to moneylenders who demand high rates of interest. In practice the urban poor are often worse off than their rural cousins. There are two reasons for this:

1 **Fewer people are living in one household**. When disaster hits one family member it has a big effect for the others. There is no extended family to turn to

Table 11.1 Common misfortunes that happen to people living in slums	
To individuals	**To communities**
Serious or fatal accidents, on the road, in the house or at work	Demolition
Fire	Fire
Flood	Flood
Electrocution or electric burns	Civil disorder
Tuberculosis	Severe weather
AIDS	
Loss of job	
Imprisonment	
Drug addiction	
Demands from creditors	

for help. For example when a villager dies, other family members will usually take care of the partner and children. But in an urban nuclear family if one partner dies or is unable to work, the other must take on the tasks of wage-earner, homemaker and child carer. In practice they are rarely able to do this.

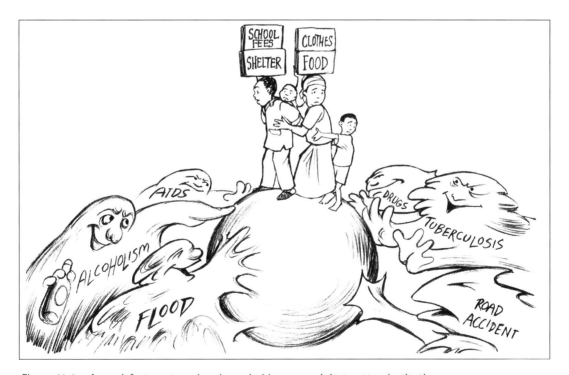

Figure 11.1   Any misfortune to a slum household may precipitate utter destitution.

❷ **The urban poor are living in a cash society**. In rural areas, people can survive for periods of time without money: free water is accessible; they can forage for food; they usually have shelter and if not relatives will take them in. In the cash economy of cities, slum dwellers must pay for everything and usually have no reserves. Loss of income means immediate loss of food – or even water.

From the field: A CHDP in Jakarta, Indonesia began working in the outskirts of the city, which was thought to be the most disadvantaged area. But soon the project realised that people in the periphery had small plots of land that were an important source of food and income. Overcrowding was less and the environment healthier – no stagnant water or blocked sewers. After a more careful assessment of need, the project shifted its effort to the city centre to serve pockets of very poor that were situated in the midst of higher income neighbourhoods and had been overlooked initially because of superficial inspection.

Lesson learned: Initial assessment of vulnerability can help to target the very poor.

Source: Authors.

Types of household that are most vulnerable for destitution

Households that are already coping with one misfortune are especially vulnerable if further problems strike. Table 11.2 lists some characteristics of vulnerable households.

Table 11.2   High-risk factors that characterise vulnerable households
Belonging to a minority group that suffers from discrimination
Headed by a woman or child
Having only one or no employed adult
Having only one or no literate adult
Having an alcoholic, gambler or drug abuser
Having one or more children under 5 years old
Having chronically ill or seriously disabled person(s)
Having a house made of cheap or free materials such as plastic, cardboard, canvas, etc.
Having no household latrine
Having no access to safe drinking water
Consuming two meals or fewer per day

What we need to do

Phase 1. Choose high-risk factors for our community

We need to decide which high-risk factors to use for our community. We can use some or all of the ones just mentioned in the previous section. Our decisions should be

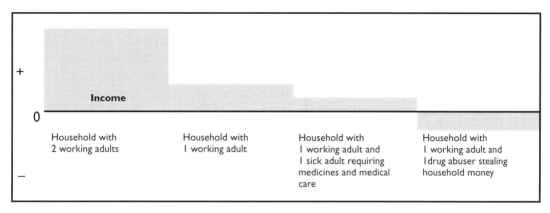

Figure 11.2   The effect of illness on household income.

based on the detailed understanding we have of the communities we are working with.

When we have our list of high-risk factors, we will assess each household to determine how many high-risk factors it has. Those households with the highest number of high-risk factors become our target high-risk households.

Phase 2. Discover which households are at high risk

We can do this in various ways:

Through the house–to–house survey

If the CHDP and community plan to conduct a house-to-house survey, information on the above categories (or whatever categories that the CHDP/community decide) can be included in the questionnaire or survey form, see page 45, Chapter 3, Initial Activities.

By special survey

If at any time the CHDP or a community group want to become involved with high-risk households, a special survey can be carried out. Sometimes a project or community group will decide to work only with one type of vulnerable household such as those headed by lone mothers or which include someone living with HIV/AIDS. In that case, the survey can be designed to obtain information relating to that particular problem.

By area or cluster

The community health volunteer or other community member responsible for a certain area of the slum can find out more detailed information about the households they are responsible for. Often they will already be aware of neighbours who are in trouble and other vulnerable households.

Labelling high-risk households on a community map helps in planning and follow-up.

> **From the field:** In the Philippines, an NGO helped the community to conduct a demographic survey, after which neighbourhood clusters of 15–25 families were organised, with an elected central Council of Leaders. Various committees were set up, e.g. water and sanitation, education, health and nutrition, and a committee for street children. The community identifies vulnerable families, e.g. female-headed households or families whose children live on the streets. These families are given specific help through scholarships, income generation loans, etc. Other projects benefit the community as a whole, e.g. paved footpaths, community toilets and washing areas.
>
> **Source:** Black, 1991.

Phase 3. Carry out specific interventions for high risk groups

When sudden misfortune strikes an individual household, our first job is to provide any immediate assistance that is needed. The Community Action Group is in a good position to do this. It can assess the needs of the affected household, provide family members with immediate assistance and possibly provide emergency funds or give a no-interest loan. They can organise emergency meals and child care via friends or neighbours until the household begins to recover.

For each household that we have identified as high-risk, we will need to develop an action plan, see Chapter 4. This section first looks at four highly vulnerable groups, and then outlines ways in which the CHDP can help, if the slum as a whole is hit by a calamity.

Woman-headed households

Women who have been suddenly widowed or abandoned often have little working experience outside the home. They are often illiterate, unskilled and frightened. They may be lone mothers, with no one to care for their small children. These factors greatly limit their work opportunities. In addition, women with no partner are more likely to be sexually, physically or emotionally abused in the community or in the workplace. It can be hard for such women to speak up at community gatherings, even when the needs of widows or lone parents are being discussed.

Here are some ways we can empower women who head households:

① **Set up vocational training programmes or income generation schemes,** based on work that can be done at home, or in a nearby safe environment with child-care facilities.

② **Help the women's Community Action Group advocate for the needs of single mothers,** for example by setting up a child-care centre.

③ **Build awareness in the community about the needs of women** and woman-headed households.

④ **Try to make it possible for the CAG to include at least one lone mother on their committee.**

Life in a slum

Maria, her husband and their young child moved to Sao Paulo about 10 years ago when a prolonged drought forced them to leave their village. They were able to rent a hut in a kebele (slum) where others from their village had settled. Maria was able to find work as a domestic. Her husband found some construction work, but often the jobs were far away. He would then stay on the site and only come home once a month. He spent most of his earnings on alcohol and gambling. He came home less and less and finally stopped altogether. In the years since, two other men have lived with Maria. She has had two more children. The last man she lived with, Lorenzo, left one year ago. Maria's 11 year old daughter Sheila cares for the younger children while Maria works. When Maria comes home in the late afternoon, Sheila attends a special school set up by an NGO that provides evening classes for girls who have to work during the day. (Brazil)

Households with many dependants and few wage-earners

With many mouths to feed and few people earning, these households are always struggling to survive. Often children will be malnourished and as a result more vulnerable to infectious diseases such as diarrhoea and pneumonia. In addition the very young and the very old will need day-time carers. All family members will be vulnerable to illness and to higher medical fees. These households are an example of how poverty generates even greater poverty.

Here are some ways of making such households less vulnerable:

1. **Help the women's Community Action Group set up a child-care centre or creche.** Young children can be cared for, and older children can be given pre-school education. All children can be provided with a nutritious mid-day meal.

2. **Community Health Volunteers can give special attention to these households**, by monitoring the weight of under 5s, ensuring the children are fully immunised, arranging for regular supplements of vitamin A and iron, and giving regular de-worming tablets every 4–6 months. They can make sure antenatal care and delivery care is available.

3. **Community members can set up support systems**. For example residents who are home during the day can look in on an elderly neighbour from time to time. Alternatively the community can help to set up a day-care centre for the elderly or disabled.

4. **The CHDP can actively promote family planning and ensure that supplies are easily accessible.**

5. **Household members can be given free or subsidised rates for medical care** at any clinics run by the CHDP.

6. **Advocacy and community support networks can be made aware of these families** and their needs.

People who are addicted to alcohol, drugs or gambling

People with these addictions often cause a downward spiral both for themselves and other members of the household. They have trouble keeping jobs. They require money to feed their addiction, and often steal from family and neighbours. Many become drug-pushers, join street gangs or get in trouble with the police who then harass the family. Serious health problems develop: these include abscesses, hepatitis, HIV/AIDS, sexually transmitted diseases, and poor nutrition, all needing costly medical treatment. The stress of unemployment, debt, and low self-esteem, often leads to physical or sexual abuse of family members. Finally the whole family may disintegrate.

Here are some ways of giving support to these households:

1. **Organise self-help support groups for addicts and family members**. Two well known groups are Alcoholics Anonymous for alcoholics and Al-Anon for family members. If such groups exist we can make use of them, if not we can start them, having first trained a project or community member on how to run such groups.

2. **Provide subsidised or reduced health care** for family members at community clinics.

3. **Advocate for former addicts with family, employers, community and authorities.**

4. **Organise needle syringe exchange programmes** to reduce the risk of intravenous drug abusers becoming infected with HIV and hepatitis B and C.

5. **Find out about good, low-cost detoxification centres, refuges for abused or battered women** and other resources which may be present in the city.

We can also concentrate on prevention:

1. **Raise awareness of the dangers of drugs and alcohol among young people** – through schools, clubs, and by using national or local sports celebrities.

2. **Help to set up sports, education and vocational programmes for young people at risk of starting addictive behaviours**. This may mean constructing a well-resourced and carefully planned programme. To be effective, the activities should be popular with the community and in tune with the needs and cultures of the most vulnerable groups. Other NGOs may be able to share their expertise or resources.

3. **Facilitate community groups who press for the closure of any liquor shops and gambling dens** located in or near the community.

Life in a slum

Lal was a 17-year-old boy, addicted to heroin, which is cheap and readily available in Manipur, near the India–Myanmar border. His mother came to SHALOM, an NGO that works with drug addicts and those living with HIV/AIDS. She begged the staff to accept him into their detoxification programme. Lal had stolen nearly all of the household goods to help buy drugs. Only the rice cooker was left: she kept it locked away. Lal's mother knows that he is unlikely to stay off drugs for good, but by going through detox, he may have a period of weeks or months free from drugs. Even if he restarts, expenses will be less at least to start with, as he won't need such high doses to satisfy his craving.

People with physical or mental disabilities

In developing countries, people with physical or mental disabilities are one of the most neglected groups of people. They have little opportunity for schooling, employment or specialised medical care. Their ability to move around is often limited.

They are often harassed, rejected and humiliated by the general public. The disabled often sink deeper into poverty making their problems even more extreme.

Working with the disabled requires skill and dedication. This chapter can only draw attention to some of the many possibilities. Any programme we start needs a careful needs assessment, the recruitment and training of skilled and compassionate staff and full involvement of the community. Here are some possible options:

① **Advocacy** for the needs of the disabled, including the blind and deaf (visually and hearing impaired) and mentally ill or disabled. We can start by helping to change attitudes within the actual communities we are serving.

② **Encourage the use of simple low-cost aids and appliances**. These can make a surprising difference if appropriately used. David Werner's book *Disabled Village Children* shows how to create low-cost aids and appliances (see Resources)

③ **Identify special schools, vocational training programmes, employment opportunities, group care facilities, and other resources.** As part of a planned programme we may be able to help set up one or more of these.

④ **Arrange for a specialist to visit the programme and make recommendations** on how an effective approach can be developed.

⑤ **Contact any government agencies or NGOs** who work with the disabled groups, e.g. an NGO or government Community Rehabilitation Workers.

Response to a community-wide crisis

If a calamity such as a serious fire, flood or earthquake strikes, the government, relief agencies or religious groups often provide water, food, shelter and latrines.

The CHDP will however be in a strong position to help. It will know, probably better than anyone else, the (original) lay-out of the slum and its facilities: also details of the slum leadership, support networks and the special needs of groups and individuals.

Here are some ways in which the CHDP may be able to help:

① **Acting as advisor to those providing the emergency relief**, so that supplies and resources can be used most effectively.

② **Offering to give practical assistance**. Health workers and others with special skills can join in the relief operation.

③ **Mobilising community members known to have special skills**. This will include Community Health Volunteers, CAG members or those who have been trained in special construction skills. The CHDP can make these people known to the emergency services.

④ **Offering emotional and psychological support to those who have been hardest hit**.

⑤ **Being aware of vulnerable households and making sure their members receive the help and support they need**.

⑥ **Helping in the transition phase back to normality once the emergency is over**. The community can be vulnerable at this time. Emergency services are no longer available but repair and reconstruction is not complete (or even started). Before the emergency services pull out, the CHDP should meet with them and draw up plans for the transition. With the help of the community the CHDP can help to guide this transition and hasten the community's return to normal.

❼ Sometimes similar calamities will have hit the community before, e.g. severe flooding. The CHDP or CAG may remember lessons from the previous occasion. **They should make themselves known as soon as possible to those in charge of emergency assistance**.

A new opportunity. Sometimes a crisis can help bring project and community closer together. Sometimes also the emergency creates new ideas, motivation and awareness which the CDHP can tap into and take forward.

Chapter summary

Those living in slums can fall into severe destitution if misfortune strikes an individual family or the slum as a whole. Certain households have virtually no reserves to fall back on if times get hard. The Community Health and Development Programme needs to identify those families and help draw up action plans to support and empower them.

Certain households are at especially high risk. These include homes headed by women and especially by lone mothers: households with many dependants but few wage-earners: those where one or more members are addicted to alcohol, drugs or gambling: and those where a family member has a physical or mental disability. Each of these groups needs a different approach. The CHDP is in a good position to assess what solutions are most appropriate. However before any major programmes are started careful assessment is needed and no solutions must be allowed to overwhelm the capacity of the CHDP. Meanwhile simpler interventions at community level can bring considerable benefits. Finally CHDPs can play a valuable role, when a calamity such as flooding affects the whole community.

Resources

1. *Nothing About Us Without Us*. D Werner. The Hesperian Foundation, 1998. Provides ideas for innovative aids for the disabled that can be made at low cost.(Available from TALC.)

2. *Poverty and Health: Reaping a Richer Harvest*. M-T Feuerstein. Macmillan, 1997. (Available from TALC.)

3. *An Agenda for Caring: Interventions for Marginalised Groups*. V Rao, H Mander. Voluntary Health Association of India, 1996. Discusses many marginalised categories of people, their problems and possible interventions.

4. *Disabled Village Children*. D Werner. The Hesperian Foundation, 1994. Comprehensive guide for community health workers and families with many ideas directly transferable to urban situations. (Available from TALC.)

Part 4

ENVIRONMENTAL IMPROVEMENTS

12 Environmental improvements: general principles

Slum dwellers live in a polluted and ugly environment. Improving their environment does two important things. First, it improves their health (usually seen by them as reducing illness). Second it raises their sense of hope and self-worth. In this part of the book we will look at the five main areas in which the urban environment can be improved:

① **housing** (Chapter 13) – which is usually crowded and cramped;

② **water supply** (Chapter 14) – which is usually unsafe in quality and inadequate in amount;

③ **excreta disposal** (Chapter 15) – which is usually unsafe and inadequate;

④ **surface water** (rainwater and household wastewater) disposal (Chapter 16) – which is usually inadequate;

⑤ **garbage disposal** and a variety of other environmental hazards, including air and noise pollution (Chapter 17).

This chapter gives a general framework relevant to any environmental improvement and gives broad guidelines that apply to each of them. Later chapters in this part look at the specific problems of each topic and the best ways to deal with them.

This chapter and the next five chapters describe four broad phases in bringing about any environmental improvement: They are headed as follows:

- **Phase 1**: Prepare the community for action
- **Phase 2**: Help the community choose which problems to solve
- **Phase 3**: Carry out the improvements
- **Phase 4**: Maintain and evaluate the changes

In reading through each of the following five chapters in this part of the book, it will be helpful to refer back to the equivalent phases in this chapter. For the sake of simplicity many of the phases are subdivided into specific Steps, which are unique for each type of environmental improvement.

In practice, the process of environmental improvements rarely follows the sequence that is outlined in this chapter. Activities in the four phases will overlap, and plans will need to be continually revised and updated. We always need to remember the importance of being flexible so that the community can be fully involved in its own way and at its own pace.

Phase 1: Prepare the community for action

Preparing a community for action is one of the most critical tasks of a Community Health and Development Programme (CHDP). The topic is so important that we have set aside the whole of Chapter 2, Working with the Community, to describe this in detail.

Our overall aim is to help communities to become self-reliant and to solve their own problems. The key to this is mobilisation, which if maintained increases the chance of turning early hopes into long-term change. This is most likely to succeed when there is **full partnership between the CHDP and the community** leading on to the **community's ownership** of the programme. Only then is there a real chance that lasting changes will occur, and be maintained.

Mobilisation of the entire community is all the more important because most environmental improvements are at a community, and not an individual level. Therefore we must ensure that the community as a whole owns the project and assumes full responsibility for maintaining it from the very beginning. Unless this happens the whole programme will gradually deteriorate – as vandalism, lack of maintenance and dwindling interest spoil all the labour, time and expectation that has been present from the start.

A critical time is when outsiders have left, the technical experts are gone, and the community is left to its own resources to use and maintain the improvement. The government may be responsible for maintenance and repair, but its services are seldom adequate. The world is full of projects built with great enthusiasm and at great cost, which then fall into disuse months or even weeks after construction was completed. Usually this is because the community felt no ownership or received inadequate training for repairs.

From the field: In a slum community in New Delhi, the government built a community-latrine complex as part of a city-wide scheme to improve civic services to slum communities. The community was not involved in the decision or in the building process. The government hired a private firm to operate and maintain the complex. The facility was poorly maintained: the government, which did not monitor the operation of the facility, continued to pay the firm regularly every month. The complex became so dirty that most of the community stopped using it. Eventually the community approached the government, which agreed to turn over the operating and routine maintenance to the community. Now users pay a small fee that covers the wages of the manager and cleaners, as well as routine maintenance costs.

Lesson learned: When the government establishes facilities without the community's full involvement, the use and upkeep of the facility usually fail. Even if this happens a CHDP can help the community realise its benefits and train them how to use it and how to look after it.

Source: Authors.

We are basically asking communities to become self-reliant and to solve their own problems. There are three Steps in helping to motivate and mobilise a community.

Step 1. Increase the knowledge and awareness of community members

This usually starts by helping community members to recognise the problems, understand their causes and consider solutions. Then most important of all, they begin to believe that they themselves can do something about the problems they have identified.

Step 2. Motivate the community for action

Changes in behaviour do not come easily, especially for the poor. We can help them overcome their lack of knowledge, but they must also convert their feelings of hopeless acceptance into a genuine belief that they can have some control over their situation. It is important to identify a few people in the community who have vision and then help them to bring that vision to the community. The process is slow, and often has setbacks.

In practice most slum dwellers are very interested in making changes to their environment, but they are often beaten by two difficulties:

1. The first lies within themselves: **a sense of hopelessness and cynicism**. Politicians, government bureaucrats, NGOs and even other community members have made so many promises, without delivering what was promised. Thus they are very reluctant to give time, labour and money to yet another cause. To help overcome this we can first work on an environmental problem that is likely to have a quick, successful outcome.

2. The second lies in the environment itself: the fact that there is **usually more than one serious environmental problem**. This can make the idea of any change at all too overwhelming, or cause different opinions to emerge. Some community members or groups may want to work on one problem and some want to work on another. It may be useful to make priority tables (see Chapter 4 on Making an action plan) to help the community come to a more united, informed decision. The process of doing this helps to bring about a change in attitude and behaviour.

Step 3. Channel motivation through organising the community: the Community Action Group

Although the entire community should have input into project activities, an action group is the best way to channel activity, and to keep the process moving. The Community Action Group (CAG) should include both community and CHDP representatives. The CAG may be called something else such as 'the Housing Committee', 'Water/Sanitation Committee', or 'Community Welfare Committee'. If no effective committee exists, one should be started. Also it is better to use the name

Action Group rather than committee as members are then primed to get things done rather than to seek privileges for themselves.

The CAG must be a representative group, including women and members of any marginalised or minority group. The CAG must be empowered to plan and implement improvements. The CAG acts on behalf of the community whose ideas and opinions it needs to understand and represent at all stages. (See Chapter 2, Working with the community, page 25)

Phase 2: Help the community choose which problems to solve

When the community feels ready to take action about its felt needs, the next phase is to decide which environmental problem(s) it wants to work on. But to make this choice in an informed way, it is helpful to follow a number of steps. Some will overlap and they will not always occur in the order listed below.

Step 1. Gather information about major environmental problems

Some of the ways we can do this are described in Chapter 3, under Make a community diagnosis, page 43.

The CAG (or other named group) should take the initiative and co-ordinate this phase of the project. But the group must represent the community's wishes and keep it actively involved or it will lose the trust of the community at large. It can do this through community meetings, on community walks, and during informal discussions with individuals and groups. It is especially important that women are fully consulted and involved: most environmental improvements will have an especially large impact on their lives.

We will need to gather information on the following:

Layout and facilities in the community

Even when looking at only one aspect of environmental improvement, e.g. water supply, it is helpful to make a detailed survey of all facilities that have any impact on the health of a community, e.g. clinics, latrines and water points. These are then documented onto a community map.

The best way to discover these is by systematically walking through the community. Here is how to do it:

1. First of all, get hold of a community map or plan. If a map is not available, then we can work with the community to make a map, adding information from the survey walk.

2. Start by making a basic map with roads, schools, government facilities, rivers, ponds, etc. Make the map on a large piece of poster board.

3. Then add information about structures and hazards that specifically affect health. It is helpful to use a key for this. For example, when putting water points on the

map, draw a green hand pump for those that are working, and a red hand pump for those that are broken. Do the same thing for water taps. The key for medical clinics could be a red cross for government clinics, a green cross for private clinics and a blue cross for traditional healers.

Sometimes a map may get so cluttered that it is hard to get a clear picture of the structures we want to highlight. To minimise this problem, first make the basic map as in point 2, above. Then cut several sheets of stiff clear plastic the same size as the poster board. Take one plastic sheet and overlay the map. Then using keys as mentioned above, draw on the plastic sheet all sources of water in the community, using the map underneath as a guide. Remove that sheet, and replace it with another on which to write drains, areas of standing water, areas that flood, etc. Another sheet can be used for areas of defecation and existing latrines. If wanting to see more than one aspect at a time, just layer the plastic sheets on top of the map. With experience we will learn to place the keys for each layer in a different spot so that they don't become superimposed when using more than one sheet.

Be sure to indicate on the map areas where the poorer residents or different minority groups live. That way it is easy to observe if they have less access to water, latrines, etc. Also when we plan where to install a new well or other improvement, it is easier to ensure that the needs of the very poor are fully taken into account.

Most slum communities are located on land that no one else wants. In most cases, this is because the land is hazardous to health. For example the land may be:

- low-lying with a high water table and poor drainage;
- situated along a river flood plain;
- steep, with the danger of flash floods or landslides during heavy rains;
- near factories that deal with dangerous chemicals or cause a high level of noise;
- next to main roads with traffic noise and pollution.

We will need to be aware of these overall characteristics as we plan any community-wide improvements. Occasionally we may find the area is so hazardous that the best solution is to negotiate relocation with community and government, especially if the colony is small.

Relevant health problems in the community

The different environmental short-comings in slums usually cause specific health problems. Therefore if we find out what the major health problems are in the community, that will suggest which environmental problems are most harmful to the health of the community. For example, if we find that malaria is common, then we should look for pools of standing water that act as breeding sites for the mosquitoes that carry malaria and for the prevalence of netting on windows and the use of mosquito nets. On the other hand, if ascariasis (roundworms) is a big problem, we

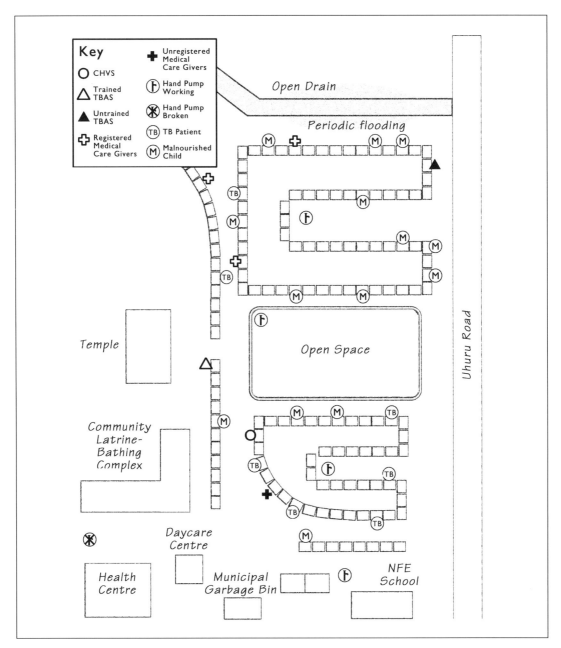

Figure 12.1   Label maps with items that are important to project activities. This project helped communities get better water supplies and also provide maternal-child health care services.

should look at where people, particularly children, defecate, what happens to the faeces, and where children play.

Knowing the health problems in the community is especially important later when the community prioritises the problems. Those problems that cause health problems should be given a higher priority when the community decides which problems to work on.

Social and cultural factors

All aspects of community living are closely bound up with the beliefs, practices and traditions of the community. This is especially true for timing and practice of defecation, ways of bathing and washing, and patterns in which houses are clustered or arranged. For example, when planning a latrine system, it is important to know how people clean themselves after defecation. If they use water for cleansing, which is the usual method in Asia, then a water seal latrine will work. If they use mud, leaves, corn husks or sticks, common in much of Africa, then the choices are more limited – but there are suitable composting and dehydrating latrines.

Within one slum community, different traditions and practices exist side-by-side because residents come from different areas and ethnic groups. This is a very different situation from most villages where people are more likely to be from similar traditions and backgrounds. Sometimes differing attitudes towards general cleanliness or open defecation by children can lead to frank disagreement between different ethnic groups living in the same community.

When we complete this situational analysis of our community, we will have a fairly good idea of the environmental problems. Often there are so many problems that it may be difficult to decide which ones to work on first. Sometimes using a ranking table can help, see page 62.

Certain health problems typically occur with specific environmental problems, e.g. roundworms and hookworms with open defecation, mosquito-borne diseases with standing water. These will be discussed in the relevant chapters that follow.

Step 2. Discover the government's willingness and capacity to take action

Most city governments in developing countries are overwhelmed by the problems they face, and often lack political will to provide major improvements for slums. The best way for slum communities to improve their environment is to take on the task themselves. City governments are often willing to work alongside those communities that are prepared to contribute to costs and which have existing community groups able to oversee improvements. (The government can then claim success but at far less cost in resources and effort.)

For relatively **minor** improvements, progress is often faster if the government is not involved. Politicians may want to serve specific interest groups, meaning there is often inefficiency or corruption that causes delay. Low-cost improvements such as window netting or safe storage of water in covered containers is best thought of as part of health promotion. It can be done at low cost and does not require government help.

With **major** environmental improvements the government must play a key role. It may be needed to:

- **Grant permission** and approval.
- **Provide funding** or revolving loans.
- **Supply technical expertise**.

- **Assist with major maintenance and repairs** that are beyond the community's ability to manage financially or technically.
- **Provide certain services**, such as connections to municipal water supplies, or vacuum truck removal of excreta.
- **Provide land** at low rent or on long-term lease for on-site rebuilding or resettlement.

Community latrines, desilting major drains and on-site rebuilding are all major environmental improvements that need a government with both the resources and political will to work with the community. Unfortunately, in many cities this is almost impossible. People are pouring into cities and completely overloading services such as water, sanitation and electricity. In addition, slum dwellers usually have very little influence with politicians and government bureaucrats. The best option is for communities to be trained how to assert their rights and how to implement and maintain any improvements.

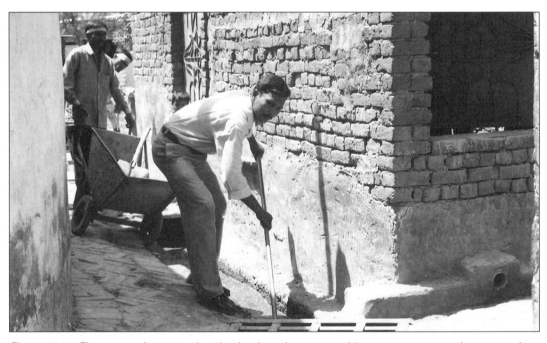

Figure 12.2   The community can undertake simple maintenance without government assistance, such as cleaning pathside secondary drains. (Godfrey Martin/ASHA)

As we work with the community in choosing options, it becomes clear that we must learn how local government operates (see Table 12.1 below). Building relationships and understanding between community and government is crucial for major projects to succeed (see Table 12.1). In Latin American countries in particular, governments are most responsive if low-income communities get together and make specific demands for improved civic services.

Table 12.1   Effects of the different types of government involvement on slum improvements

Type of government involvement	Advantages (+) Disadvantages (−)	Result
Facilitating: Government is looking for community partners to work together towards environmental improvement	+ Community shares in decisions and in providing resources + Community feels ownership	Most likely to be successful and sustainable. The community will use, monitor and maintain the facilities. But it requires an organised, cohesive community
Reluctantly involved: When pushed, the government is prepared to give some assistance in granting permission/ licences, provide expertise and services. It is not usually willing to provide financial assistance	+ Community may get some government assistance + Community may be able to link up with existing government services (drainage system, solid waste disposal) etc. − Progress is limited by lack of funding, expertise and bureaucratic delays	With a very motivated and organised community, progress can be made. However, bureaucratic delays and lack of funding may slow down progress
Not involved: Unwilling or unable to participate or co-operate	− Community is denied source of expertise and funding − Difficult to link up with existing civic services	Very difficult to make any major community-wide improvements
Dominating: Government carries out 'improvements' with little input or involvement from community	+ Something is being done − Community feels no ownership of facility − Facility may be culturally or otherwise inappropriate	Community has physical plant (community latrine, drains, etc.) but does not use or maintain so it falls into disuse and disrepair. Money is spent with no gain

Step 3. Obtain technical advice

Because environmental improvements are so technically complex, expert advice is needed at an early stage to know if and how we can make improvements. Without this we can waste a lot of time, money, interest and hope.

Two of the most useful technical experts are engineers and architects. There are several places to look for such people – government departments, universities, NGOs, the private sector, or recently retired experts with an interest in helping the community. It is ideal if these people consider their involvement as 'community service' and offer their time free of charge or at a reduced rate.

It is most important that experts do not dominate the project. They should help inform the community so that the CAG, as the community's representatives, can make the best decisions. Experts from NGOs are often more sensitive to community issues and better able to give their advice in a non-technical way which the community can understand. Also they are more willing to act as facilitators rather than directors.

Step 4. Consider various cost options

No one will want to spend money unless there is a good chance the project will succeed. This applies to government departments and donor partners. But it applies as much if not more to community members, who will want to make sure they get the best possible returns for what they spend.

Two approaches will help the community:

❶ **Offering a choice of options**. One problem, especially with community financing, is that some people are able or willing to pay more for improvements than others. One way of dealing with this is to have a range of options, each with a different cost. People can then choose what is best for their particular situation.

> **From the field**: In an urban sanitation project in Brazil, groups of households in poor urban communities have a choice of three different options of connecting to the sewer system at varying cost to themselves, and also the choice of not connecting at all. The residents themselves choose the project designs. Low-cost technology is used and construction costs minimised by using local contractors. The community maintains the secondary sewer lines.
>
> **Lesson learned**: Often the quality of service is so low that many are unwilling to pay for it, or too expensive so that many are unable to afford it. By giving informed choice, each household can bid into the level or cost of service most appropriate for its own situation.
>
> **Source**: Authors.

❷ **Designing options so they can be upgraded later**. For example in Hyderabad, India, sewer lines were laid in slums so that residents had the option of connecting to the sewer system. Those who elected not to connect at the time could easily do so later.

Step 5. Ensure the project is sustainable

Sustainability is a key issue for all projects (see Chapter 19). The long-term future of any development activity must be central to all the plans we make. This is especially true of community level improvements because individual residents are less likely to care for a facility that belongs to the whole community, rather than to their particular household.

One secret for this is building the community's capacity to deal with problems in the future. Community members must learn the processes described in this and other chapters, especially Chapters 3 and 4. Asking some key questions can help raise the issues. For example can the community:

• Recognise and define problems?
• Discuss problems giving voice to all members of the community?
• Prioritise its problems?

- Plan activities to fix problems that arise?
- Implement a plan?
- Monitor the progress of its activities?
- Operate and maintain communal facilities?
- Evaluate its activities?

A CAG that has interested, capable and trustworthy members is the key to sustaining a project. The goal of the CHDP should be to empower members of the CAG and community to be able to manage their own activities from start to finish.

When dealing with major environmental improvements in slums, there are two major challenges to sustainability:

❶ Who will pay for the **on-going maintenance and repair costs**?

❷ Who will be **responsible for operating and maintaining the improved facility**?

Success is most likely when the community has been involved as a major partner in any planning and construction. Also when it has taken on responsibility (after appropriate training) for keeping the facility in working order. For any project to have a long-term future, residents must be fully convinced of the benefits of the change. A very good indicator of this is the amount of money and labour they are willing to provide during construction.

Step 6. Choose the best way forwards

Having worked through these steps, the community should now be able to decide which broad type of improvement it wishes to follow, e.g. excreta disposal, safer water supply or house improvement. It will also need to decide on the best ways of tackling any improvement it decides on. For example, if the environmental problem is unsanitary excreta disposal, community members will need to choose between different models of latrine, whether to opt for community, group or individual latrines, or even whether to choose a simpler method of excreta disposal.

In making these choices CAG members and others with a special interest can visit other communities to see the various options that are being used. A SWOT analysis (Chapter 4) can also be helpful at this stage. After deciding which way or ways it wants to deal with the problem, the community moves into the implementation phase.

Phase 3: Carry out the improvements

Again the process of implementation will not necessarily follow the order given below, and one or more activities may be happening at the same time. For example, when carrying out a pilot study comparing the use of lined and unlined drains, the community will be starting to look for outside funding. However, most environmental projects will at some stage be involved in the following steps.

Step 1. Mobilise skills

From the very beginning we will need to help the community identify sources of help, both from inside and outside the community.

From inside the community

- **Skilled community members**: masons, plumbers, electricians, etc., who can guide and assist in the construction process, and at a lower cost than people from outside.
- **Informed slum leaders, teachers, and other informal opinion makers**. If they are convinced that something new will be good for the community, they can help to inform and convince the others.

From specialised NGOs, the private sector and universities

These organisations can provide valuable human and technical skills, from engineering and architecture to advocacy and training.

- **NGOs**: Some NGOs specialise in particular tasks, such as digging wells, building low-cost latrines, starting kitchen gardens and extending low-interest loans. Others are involved in advocacy issues and helping poor communities to obtain services which the government is legally supposed to provide.
- **Local industrialists/employers/technical consultants**: Slums are often located near factories or other sites which use unskilled labour. Could major local employers donate resources to the community and in return benefit from healthier and more productive employees?
- **Local university or vocational schools**: Would a local university or trade school be willing to donate the services of students and faculty in exchange for real-life

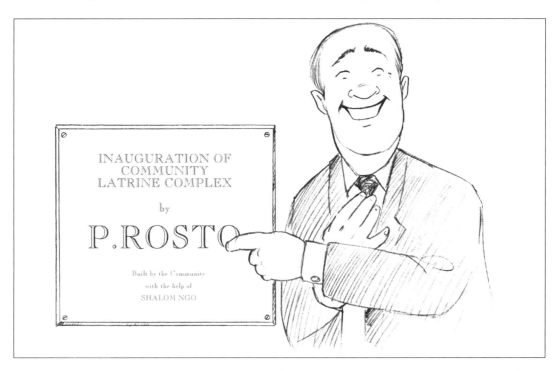

Figure 12.3   Politicians may be quick to take credit for a success story, whether deserved or not. If their future co-operation can be gained this may be a price worth paying.

learning experiences? For example, students of architecture could help plan and provide architectural drawings of the future homes. Engineering students could help plan civic services.

- **Local politicians**: Sometimes government schemes exist, but are hard to access. Could local politicians use their influence to pressurise the government to release funds for a specific need? Sometimes politicians have special funds to help the people living in their area. Could they be convinced (e.g. by seeing this as a popular move) to allocate a portion for housing improvements?

From the field: In the Orangi Project in Karachi, Pakistan, students from local universities assisted by community members, conducted a survey of the community as part of a sanitation project. They plotted the slope of the land, number of houses, number of lanes and the existing drainage situation. Each surveyed area was the political unit of one elected government representative. The representative then used the information to advocate for his constituency.

Lesson learned: Government help may come easier if government politicians can be involved at an early stage.

Source: Tabibzadeh, 1989.

Step 2. Approach government officials

Approaching the right government officials is a key aspect of most work in urban development. Chapter 18 looks at this in more depth. The community must now approach the appropriate government agencies for the following reasons:

- **To obtain necessary approvals**, sanctioning, etc. for land use.

- **To obtain any co-operation promised in earlier discussions**, such as government willingness to extend the municipal water supply, connect to the sewage system or bore deep tube wells.

- **To access relevant government programmes**. Common community-wide programmes include putting in water points, community latrines, drains and roads, but pressure will still be needed from the local community. Examples of schemes for individual households include providing individual latrines, tin roofs, and mosquito nets. Sometimes the government will pay part of these costs, if the household provides the labour and guarantees to pay a percentage.

At some point the community will be left to fend for itself. Learning how to interact with the government is a skill that will strengthen its hand for the future. As government comes to know the community it may be more willing to work with it again.

A small team often comprising one or two members of the CAG and a community chief along with a couple of CHDP members is usually suitable for meeting with government and other agencies. Forming a team helps to ensure continuity in any future co-operative schemes.

Step 3. Mobilise funding

The CHDP can help the community to identify and access sources of funding. Government, NGO, the private sector and citizens groups are common sources. But the community should also consider covering some of the costs itself.

Why should the community pay for parts of the costs?

When a community is informed and motivated, it may be willing to provide a proportion of the start-up and running costs. In fact the willingness to contribute towards an environmental project is a good indicator of how much the community owns the programme and is likely to see it through. This contribution by the community has several major advantages:

❶ **It encourages outside donors to come forward.** NGOs are often willing to provide financial and other resources to a community that has already paid up its own share.

❷ **The community does not have to wait until the government (if ever) gets around to paying for the improvements.** But as with private agencies, the government may be more willing to contribute if the community is prepared to give its own resources. This becomes more important all the time, as governments have less resources to pay for ever increasing numbers of the urban poor. They are often only willing to help fund improvements that are being partially paid for by the community or from other sources.

❸ **A community is likely to have more options if residents provide some of the funding.** There can be a choice of improvements so that those who can pay more can get better improvements

❹ **A community is more likely to look after improvements that they have chosen and paid for.** This is especially important because governments are not usually willing to pay for the upkeep of services in low-income areas.

How can the community help pay for civic improvements?

This section of the book is deliberately emphasising ways in which communities can be self-sufficient as far as possible. Here are some practical ways in which the community can help pay for civic improvements.

❶ **Savings/loan schemes**: The main challenge for slum dwellers is their lack of funds to pay for the high capital costs of an improvement project. Slum dwellers don't have a large chunk of money that they can give at one time for the capital costs. Also, the costs are usually highest at the beginning, but benefits are delayed. This 'delayed gratification' in which money must be paid at the beginning but the felt benefit is only experienced later is especially difficult for slum dwellers to commit to.

To deal with this problem, savings and loan schemes can be used. The residents earn interest on their deposits, and can borrow money at reasonable rates. The approach can run hand-in-hand with seed funding from an outside agency, usually an NGO.

From the field: In Bangkok in 1985, a fire in the Klong Toey Slum left thousands of people homeless. Overnight the residents put up makeshift houses even while the ashes were still warm. They knew that the government did not want them to return. Despite fires and eviction notices, the community continued to live there and to pressurise the government to give the land to the community. A local NGO, the Human Development Centre, helped residents negotiate with the government. After 2 years the government gave the land to the community so that residents could rebuild their houses.

However there was no money to pay for construction materials to build the houses. The Human Development Centre provided seed money and helped the community to set up a savings and loan association. Community members deposited money. Then on the first day of building they were paid back their deposit plus 18% interest. Alternatively they could receive back twice the value of their deposit in building materials, and take out a small no-interest loan repayable after 3 years.

As the loans were paid back, the money was used to make improvements in the slum. Very few residents defaulted. The Human Development Centre has facilitated similar projects in three other communities since.

Lesson learned: Slum communities can pay for their own housing when they can borrow money and pay back over time at low or no interest. Loans are likely to be repaid when the residents see that repaid money is actually used to improve their community. They consider the money as belonging to the community and not to some rich outside donor.

Source: Author visit.

One way we can encourage residents to pay back loans: no new loan can be taken out by a community member until all outstanding loan payments from others have been repaid.

❷ **Loan programmes from outside agencies**. Sometimes government will provide partial costs, e.g. for the purchase of materials. Governments may also give grants and tax benefits to banks to encourage them to extend loans to people with low income. NGOs may provide seed money to set up a revolving loan programme or they may grant loans directly to community members.

❸ **User-pay schemes**. Here community members pay for the cost of a service or facility as they use it. Alternatively they can pay per household on a monthly basis. One example is where users pay a small fee each time they use a community latrine, the income made being used for cleaning and repairs. User-pay schemes are good for maintenance programmes. But usually fees would need to be set too high in order to pay for any capital costs.

Step 4. Train people in skills and tasks

Training is an important area that is often neglected. Nearly everyone involved in an environmental programme will need training of some sort. Here are some examples:

- **Health workers** (staff and CHVs): Health education must go hand in hand with environmental improvements. Health workers need to be trained in effective teaching methods as well as health education topics.
- **Skilled construction workers from the community**. They must be identified and trained in areas that require new knowledge and skills. A list of community craftsmen who have been trained should be maintained and made available to residents.
- **Unskilled community members, including women** should be given the opportunity to gain new skills relevant to the project being carried out.
- **CAG members** need to be trained in bookkeeping, budgeting, management and leadership skills.
- **Schoolteachers** need training in the purpose and design of the project, and also the way in which it works in practice. They can pass this on to their students who in turn reinforce the understanding of the community.
- **Community members** need skills and knowledge to accomplish tasks for which they are responsible. Construction, cleaning and maintenance are common examples. In addition is the need for behavioural change in order to sustain any improvements in living conditions.
- **CHDP staff members** need training in how to manage a project, and how to mobilise and share information with a community.

From the field: In Zambia an NGO was able to assist slum communities to upgrade their housing at low cost by concentrating on skills training and income generation. Community members were trained to produce housing materials, which could then be sold at low cost to community members. Others were trained in building skills to provide low cost semi-skilled labour.

Lesson learned: Community-provided labour and materials are cost-effective and provide income for the community. And the transfer of skills is empowering.

Source: Harpham *et al.*, 1988.

Step 5. Carry out pilot studies

Doing pilot studies helps to answer important questions at an early stage before time and money is wasted on methods that are unlikely to work. Here are some questions which pilot studies may help to answer:

- Is the chosen option likely to be cost-effective?
- Is it socially and culturally acceptable to the majority in the community?
- Are the materials and techniques appropriate and workable?

Sometimes one or more pilot studies can be run together, especially if ideas or materials are new to a community. Alternatively, if a system is known to work in a neighbouring community, pilot studies may not be needed.

Step 6. Build demonstration system(s) and promote their use

The next step in many projects will be to build a demonstration system using the most appropriate methods and materials as revealed by the pilot studies. This is a critical time in which everyone must feel free to give their ideas and suggestions: community members, the CAG, CHDP staff members, technical experts and government officials. Any helpful suggestions can be added into the plan. The CAG can help, both in improving the design and promoting the improvement. They can organise community meetings, which give an opportunity for brainstorming ideas and for community members to make suggestions and to respond to the plans. Individual members can often make important cost-saving contributions to the design plan. These meetings help the community to feel closely involved during the construction stage.

We must make sure that the demonstration system is located within the community so that residents observe it, see how it works and can even try it out. If it is a home improvement, it should be installed in the home of a health worker, CAG member, or community leader who is enthusiastic about it and who will use and maintain it properly. Demonstrate several different options so that households of differing incomes can consider one(s) they can afford.

Demonstration units can generate a demand for its use. As community members are able to see the benefits it brings and make comments on how it can be improved, they begin to feel ownership, and start acting as agents of change. What usually happens is this: when a community is exposed to a new idea, such as improved technology, or a new way of doing things, a few adventurous people are willing to try it out. Most community members will remain cautious until they are convinced of the benefits that it will bring them, especially in terms of time saved, improved living conditions, or cash savings. They may have a neighbour who tries it out and persuades them to try it also.

Even if a new technology works well and is cost-effective, it still needs to be promoted within a community over a period of time. In general, consider the implementation to be successful if about 80% of the population accept the new technology. The time will hopefully come when other residents will see that the change is fashionable and it will become a status symbol to approve of it or use it. Introducing anything new needs social marketing, just like the promotion of a new consumer product, such as a television or cassette player. Here are some points to explain when 'marketing' environmental improvements to the community:

- How they will improve health (or reduce the likelihood of illness).
- How they will make the environment more pleasant to live in.
- How they will make the community a safer place, especially for children.
- How the changes might increase the value of their property.

Step 7. Set up the improvements or build the facility

This phase of the project obviously needs a great deal of careful planning – and communication. Although the set-up phase will be unique for each type of improvement (and will be discussed in later chapters), there are some general guidelines that apply to most planning activities. Here is a summary of important areas for environmental changes.

1. **List objectives** using a 'SMART' framework: Specific, Measurable, Achievable, Relevant and Time-bound, See Chapter 4, page 64.

2. **Make 'Who? What? Where? When? and How? plans'** for each phase of the project and for all main groups and individuals who will be involved. Some tasks will be the responsibility of each household, or group of households, or of certain unskilled or skilled workers. The community workforce for some tasks may be organised through a rotating system. School children and the elderly may be included and will need careful managing.

3. **Make estimates of the time required to complete each task.** By knowing how much time different tasks are likely to take, the CAG can monitor the project. It can quickly see where the delays are occurring and then try to overcome their causes. Technical experts can help to estimate how much time different tasks or phases will take, especially for larger scale improvements such as on-site rebuilding.

4. **Find and prepare storage facilities, work areas and sources of water and power.** Slums are usually crowded with very limited open space. Water and electricity sources may be hard to access, especially at the times they are needed. This means that the community will need to release space, facilities and power, ideally through voluntary encouragement. Often rights-of-way along streets can be taken over and fenced temporarily for the duration of any construction period.

5. **Purchase materials and equipment.** People from the community who are skilled workers in construction can be trained to carry out these critical tasks with technical guidance from project staff as necessary. The CHDP can arrange to provide special tools, moulds or other vital equipment either on loan or for hire at nominal cost. The CHDP can encourage local small-scale manufacturing of pre-cast slabs, water seals and other similar materials.

6. **Encourage community members to take part in each of the implementation phases.** This may slow progress, but it will empower individual members through developing new skills and self-confidence. This 'transformation' forms the basis for further progress and growth in future community programmes.

7. **Keep supplies and equipment secured and monitor their use.** Theft can be a demoralising problem. Set up a monitoring system to make sure that materials are accounted for and equipment is returned.

8. **Keep accurate records and accounts for all costs and expenses.** The community should handle the finances from start to finish. One or more community members with experience or training in finance should be selected by the committee to manage the accounts. The NGO can provide additional training. We need to ensure that systems are set up to prevent the misuse of community funds.

⑨ **Make a policy at an early stage on how to deal with people who receive benefits but refuse to contribute**. Some households may give cash or materials in place of labour. However, pressure or sanctions against those who contribute nothing will be easier to apply if they were decided ahead of time.

Phase 4: Maintain and evaluate the changes

Maintenance

It is the people who will directly benefit from any improvement who should be responsible for operating it and looking after it.

The project is not complete when the facility has been built and becomes functional. The CAG (or another designated group) needs to be trained and empowered so that the facility can serve the community for years to come. The CAG will have the following key tasks:

❶ To organise, supervise and monitor how the facility operates, and is maintained and repaired. Even if the municipal government apparently does this, an organised community group needs to keep close watch in order to report and deal with any poor service.

❷ To collect and manage monthly or other agreed fees to cover maintenance costs.

❸ To advise, troubleshoot and arbitrate over problems or disputes, including dealing with residents who fail to contribute their share, or who do not abide by the rules.

Evaluation

It is important for a community and a CHDP to find out if progress is being made towards their goals. The best way to do this is to:

❶ **Set a SMART objective** (see Chapter 4) that when met, is evidence that progress is being made towards the goal.

❷ **Choose an indicator** to measure this. **Process indicators** to measure the amount of effort put in, and **impact indicators** to measure the benefit to the community. Every year monitor progress and every 3 years consider having a wider-ranging evaluation using impact indicators.

It is best when the community decides on the goals and indicators and collects the information needed to monitor progress. That way, the community becomes involved in the whole process. The objectives and indicators will depend on goals set and activities being carried out. Here is an example using a very simple environmental improvement:

A community set the goal that malaria deaths should decrease by 50% over a 2-year period. There are several ways to reduce these deaths, but a key method is the use of insecticide-impregnated bed-nets. Children in the 5th class from the local government school did a house-to-house survey and found out that only 5% of the households had a mosquito net. They presented their findings at a community meeting. The community then made the following objective: within a 2-year period, 80% of households should own and be using a treated mosquito net. To monitor progress towards that objective, the school children would re-survey after a year to see how many households are using treated mosquito nets. To evaluate progress towards reducing malaria deaths, the community is keeping records through the Community Health Volunteers. At the end of 2 years the numbers of malaria deaths will be tallied, and the community will know whether they have reached their target.

> **From the field**: The Curitiba Municipality in Brazil started a programme in which community members go through a process of making a community diagnosis and action plan for environmental problems. Part of this process is a 'community stroll' in which the local people carefully plan a walk through the community to determine the environmental problems. During this walk, a video is made to document the situation at that time. When the stroll is repeated at a later date, it is video taped again in order to compare the first and subsequent strolls and highlight the improvements that have occurred during the intervening period.
>
> **Lessons learned**: When improvements are made we often forget how bad things used to be. A video can remind us by documenting the 'baseline' situation, so that when it comes time for evaluation the community can be helped to appreciate how much progress has occurred.
>
> **Source**: Author visit.

Chapter summary

There are four phases in bringing about environmental improvements in the community. In the first phase, the community prepares for action. It gains information and understanding so that it becomes motivated for change. The Community Action Group (CAG) is set up as part of this process and then leads the process forwards. During the second phase, the community chooses which broad improvements to make and the specific options it wants to follow. Its choice will depend on gathering information from the community, discovering what help is available from government and considering relevant costs. Having chosen which facility to build or improvement to make, the community, helped by the Community Health and Development Programme (CHDP) and working through the CAG, follows a series of logical steps. These include: mobilising skills and funding, providing training, carrying out pilot studies, building a demonstration system and finally implementing the project. The final phase, follow-up, underlines the need for ongoing maintenance by the community, with regular evaluation. In all these activities the CHDP helps by building the capacity of the community to become self-reliant.

Resources

1. *Health and Environment in Sustainable Development*. WHO, 1997. A very comprehensive review of the effects of the environment on health with many mini-case studies.

Improvements in housing

13

In this chapter, we shall consider:

What we need to know:

How does slum housing affect health?

What is needed for a safe and healthy house?

How can housing be improved?

What we need to do:

Phase 1: Prepare the community for action

Phase 2: Help the community choose which problems to solve

Phase 3: Carry out the improvements

Phase 4: Maintain and evaluate the changes

What we need to know

Most of us take for granted that our houses are safe places to live, reasonably secure from theft or attack and supplied with water, sanitation and electricity; and also that our urban housing is legal. The United Nations estimates however that between 30 and 60% of housing units in developing countries are illegal, either because they have no legal right to occupy the land or because they do not comply with housing codes (or often, both). The situation is becoming worse: the majority of **new** urban housing units in developing countries are thought to be illegal or unauthorised units.

How does slum housing affect health?

Slum housing causes poor health for a number of reasons:

1. Housing is located in dangerous places:
   - Slums tend to be located in areas prone to the collection of stagnant water, flooding or landslides.
   - Slums are often near open drains or in areas where there is noise, or pollution from traffic or industry.
   - Dwellings are crowded together with poor access to roads.

2. Dwellings are shabby and poorly constructed:
   - They are usually made from materials such as cardboard, plastic and straw that can easily catch fire.
   - Dwellings do not protect those living in them from the heat, cold, rain, nor from noise or air pollution.
   - Shabby dwellings fail to keep out dust, insects or small animals such as rats or mice.

- Dwellings are small, and, for security reasons, may have a small door and no windows.
- If they have windows, they usually have no protective netting.

③ Dwellings lack civic services:
- They have no running water or toilets.
- Electricity connections, if present, are usually illegal and unsafe.
- The areas that surround the dwellings usually have poor drainage.

④ Dwellings are dangerous inside:
- Slum-dwellers often use open fires for cooking.
- The dwelling has little space for safe storage of food and dangerous materials.
- The dwelling may also be used as a workplace, with tools and supplies left lying about.
- The dwellings have high levels of air pollution because of indoor tobacco smoking and cooking fires, poor ventilation, and high levels of surrounding outdoor air pollution from neighbour's houses, motor vehicles and factories.

⑤ Dwellings lack security:
- Slum-dwellers feel insecure because they do not own the land they live on. They realise that at any time bulldozers could come to demolish their homes. Not only could they lose belongings and shelter, but their jobs could go as well, especially if they had to move to a different location.
- Theft and vandalism is a constant threat, especially if they are unable to make regular payments to the landlord.

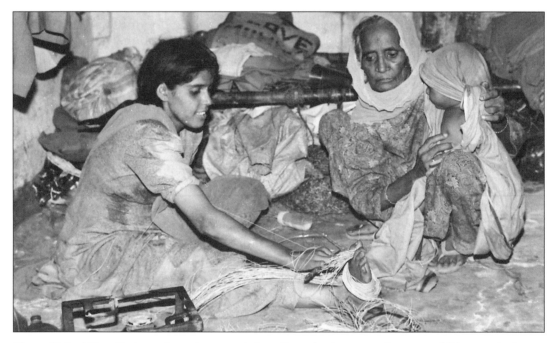

Figure 13.1   When the home is used as a workplace, it can be dangerous for young children, and take up a large amount of living space. (Godfrey Martin/ASHA)

Life in a slum

Sarah lived in a Nairobi slum with her two daughters and two sons. Her house was too small for all to sleep in it, so her two sons slept just outside. But when the boys became teenagers, Sarah didn't like them to be sleeping outdoors because sometimes they would sneak out at night to carouse with older boys without her knowledge. One night they both came home drunk. Because Sarah had a regular job as a cleaner, she was able to get a loan and was able to extend her house another few feet which gave enough space so that her sons could sleep indoors. (Kenya)

What is needed for a safe and healthy house?

A healthy house provides shelter, a regular supply of clean water and adequate sanitation (Table 13.1). It is located in an area with good access for work, schools and health care. A healthy house minimises the chance for injury or illness and contributes to the physical, social and mental health of those who live in it. Slum dwellers usually live in unhealthy houses, making them much more prone to illness, especially to infectious diseases. **But simple improvements can greatly reduce the chance of catching these diseases.**

Table 13.1 What makes a healthy house?	
A healthy house provides:	**Which helps to protect against:**
1. A safe, adequate and accessible supply of water nearby 2. A clean, safe place to store food and water 3. Adequate bathing and washing facilities 4. A sanitary way of removing human and household waste 5. Drainage of surface water 6. Netted windows and doors that can be closed 7. Sufficient space and ventilation	**Infectious diseases** Diarrhoeal diseases, including cholera; typhoid; hepatitis, polio, trachoma, skin infections (1–5) Schistosomiasis, intestinal parasites such as hookworm and roundworm (ascariasis) (1,3,4,5) Plague, typhus, rabies and leptospirosis (4) Malaria, yellow fever, dengue fever, Japanese encephalitis, filariasis (5, 6) Tuberculosis, measles, influenza and other acute respiratory infections (7)
8. A location away from roads, steep hillsides or land prone to flooding 9. A protected place to store dangerous household materials 10. A separate place for work-site, tools and supplies 11. A cooking fire source that is protected	**Injuries and poisonings** Vehicular accidents, drownings, falls (5, 8) Accidents and accidental poisoning and effects of toxic chemicals (9–10) Accidental burning (9–11)
12. Walls and roof that protect from rain, cold and sun, animals and insects	**Exposure** Exposure, heat exhaustion, Chagas' disease, plague (12)

Table 13.1　Continued

A healthy house provides:	Which helps to protect against:
	Air and noise pollution
13. A suitable location away from roads, airports, factories	Deafness (13)
14. A smoke-free cooking source	Chronic respiratory diseases; conjunctivitis; lung cancer (13–14)
	Poor access to supportive services
15. A location that is near schools, health facilities, and jobs	Illiteracy, illness neglect, unemployment (15)
16. Roads for access of emergency vehicles	Fire, illness, neglect (16)
	Mental stress
17. Adequate living space and comfort	Mental illness (17–19)
18. Provision of cultural and recreational facilities	Intimidation; murder, rape and robbery (19)
19. Adequate security	

How can housing be improved?

The community can provide healthier housing in three different ways:

Option A: On-site rebuilding with improved services

This option usually includes:

- rebuilding the existing dwellings;
- setting up an electricity supply and access roads;
- improving the water supply and sanitation, including latrines and drains.

Improving both housing and services is sometimes known as '**upgradation**'.

On-site housing rebuilding is usually only possible when:

1 **The land is government-owned.** Private owners are usually not willing to allow permanent rebuilding or to sell the land at a price that the community can afford. One exception is **land-sharing**. Sometimes the owner (which may be government, corporate or private) has urgent need of some of the land and repeated attempts to evict the slum dwellers have not been successful. Through land-sharing, people agree to swap some of the land to the rightful owner in exchange for legal tenancy or outright ownership of the remaining portion at low cost.

2 **The government or another agency contributes some of the funds needed for major improvements.** Community members contribute financially through long-term loans, or through rent if the housing is built and kept under government control.

The most ideal solution is for members of the community to build their own houses and then become owner-occupiers. There are several reasons:

- Houses built by their owners are likely to be of better quality and cheaper to build than those provided by the government.
- Building is faster if owners are responsible for the construction, especially if temporary housing is uncomfortable or inconvenient.
- The security of owning their own home encourages residents to take better care both of their homes and their surroundings.

From the field: In Cebu City, Philippines, a national programme called the Community Mortgage Programme was started in 1988. It helps poor urban communities to organise themselves and to obtain credit to purchase the land where they live. The programme informs communities about laws and regulations. This helps to empower them to assert their rights regarding land ownership and civic services to which they are entitled. Nearly 10,000 families are now living in more secure housing and with better services through this programme.

Lesson learned: A motivated government can help the urban poor to become owner-occupiers with improved security and services.

Source: Shubert, 1996.

Option B: Resettlement to a different site

When resettlement occurs, the community moves to another site, either because the owner demands the land, or because On-Site Rebuilding is not possible. After resettlement, slum-dwellers are less likely to be evicted because the resettlement usually has government support.

Resettlement makes it possible for community members to own their own homes, providing the government is willing to give the land outright, or lease it long-term to the residents at low rates.

Voluntary resettlement often takes place when there is a serious health problem or one that frequently recurs. For example, the slum may be located on a riverbank that floods every 2–3 years or be next to an open drain that cannot be covered. Or the slum may be so densely populated that on-site improvements are impossible. In this situation we can sometimes help the community to approach government officials and ask to be resettled on a more favourable site.

Forced resettlement, a nightmare for those living in slums, is when the government or legal owners demand the land and forcibly evict them. They may lose not only their home and possessions but their network of friends and neighbours. There may be resistance leading to injury or death. Often when forced evictions are carried out, the people are left to fend for themselves and to find new housing. If they are offered a new location, it is likely to be on the outskirts of the city with poor transport, health care and job opportunities. Often this move happens before any services or even new houses are in place. The people literally have to start living again from scratch.

The reason given for forced resettlement is usually one of the following:

- The government or rightful owner urgently needs the land.
- It is part of improving the image of the city.
- The site is too unhealthy for its residents.

But in practice, demolition usually occurs when political and commercial interests demand that the site should be used for other purposes.

Option C: On-site improvements

When On-Site Rebuilding or Voluntary Resettlement is not possible, the community has only one choice: to try and improve existing conditions. Major improvements like providing safe water or improving sanitation are so expensive that they can usually only be done with the help of major grants from government or larger agencies. The government may be willing to give these if it has no obvious need for the land and is willing to recognise the settlement as semi-permanent. However there are other options that cost less but still help to improve the health and safety of housing.

Improvements to individual houses

Some improvements to the house can be done at low cost and bring significant benefits. Here are some examples:

- covering vessels for storing water in order to discourage hand dipping;
- providing locked storage space for dangerous chemicals and equipment, especially in houses where young children live or visit;
- building a chimney for indoor cooking fires;
- screening windows;
- planting a garden on a windowsill or rooftop;
- building a household latrine;
- adding a household water point.

Some of these improvements cost more than others, such as building a latrine or adding a chimney. Sometimes the government, a supporting NGO or other donor may provide a proportion of the cost of materials, in return for the family providing the labour.

Making simple improvements to existing houses can help 'set a fashion'. This encourages other families to do the same, so eventually leading to a healthier community. This works especially well if a group of families or a community leader start making improvements.

Area improvements

Making improvements that benefit the community as a whole can help to raise the standard of health. Because they are usually expensive to carry out, financial help is needed from the government, development agency or donor. Here are some examples of effective improvements:

- installing drains and roads;
- creating more community water points (if water flow permits) or drilling deep tube wells;
- erecting multi-family or community-wide latrines and bathing complexes;
- building safe recreational areas for children.

For all these activities, the interest and co-operation of the community are essential. The community itself should approach the government or other agency to obtain funds or materials. They should also take responsibility for maintaining the new facility once it is installed. The Community Health and Development Programme can provide encouragement, training and advocacy.

What we need to do

Broad guidelines for each of the four phases in making environmental improvements, follow.

Phase 1: Prepare the community for action

Community Health and Development Programmes must resist the temptation to start making plans without involving the community. To do so runs the risk that the CHDP rather than the community ends up 'owning' the project.

Step 1. Increase the knowledge and awareness of community members

The first step is to help the community understand the issues. Community members will need to learn about:

1. the main health problems in their community;
2. what safe and healthy housing means in practice;
3. options available for making their houses healthier places to live;
4. who actually owns the land and what they plan to do with it in the future;
5. the names of government agencies and officials that deal with housing issues;
6. the government's responsibilities for each of the following:
   - providing water, sanitation, drains, roads and schools,
   - cleaning streets and drains,
   - details of any compensation available if forced resettlement occurs, including relocation expenses.

Step 2. Motivate the community for action

Our aim here is to show clearly the value of improving homes, so that residents will be convinced.

Slum dwellers are often eager to improve their water supply or sanitation – in many cases they will make this quite clear. However they may be much less ready to improve their housing. They do not own their homes and may be under threat of forced eviction. They will not want therefore to waste money on improving their houses, unless they can be sure of the future. The best option is to become owner-occupiers through being offered legal ownership. If this is likely they will be much better motivated to improve the quality of their houses. There are several ways we can help people see the value of improving their homes:

❶ explaining clearly how poor housing contributes to poor health;

❷ helping them to understand their rights as city residents;

❸ by arranging visits to other slums where successful improvements have been made;

❹ helping them to see that by improving their houses they will increase their value – either to sell or to rent out to others;

❺ explaining they will live in nicer surroundings. This will add to their quality of life and to their status.

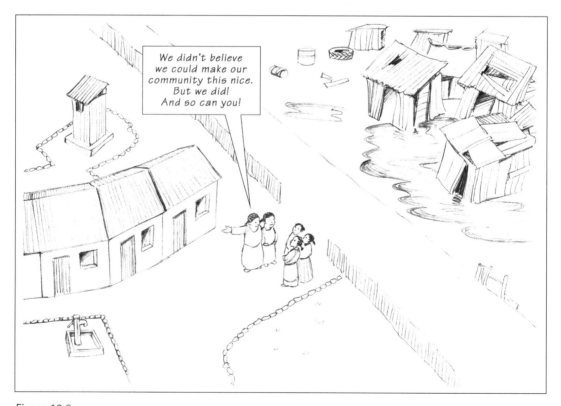

Figure 13.2

Step 3. Channel motivation through organising the community: the Community Action Group

A strong and active Community Action Group is essential for any rebuilding programme. A CAG may be expanded into a Housing Society or Co-operative or these may need to be formed separately. If a Society or Co-operative is set up it will need to be legally registered if at all possible. Whichever group is formed must fully represent women and minorities, along with any officials who have key functions. There should be one or two CHDP members attached to it.

Phase 2: Help the community choose which problems to solve

There are various steps to follow that will help us make the right choices.

Step 1. Gather information about major housing problems

Before deciding what improvements to make or which rehousing option to follow, the community must first gather information. It should aim to understand the problems, strengths, weaknesses, threats and opportunities that exist in the community. We need to gather information on the following:

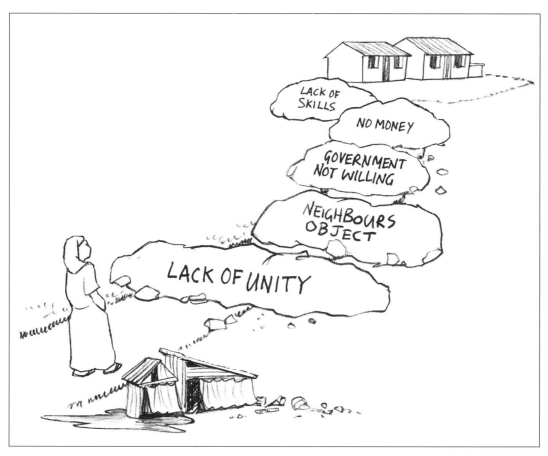

Figure 13.3   The path to On-Site Rebuilding is a long one, with many challenges along the way.

Lay-out and facilities in the community

① During a systematic survey walk of the entire community:
- **Identify areas of different land use**: for example areas that are residential, commercial, or belong to the community (e.g. roads, paths, drains, etc.). List schools, places of worship and other key buildings. Label those that are permanent and will need to be preserved if On-site Rebuilding becomes the preferred choice.
- **Identify water sources**: drains, bodies of water, areas that flood, areas of natural drainage.
- **Identify hazards**: busy streets, factories, open drains, steep areas prone to landslides, etc.
- **Look for common defects in housing**: lack of netting, indoor cooking sources that generate smoke, etc.
- **Estimate the size of existing houses**: We can do this by conducting a rapid survey. Measure the area of 20–40 houses randomly selected from the entire community (see page 47 on how to do this). Measure the area of each house (overall length multiplied by overall width), and calculate the average size. Members of the community should be trained to do this themselves.
- **Measure the size of the entire area** to discover if there is enough space for On-site Rebuilding.
- While on the survey walk, **chat with community leaders and other residents**, especially women. Find out any housing problems that are important to them. See if they have any ideas about changes they would like to make.

② **Make a map of the community**: First see if a map is available from the government. If not we will need to help the community construct a map. The map should be large and accurate enough to record the areas occupied by the main blocks of housing. Important structures and buildings should be marked and labelled.

③ **Other information needed**: To help decide which option to follow, the following information is also needed:
- **The total population of the community**. If On-site Rebuilding is seriously being considered we will need to know the total number of people and households within the colony. This will help us decide whether there is enough room for everyone to be rehoused and whether housing would need to be one, two or multiple storeys high to fit everyone in.
- **Any future plans by the legal owners**.
- **Willingness of the owner (often the government) to provide the land at low cost**, so that community members could become owner-occupiers.
- **Availability of an alternative site** and whether it has good access to employment, schools, health care and civic services.

Relevant health problems in the community

We should have already carried out a community diagnosis, see page 39. We can look at the problems which came to light see how these tie-in with housing design. Table 13.1 (What makes a healthy house?) will help us to do this.

We may also have started community clinics, trained Community Health Volunteers, and set up a woman's Community Action Group. These will all provide detailed information about common health problems and how they relate to poor quality housing, water and sanitation.

Social and cultural factors

We need to find out the opinions of residents on the implications of possible changes. For example what do they think about:

- multi-storey housing that could provide each family with a larger living area;
- households sharing bathrooms and kitchen areas;
- redesign of houses either to include safe work areas, or to transfer work from the home to specially designated areas in the community;
- houses being owned by women (an option which can work well in practice, providing initial objections are overcome).

From the field: In Curitiba, Brazil, a project to rebuild housing included bringing the workplace and living area together under the same roof. Family trades and small scale commerce were established in two storey townhouses. This helped to deal with two crucial problems for the low-income population of the city: housing and employment.

Lesson learned: Providing for employment as well as housing helps the community to dig out of the quagmire of poverty.

Source: Author visit.

Step 2. Discover the government's willingness and capacity to take action

Many housing improvements are so expensive that the community and CHDP cannot afford them without help from outside. In practice the government is usually the main source of this help. Government approval will also be needed for major improvements. On-Site Rebuilding and Voluntary Resettlement are huge projects, which will require major support from different government departments.

An important part of our preparatory work will be making links with government and finding out the type of help they might give. We must remember the constraints and problems, and find the best ways to overcome them (see Chapters 12 and 18).

From the field: In Rio De Janeiro, Brazil, the government and the community transformed their slum in the Favela Barrio Programme. Informal housing on the river bank was subject to frequent flooding. The government and the community decided that the river should be re-channelled and the recovered land used for a football field, community market and flats for re-housing the residents who had previously lived along the riverbanks.

Lesson learned: Governments and communities that genuinely work together can bring impressive changes.

Source: Author visit.

Step 3. Obtain technical advice

In addition to experts from government, universities and the private sector, some specialised NGOs can provide excellent professional support. Often this will be information and consultancy on low-cost housing designs that use appropriate technology and on long-term loans.

Steps 4 and 5. Consider various cost options and the sustainability of each

The community must fully understand the costs of various options, as well as having information on funding or loans that might be available from outside agencies.

If the community is considering on-site rebuilding or resettlement, the issue of who actually owns the new house is important. Linked with this is who is responsible for maintaining them. Usually the only way that on-site rebuilding or resettlement can take place is with the help of the government. Here are some ways in which governments can help with the cost of housing:

❶ **The government may build improved housing and continue to own both the land and the housing**. In effect the slum becomes a government owned housing estate, and residents pay a low monthly rent.

❷ **The government may sell the land to the community** at a reduced price, or it may occasionally give the land to the community or to individual community members.

❸ **The government may arrange a long-term lease of the land to the community** or its members, for low monthly or yearly fees.

Residents are likely to care for their houses better and reduce the damage through vandalism if they own their own properties. The community should make great efforts for this to be possible.

Step 6. Choose the best way forwards

Once the community has collected sufficient information and looked at each option in depth it will be able to decide on the best way forwards. The main role of the CHDP should be to inform and guide the community in coming to an appropriate decision. As we have seen earlier there are three broad options to choose from:

Option A. On-site rebuilding

This is a very major project requiring great skill, time and persistence. If successful the gains are great. On-site rebuilding involves the rebuilding of houses along with an improvement to all local services including water, sanitation, roads and electricity. Experience has shown that this is only likely to be successful if the following conditions can be met:

❶ **The community is united, or has the potential to become united**. People of different religious, ethnic and political groups often live in the same slum community. If these groups fail to get on with each other or cannot find ways of working together it is unlikely that this option will work. Trust between community members is an essential component of On-site Rebuilding.

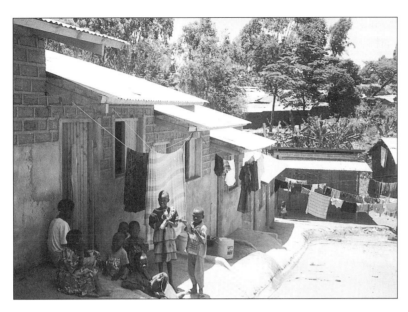

Figure 13.4   Upgraded housing can markedly improve the quality of life of the urban poor. (Kiran Martin)

➋ **The majority of community members are committed to this approach**. By the time construction starts, the entire community must be willing to go for rebuilding. Certain members of the community are likely to oppose this option, especially the following:
  • **People who occupy more land than most**. They may be unwilling to exchange their present larger plot for a smaller one that is the same size as everyone else's. This group includes not only better-off or land-greedy residents, but those who need plenty of workspace such as rubbish recyclers or home-based assembly workers.
  • **People who occupy land in strategic places**. This group includes shopkeepers whose income may fall if they move to a less suitable site.
  • **Slumlords who may currently 'own' more plots than the average person**, and so have more to lose when each family receives only one plot of land. Often such landlords receive payment for providing electricity, water or other favours. On-site rebuilding threatens their income, power and control over others.

➌ **Most families in the community are eligible for rebuilt houses**. The government may be willing to provide housing only to families that have lived in the slum for a certain number of years or whose income is below a certain level. A past date of residency or specific income level is chosen as an arbitrary cut-off point. Residents may need to offer legal proof of length of stay, e.g. a voter registration card. Inevitably some will not be eligible if rigid conditions are set, but it may be possible to negotiate different terms.

➍ **The population density is not too high**. New houses will need to meet certain standards, and are likely to occupy more space than the original ones. Rebuilding may not be possible unless the new houses are multi-storey/multi-family dwellings, or there is additional land nearby.

⑤ The government is willing both **to sell or lease the land**, and to **construct and provide basic civic services**.

⑥ Low-interest loans are available **for building materials**.

Only when all these factors are favourable, should the community consider On-Site Housing Rebuilding.

> **From the field**: In an informal slum settlement of 350,000 inhabitants in Cali, Colombia, community members struggled to improve their housing but met several obstacles: very expensive building materials, lack of knowledge about how to draw up house plans, no access to loans, and difficulty in getting building construction licences. An NGO, the Carvajal Foundation, assisted the community by setting up vendors of building materials in the middle of the community; because they sold direct to residents their prices were cheaper. The Foundation also arranged for students from two schools of architecture to help the people draw up plans. They also encouraged the government to open a small office where people could obtain building licences and persuaded a branch of the government bank to encourage people to save money and take out low-interest loans for constructing their houses.
>
> **Lesson learned**: The value of an NGO facilitator that recognises and addresses the main hold-ups to progress.
>
> **Source**: United Nations Centre for Human Settlements, 1996.

Option B. Voluntary resettlement

With voluntary resettlement, the people decide, after careful consideration, to move to another site. As with On-Site Rebuilding, certain conditions must be met for this option to succeed:

① **The community is united, or has the potential to become united.**

② **Most community members favour resettlement.**

③ **A suitable resettlement site is available.**

④ **The government co-operates**, especially by paying for resettlement costs.

⑤ **The option must not be too costly.** If the government is willing to sell plots at the new site, the price must be low. If the land is to be rented on long-term lease, the terms must be favourable and the lease must be affordable. In all cases, low-interest loans must be available to buy/lease the land and to purchase building supplies.

Option C: On-site improvements

When houses cannot be rebuilt, valuable small scale-changes can still be made. In practice this is the commonest option to choose, especially in the early stages of a project.

From the field: A housing co-operative society was formed in Nairobi, Kenya in a resettlement colony. The members were former squatters who now had plots in the resettlement colony. They were poor with few skills and little education. But there was a strong sense of solidarity. Local politicians, realising the number of votes that the group represented, came to their aid by ensuring that the society qualified for a government loan programme. The loan eventually came through after 2 years of persistence by members of the housing society.

Lesson learned: Clearly defined and attainable goals with strong community motivation can enable a group of slum residents to obtain the outside support that fulfils their hopes.

Source: Author visit.

Minor improvements such as putting netting on windows, covering water containers or making a smokeless indoor cooker can be done at little expense. These individual house improvements can be an excellent starting place when funds are limited, community participation is not widespread or when there is little government support.

AN OPPORTUNITY FOR PARTICIPATORY LEARNING
Story with a Gap

Purpose: To train community members to solve a problem.

Materials needed: Three or four identical sets of 'before' and 'after' pictures. The 'before' picture shows a problem situation, such as a slum scene with houses made of plastic, plywood and tin, with a small child defecating on the path, and household waste being dumped outside the dwelling. The 'after' picture shows a clean house with brick paths and a covered drain. A staff (or community) member with drawing skills can help to draw these before the session.

How to play:

Divide the participants into small groups of three to four people each.

Give each group a set of the pictures. Ask each group to look at the 'before' picture and discuss what the problems are and why they are caused. For example they may say that the little girl is defecating because there is no latrine, or the latrine is too far away for her to go alone, or that she is afraid that she might fall in.

Next ask each group to discuss the 'after' picture. Ask them what steps they think the community might have taken to change conditions in the slum, what obstacles they may have met and what resources they needed.

It is more difficult to make **major improvements** such as building household latrines or obtaining licensed low-cost electricity connections. These involve community support and agreement, not just the decision of a single household. For these more major changes to work in practice, two conditions must be in place:

❶ A degree of community organisation to approach the government or outside funding agencies for financial support and technical assistance.

❷ A government that is willing to provide permissions, and where possible, funds and technical help.

Phase 3: Carry out the improvements

The community may not follow the steps described in strict order but each one must be included. It goes without saying that this phase of the programme needs skilful management, and that everyone involved must understand what their own jobs entail and how they fit into the overall programme. Leaders who are good at communicating and at sorting out disputes are essential!

Step 1. Mobilise skills

Wherever possible, skilled and unskilled workers from the community should carry out most tasks. This has three advantages:

❶ It reduces project costs.

❷ It gives community members a deep sense of involvement.

❸ It is an opportunity to empower community members through training in new skills, which may improve their job prospects in the future.

In addition to construction skills, some community members should be trained in leadership, accounting and management.

Women and Housing

Women, and woman-headed households are often sidelined in housing improvement schemes. When planning a housing programme, we should ensure that:

- Women are allowed to participate, including heads of household. In many schemes only male heads of household are are permitted to participate in the programme.

- Ways are made for women to fully participate, use their skills and receive training. This means being flexible so that their responsibilities in the home and caring for children are fully taken into account.

- Women are trained in construction skills that will help them find better employment.

- Childcare facilities such as crèches are provided so women can attend meetings and take part in training and construction.

- Unskilled people working in the informal sector, e.g. day labourers, are fully involved. In some schemes, loans have only been given to those working in the formal sector with more permanent jobs.

Step 2. Approach government officials

Government input is essential for any major improvements but it can be complicated and time-consuming. Rehousing schemes often involve several different government departments. For example, one department may own the land and must transfer it over to another which is responsible for resettlement colonies, which in turn must deal with the department that handles water and sanitation and another department that handles roads. Sometimes these departments will be unaware of others they should be working with, or worse, there may be disputes and jealousies between them. This can make it very difficult for communities and CHDPs to obtain licences, funds or even basic co-operation. The secret often lies in taking time to make high-level contacts through establishing credibility and refusing to take no as an answer.

In the meantime we need to be open and frank with the community so that we do not raise unrealistic expectations. Comunity members must understand the difficulties, have patience, and become motivated to exert influence through their own well-organised pressure groups.

If forced resettlement seems possible, urgent action must be taken. The government may hope it can act before the community has time to organise a response. But community action may still prevent forced eviction. Residents need to know their legal rights, draw up an action plan and make a united response. This may not prevent demolition, but it may buy time so that a more orderly move can be undertaken later, bearing in mind the needs of the people.

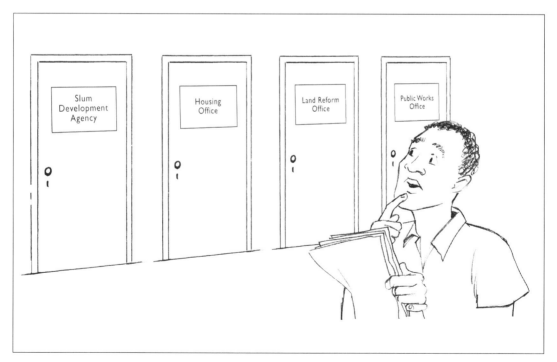

Figure 13.5   On-Site Rebuilding: the process of getting through the bureaucratic maze needs great persistence.

In the case of small on-site improvements, dealing with the government is simpler because fewer departments will be involved. It is still worth approaching the government for help, especially if the government is legally required to supply the services that the community is seeking.

Step 3. Mobilise funding

In the case of On-site Rebuilding or Voluntary Resettlement huge sums of money will be needed. We have already looked at ways to mobilise funding, page 208.

Banks and other lenders consider slum residents high-risk clients – there is no guarantee at all that they will repay loans. NGOs may be prepared to set up loan schemes if they can find ways of encouraging residents to pay these back. Sometimes banks will give loans, especially if the government agrees to act as guarantor, or gives grants and tax benefits to protect the bank against defaulters. In this situation the bank may actually do better by taking the benefit rather than by chasing defaulters.

As far as the community is concerned this has the effect of turning a loan into a free gift. This may seem a good idea but is usually perceived as a handout. This is not in the real interests of the community, which comes to expect free gifts rather than to depend upon its own resources. In contrast, NGOs that extend such loans usually consider repayment as an important way to discourage dependency. They will insist on a regular repayment schedule and be robust in their follow-up of defaulters. This may seem tough but in the end creates self-reliance.

Step 4. Approach people living in surrounding neighbourhoods

(This is necessary for On-Site Rebuilding.)

Make contacts with neighbouring communities as early as possible. This will help to minimise rumours based on fear and wrong perceptions. Richer neighbours may lead opposition to any improvements by lobbying officials and politicians. Imagine how neighbours may feel (however unjust this may seem to us). They have tolerated the slum as an eyesore for years, hoping that one day it would disappear. They have put up with the fear of theft and vandalism: they have dreaded the spread of a drug culture, prostitution and AIDS into their area, hoping things would change for the better. Now this very settlement is going to be made permanent! In addition, the value of their property will probably fall.

We should therefore meet with neighbours as early as possible to explain the proposed action and point out the advantages for them: the eyesore will disappear, the smell will lessen, and the cheap source of local labour (probably healthier and more

Seek out members of nearby communities who are sympathetic to the needs of the urban poor: encourage them in advocacy and support for the cause.

productive) will remain available. With owner occupation, the rebuilt colony will probably improve in standard and appearance, so increasing property values in neighbouring communities.

Step 5. Investigate the proposed site
(This step only applies to Resettlement.)

If resettlement seems a likely option, encourage the community to be fully involved in the choice of any new site. Community members should learn about their legal rights, and this in turn will empower them to negotiate robustly with the government. Some NGOs specialise in legal issues and advocacy; we can link them up with the Community Action Group.

The community should press for a site where water, sanitation and electricity will be available, and where schools, health care and employment will be near at hand.

Step 6. Design the layout
(This step applies to On-Site Rebuilding and Resettlement.)

Area design
The Community Action Group or Housing Committee will be the centre of activities. They will be representing the wishes of the community and co-ordinating the work of architects and engineers who will be giving advice on the design of new housing and the layout of the new community, bearing in mind the limitations of cost and space. The Housing Committee will need to monitor and guide decisions on the following:

- The location of roads, paths, toilet/bathing facilities and drains.
- The preservation of certain community structures, e.g. shade-providing trees, and possibly existing sites for worship.
- The layout of the houses: whether houses should be in clusters or in lines; single houses or multi-storey/multi-family buildings, etc.
- How water supply and electricity will be provided.
- How communal work areas and play spaces for children can be built into the plans: many people living in slums work in their homes, e.g. in assembly work. The needs of children for safe play areas will be important in the permanent new colony that is taking shape.

Individual housing
The future occupants will need to agree with basic designs that are suggested, and have an opportunity to make their own suggestions and express their preferences. For example:

- What is the best design of the individual dwelling?
- If individually owned, how much freedom should individuals have in planning and building their house, or in being able to modify a standard design?

- Will there be space for an individual bathroom/toilet in each dwelling? If not, which is better, a cluster arrangement (one unit per so many families) or a shared community bathing/toilet complex?

Step 7. Train people in skills and tasks

There will be two main areas where training will be essential:

① In **constructing homes and other facilities** in the new colony.

Community members will usually build their own homes, or if this is not possible pay a small fee to those with the skills to help them. We should identify skilled construction workers in the community and teach them how to train others in the basic skills of house building.

② In **management and co-ordination**

The CAG or Housing Committee will play the lead role and members will need to be trained in a variety of skills: how to run meetings, do simple accounting, keep minutes, write letters, talk to government agencies and motivate the community. The CHDP can arrange this training and give support and encouragement throughout the process.

Step 8. Carry out pilot studies and build demonstration system(s)

Any design that has been suggested needs building, testing out and demonstrating to make sure the community will be happy with the finished product. Demonstration units will need to be carefully built. It may be useful to have two different designs and invite comments on each. They can include new features such as smokeless cookers and rooftop gardens. Choosing a marginalised family, such as a widow with small children to receive one of the pilot units, can reinforce the message that the poorest families should receive priority.

Many slum dwellers will need a great deal of encouragement to invest in their homes. By building demonstration units and using other promotional activities we can speed up this process. Sometimes a group of people will hold out and delay the whole scheme. To prevent the majority from losing their enthusiasm, those holding out need to be persuaded, often by gentle group pressure, to change their minds as quickly as possible.

The remainder of the steps, 9–11 applies only to On-Site Rebuilding and Resettlement Schemes.

Step 9. Allot the housing sites

When people see that new housing is going to be built and they may become owner-occupiers, word will quickly spread and friends and relatives may start moving in with the hopes of being included.

Our first job therefore is to make sure which families genuinely qualify. The government will probably have rules that we can follow based on how long people have lived in the community. Take great care to include only people who truly qualify, separating out those with false papers, or several people from one family claiming to be residents in order to obtain more land for the family.

> **From the field**: After a fire had destroyed one-third of the homes of 350 families in a slum community in Nairobi, a local NGO, the Undugu Society, helped the families to build new shelters. However, outsiders took advantage of the confusion and built their own houses on the same site. At the end, the number of families living in the area had tripled, which caused severe over-crowding as well as a loss of a sense of community.
>
> **Lesson learned**: As soon as possible after the decision for On-Site Rebuilding or Resettlement is made, determine who qualifies so that false claims are minimised.
>
> **Source**: Harpham *et al.*, 1988.

The fairest way to allot specific housing sites is by lottery. If the housing is by cluster, those families who have elected to live together will occupy a cluster of houses as a unit. In that case, the lottery will be by cluster, and not by individual households.

> **From the field**: In an On-Site Rebuilding project called Ekta Vihar ('Unity Colony'), facilitated by ASHA, an NGO in New Delhi, India, the women in the community became the legal owners of the houses. Initially there was great opposition but with patient explanation and persistence, the entire community eventually owned this approach.
>
> **Lesson learned**: With persistence, women can be empowered despite initial resistance. Female ownership of building plots increases both the status of women and the stability of the family and the colony. Women are less likely to sell the house. A woman owner and her young children will also have greater security if she is abandoned by, or outlives her husband.
>
> **Source**: Authors.

Step 10. Vacate the current housing

> The levelling of the slum, even when residents know that better homes will soon be built, is a difficult time for everyone, both physically and emotionally. It needs to be very carefully planned ahead of time to minimise stress.

Temporary housing will be needed after demolition and before permanent houses are built. The ideal solution is to use nearby unoccupied land, but this is rarely available. One option is to rebuild in two stages. In the first stage, half of the slum is rebuilt with the people living in crowded temporary housing (tents) in the other half. Then, when the first half is finished, the whole community lives temporarily in the finished portion while the second half is rebuilt. During this rebuilding phase, the CAG will have to handle a wide range of complaints, frustrations and bureaucratic snags. They will need support and technical help to do this fairly and effectively.

Epidemic illnesses are more likely to occur at this stage because of overcrowding and the lack of amenities. Health workers must monitor the situation closely, and clinic opening times may need to be extended. All these problems will be minimised by rebuilding at the most favourable time of the year, when the weather is dry, and not too hot or too cold.

When On-Site Rebuilding is planned, bricks and other materials that can be used in the building of the new homes should be salvaged from the debris of the original structures.

With Voluntary Resettlement, it is ideal if the community can stay in the original housing until roads and civic services are in place, and the plinths have been laid.

Step 11. Begin construction

By this stage basic designs have been approved, the lay-out planned and skilled workers have been identified and trained.

A compromise may now have to me made. The government may have regulations about the quality of new housing that may be too expensive or complicated to follow. Community members may want to use the cheapest materials they can and cut costs in the way they construct their homes. A balance must be struck between what regulations demand and what the people can afford. This may mean negotiating a compromise with the government, and encouraging residents to use the very best materials and methods of construction that they possibly can. The Housing Committee will be central in these discussions. It should also monitor the construction of houses to make sure that any standards agreed to are clearly being followed.

During this implementation phase, it is helpful to make a specific plan that breaks down the process into specific tasks (as objectives), defining Who? What? Where? When? and How? as described in Chapter 12.

Phase 4: How to maintain and evaluate the changes

Once the houses are built and people move in, or more simple improvements have been made, there will still be tasks to carry out. A permanent Housing Committee will be needed to manage this process into the future.

Maintenance

The major tasks will include:

1. **organising the cleaning, maintenance and repair of community facilities** such as the latrine complex, drains, roads, and water sources;
2. **collecting fees**, monthly or otherwise, to cover community expenses;
3. **managing community accounts**;

④ **advising and arbitrating** over problems or disputes relating to housing;
⑤ **monitoring the selling and renting** of property.

In Rebuilding projects, house-owners often chose to live off-site and rent out their new homes to others for extra income. This defeats the whole object of the rebuilding scheme. Clear rules to outlaw this practice need to be agreed by the community before the rebuilding starts. The housing committee must be empowered to take action against residents who break this code of practice.

Evaluation

Whether we have been involved in minor improvements to individual housing or a major resettlement scheme, it is still useful to have indicators to make sure we have reached our objectives and that progress is being maintained. The Housing Committee should be guided in choosing simple indicators to do this. Here are two simple examples:

① **Activity**: To promote the use of smokeless cooking stoves. **Process Indicator**: number of demonstration stoves installed and used. **Impact Indicator**: perceived

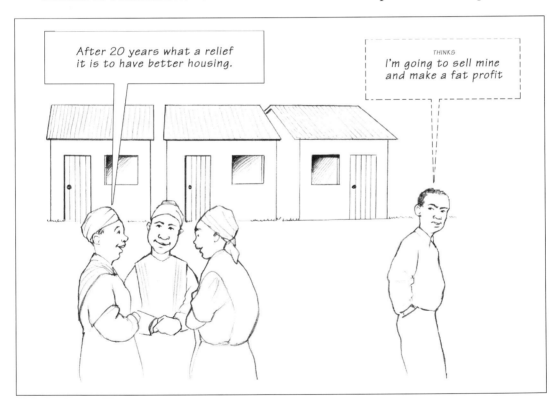

Figure 13.6   The land on which On-Site Rebuilding occurs is often of high commercial value. Thus property dealers may entice or even force the residents to sell their propertly. The community, through the CAG, should monitor this possibility and set up methods for control and protection.

or measured frequency of respiratory infections, and conjunctivitis before and after installation, or between houses with or without new stoves.

2. **Activity**: Promote women for active leadership in On-site Rebuilding. **Process Indicator**: the number of community women who were trained in leadership and administrative skills. **Impact Indicator**: the proportion of women in the Housing Society, and proportion of new housing units registered in women's names.

(For more information on indicators, see Chapter 4 on Making an action plan.)

Chapter summary

Common problems with slum housing that affect health include: hazardous location, shabby dwellings, lack of civic services, overcrowding, and lack of security. Slum communities have three options to make their housing healthier:

- **Option A: On-Site Housing Rebuilding**, the best option, in which the houses themselves are rebuilt and at the same time, civic amenities are improved;

- **Option B: Voluntary Resettlement** in which the people move to another location; and

- **Option C: On-site Improvements** in which basic housing cannot be improved so less major changes are made.

Once a community decides on which of the above approaches to take, it must prepare for action through increasing awareness, motivation of community members and the organisation of a CAG. The next phase is to plan and implement the approach through a series of steps including assessing resources, approaching government officials, neighbours and lending agencies, looking at the site and designing the layout of the colony and the individual houses, building demonstration units, allotting the housing sites, vacating the current housing, and construction. The final stage is to monitor, evaluate and maintain the change.

Resources

1. *An Urbanizing World: Global Report on Human Settlements 1996.* United Nations Centre for Human Settlements/Oxford University Press, 1996. A very extensive review of housing, including urban with case studies.

2. *The Community Health Worker: Working Guidelines for training, Guidelines for adaptation.* WHO, 1990. Unit 3: Housing, pp 29–35. A good review of what a healthy house is.

3. *Cities, Poverty and Development: Urbanisation in the Third World.* A Gilbert J Gugler, Oxford University Press, 1992. Chapter 5: The housing of the urban poor, pp 114–154. A good discussion of various options to house the urban poor.

4. *In the Shadow of the City: Community Health and the Urban Poor.* T Harpham. Oxford University Press, 1988. Chapter 10: Housing, pp 134–148. An overview of housing for the urban poor, with some case studies.

14 Improvements to the water supply

> *In this chapter, we shall consider*:
>
> **What we need to know**:
>
> What makes a good water supply?
>
> What are the usual water sources in slums?
>
> How is water supply related to illness?
>
> **What we need to do**:
>
> Phase 1: Prepare the community for action
>
> Phase 2: Help the community choose which problems to solve
>
> Phase 3: Carry out the improvements
>
> Phase 4: Maintain and evaluate the changes

What we need to know

The World Health Organization estimates that nearly one quarter of the world's population has no access to safe water and adequate sanitation. At any one time half of all those in developing countries are suffering from one of the main illnesses connected with poor access to water, and 5 million people die each year as a direct result. Every 8 seconds a child dies from a water-related disease.

These figures make improving the slum's water supply and sanitation a top priority for all health and development programmes.

What makes a good water supply?

A good water supply is **adequate** in amount. There needs to be enough water both to drink and to wash. When supplies are low, personal hygiene is first thing to suffer. Many cities have already outgrown their water supplies.[1]

A good water supply is **accessible**. It should within easy reach of homes (less than 100 metres from each household). It should also be affordable in terms of the cost, time and energy to collect it.

A good water supply is **reliable**. It should be present throughout the day and throughout the year, including during the hottest, dryest seasons.

A good water supply is **safe**. The water should not contain any organisms that cause disease (parasites, bacteria or viruses), nor any harmful chemicals.

[1] To avoid confusion the term bathe when used in this book refers to body-washing, i.e. personal hygiene: the term washing generally refers to clothes and utensils.

What are the usual water sources in slums?

Only rarely do slums have an **adequate, accessible, reliable** and **safe** supply of water. The government or other owners have no interest in improving an area that is illegally occupied by slum dwellers. As a result, poorer occupants are often forced to pay for water brought in by water vendors or obtained from richer neighbours with access to taps or hand pumps. In fact, slum dwellers may pay up to 100 times more for these unsafe, unreliable supplies than their richer neighbours pay for a municipal piped water supply.

From the field: In a certain Nairobi slum, the lack of any other source of water forces residents to purchase water from a vendor, paying ten times the rate of wealthier neighbourhoods with private connections. A prominent politician owns the water concession. He has no interest in providing the community with a better water supply.

Source: Author visit.

Slum communities often use more than one type of water supply. Individual households may use tanker water for drinking, water from hand pumps for washing dishes and river water for bathing and washing clothes. When working with the community, it is important to know which water sources are used for which activites.

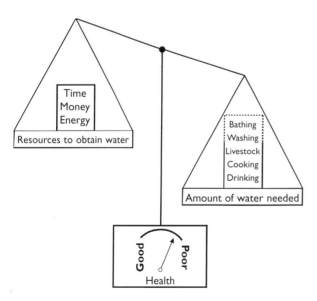

The amount of water that a household uses is a balance between two things. The **need of the household** in terms of drinking, cooking, bathing, washing and caring for gardens and livestock and the **cost to the household** in terms of money, time and energy spent in obtaining the water. As the balance tilts unfavourably compromises are made, putting health at risk.

Slum communities get their water from one of more of the following sources:

Figure 14.1   Water supply and health: a delicate balance.

Municipal water supply

Through a piped water supply

Is it adequate? Sometimes hundreds of slum dwellers depend upon a single water tap. Long queues form, made even longer by the slow flow of water. The supply often dries up or is turned off before everyone has been served. Increased demand during the hot season often means less water for slums, to safeguard supplies for richer neighbourhoods.

Is it accessible? When there are not enough taps, slum dwellers have to walk long distances and spend many hours queuing.

To preserve water, municipal supplies are often switched on for just a few hours a day. This is not a problem for wealthy people with storage tanks, but few people in slums will own these. In practice residents must arrange daily routines so that one member of a household is free to wait in line for the time when the supply is switched on. Otherwise the household gets no water.

Is it reliable? The municipal supply may not flow regularly for a number of reasons:

- power failures,
- breakdowns,
- poor maintenance,
- water theft up the line,
- vandalism or theft of taps,
- illegal connections that decrease water pressure,
- leakages for a variety of reasons, sometimes wasting huge amounts for prolonged periods.

Is it safe? Municipal water supplies are usually treated at the source to kill most disease-causing organisms. But in situations of extreme poverty or civil unrest this may not happen. Water pipes usually run underground, often alongside sewer pipes or near the surface. Broken or leaking water pipes allow sewage or surface water to enter the pipes sometimes through a suction effect. An outbreak of cholera in Kathmandu was traced back to this cause.

Through tanker trucks

Is it adequate? Delivering water by tanker is very expensive. Often slum dwellers will use this supply for drinking only, and continue to gather water from less clean sources for bathing and washing.

Is it accessible? The delivery point for tanker water is usually restricted to a paved road alongside one edge of the slum: most roads into slums are too narrow for trucks to enter. Those living at a distance from the access point may have a long walk, tanker times may be variable or they may not arrive at all, wasting valuable time for household water collectors.

Is it reliable? The process of regular delivery to large groups of people is quite complex. Often breakdowns, the unreliability of tanker drivers, strikes and inefficiency, mean that supplies cannot be depended on.

Is it safe? Although the city government intends this water to be treated and the tank to be kept clean, this will often not happen. The infrastructure needed – personnel, equipment and supplies – is just not there. In practice water may be drawn from a river or from some other unclean source. Germs from an unclean source can contaminate the next tanker full of water, even if this is collected from a safer municipal supply.

Surface water (ponds, rivers, ditches, etc.)

Is it adequate, accessible and reliable? The main advantage of surface water is that it is often nearby and easily available. There are no queues nor time wasted in collecting it. However during the dry season supplies may dry up.

Is it safe? Surface water in slums mostly originates from rainwater and water from household waste. This becomes quickly and severely contaminated, especially when open defecation is widespread. High concentrations of people who use this water for bathing, washing clothes and dishes, will often be forced to use the same supply for drinking, because an alternative source is not available, or is too expensive. Often the edges of ponds and ditches are also used for defecation.

Water vendors

In some slums, supplies can be bought from water vendors. Water purchased from these vendors is usually very expensive. Sometimes neighbours who have a water tap or hand pump are willing to provide water. They may be willing to do this free, but will often see it as a source of income for their family and charge high rates.

Is it adequate? If purchased water is the only source available, its high cost may prevent households from getting enough water for all of their needs.

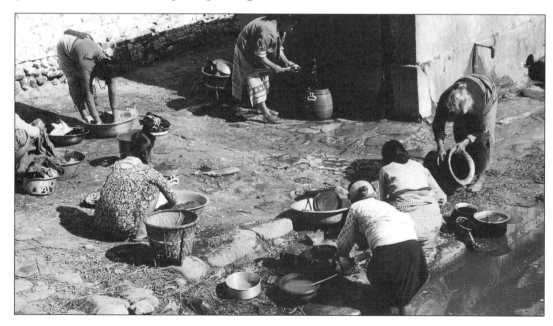

Figure 14.2   Even though surface water is often contaminated, sometimes there are no other practical options. (Beverley Booth)

Is it accessible? People usually buy water from a vendor because it is convenient, especially if the water is delivered to the home. In woman-headed households for example, there may be no one available to fetch water at the time the municipal taps are flowing. In some areas, unaccompanied women are not able to collect water outside the home for cultural reasons, and so must depend on vendors delivering water to their house.

Is it reliable? Since vendors are being paid for the water, this service is often quite reliable.

Is it safe? Water purchased from vendors is often contaminated, either through its source, or because of storage in transport tanks or containers that are not properly cleaned.

Groundwater

Sometimes the community, authorities or other agencies sink a well to access water that is below the surface (groundwater). There are several layers of groundwater, separated by layers of soil or rock. These layers are usually impermeable, i.e. they don't allow water from one layer to mix with water from another layer (see Figure 14.3). The top level of the first layer of groundwater is known as the water-table. The level of the water-table changes, becoming higher during the rainy season. In many cities of the world the water-table is falling, meaning that less groundwater is available and wells have to be sunk ever more deeply.

Through a shallow well

A shallow well is a well that uses the top groundwater layer as its source. Shallow wells can be dug by manual labour. In urban areas, most shallow wells are covered and the water is obtained using a handpump.

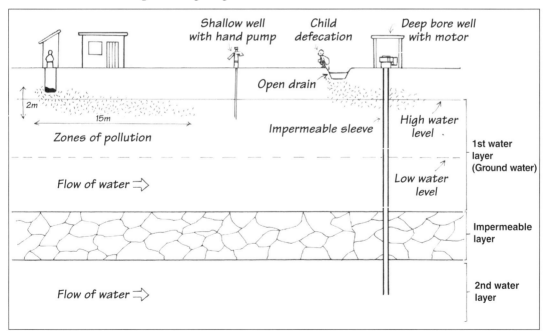

Figure 14.3   The water-table and ground water levels in relation to wells and latrines.

Is it adequate? Shallow wells alone may provide enough water for small communities. Larger slums usually need additional sources.

Is it accessible? The water source is within the community itself, meaning residents are not dependent on outside sources. If a municipal supply is not reliable, shallow wells with handpumps are a good way to make water more accessible.

Is it reliable? Shallow wells may fail during the dry season or after a few years, especially in areas where the water-table is falling. A serious problem is the breakdown of handpumps.

Is it safe? The water from shallow wells can be contaminated with disease-causing organisms in two ways.

1. **Surface water** can seep through the soil into the underground water supply (see Figure 14.3). Organisms can seep through 2 metres of soil. Therefore if the lowest part of the body of surface water is less than 2 metres above the groundwater source, contamination can occur.

2. **Fluid from pit latrines, aqua privies or septic tanks** can seep through the soil into the underground water supply if the bottom of the latrine pit is less than 2 metres above the groundwater source.

In slum communities, shallow wells are often contaminated because:

- **Open defecation contaminates the surface water**, which in turn contaminates the groundwater. This surface water can travel far, meaning that open defecation a considerable distance from the shallow well is still able to cause contamination.

- **High population density** makes it very hard to find a site for a shallow well that will not be contaminated by either surface water, a pit latrine, or leaking sewer pipes. If all potential sources of contamination are more than 15 metres from the handpump, the water from that pump is likely to be safe since groundwater usually becomes free of contamination after it has travelled 15 metres or more from the source of contamination (see Figure 14.3).

- **Slum communities are often located in low-lying areas**. The high water-table allows the groundwater to become easily contaminated from surface water or unclean soil.

Through a deep well

A deep well is a well that taps into a supply of groundwater below the top level (see Figure 14.3). Deep wells are made by boring, usually by machine, occasionally by hand. In slum communities with deep wells, an electric pump is usually needed to draw up the water, although handpumps can sometimes be used.

Is it adequate? Since deep wells come from a lower water layer, they have more reliable supplies than shallow wells, unless there is a very severe spell of dry weather.

Is it accessible? The same applies as for shallow wells.

Is it reliable? If an electric pump is used to draw water, there will be no supply whenever there is a power cut or low voltage, both very common in slums. In addition electric motors often break down or burn out. This problem can be helped by building a large water tank into which supplies can be pumped when the electricity supply is working.

Is it safe? The water provided by deep wells is safe because disease-causing organisms from contaminated surface water or soil cannot reach it. Care must be taken however, to make sure that water does not become contaminated on its way to the user. For example, water may be connected to a piped system that provides water through taps at several locations. Pipes and connections must be kept in good repair.

How is water supply related to illness?

The water supply cause illness in several different ways:

The water supply is inadequate

This can occur because supplies are unreliable, inaccessible or insufficient. Drought, falling water-tables, up-stream diversions of major rivers along with rapidly growing population are usual causes, though the real reason is too many people living in one area without sufficient resources, their own or the government's, to compete for a fair share of the region's water supply.

When the amounts of water are insufficient, people tend to wash hands and bathe less frequently. Regular hand washing and regular bathing prevent the spread of many diseases. Therefore people who wash hands and bathe less frequently are more likely to get certain diseases that are spread in the following ways:

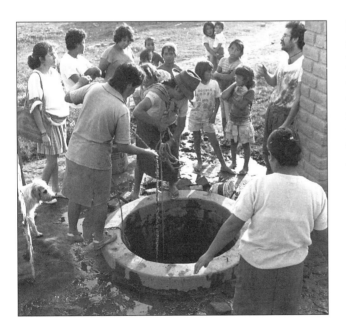

Hands spread disease-causing organisms to the mouth

Hands contaminated by faeces are used to eat or prepare food or are placed directly in the mouth. Children are at special risk from this means of spread. They may come into contact with human faeces when playing outside, especially if open defecation is common practice. Children tend to put their fingers into their own (and other children's) mouths.

Figure 14.4   When water is scarce, bathing is a luxury.
(Ph. Merchez/WHO)

Common diseases spread in this way are: **diarrhoea and dysentery, typhoid fever, hepatitis, roundworm (*Ascaris*) and pinworm**. The prevention of these diseases is to wash hands after defecation and cleaning children, and before eating or preparing food.

Hands spread disease-causing organisms to the skin or to the eyes

Certain diseases can be spread through skin-to-skin contact, scabies, ringworm (tinea) bacterial skin infections and, in very crowded conditions, louse-borne infections. Rubbing eyes with dirty hands spreads trachoma, especially if the face is also dirty. The prevention of these diseases is regular bathing of the whole body, including regular hand washing.

Disease-causing organisms are in water taken in by mouth

Parasites, bacteria or viruses are spread from infectious human urine and faeces that contaminate the water in the ways described above.

People ingest contaminated water in two main ways:

1. **Through drinking water**. Many diarrhoeal diseases, including cholera, as well as typhoid fever and hepatitis (A and E) are commonly caused this way. However, these diseases can also be transmitted in other ways (such as by food or hands) so the presence of these illnesses does not always mean that the water supply is at fault.

2. **Through eating food contaminated by unclean water**. The organisms mentioned above can also be spread this way. Cysts causing amoebic dysentery and giardiasis are commonly spread through eating contaminated fruit and vegetables, especially when washed or kept moist by street vendors, using unclean water. The liver fluke – *Fasciola*, spread by eating contaminated water vegetables, especially watercress, is common in certain cities in South-east Asia.

Disease-causing organisms are in water used for bathing and washing

The main illness caused this way is schistosomiasis (bilharzia). Though often thought of as a rural disease, this is spreading into cities in many parts of Africa and some cities in South-east Asia. This blood fluke enters through the skin via a stage of its life-cycle, when it is known as a 'cercaria'. The adult worms develop and then live in the veins lining the bladder or large intestine, producing cysts which are then passed back into the water supply through urinating and defecating. People bathing or washing in ponds or rivers are therefore at risk.

Insects that breed in standing water spread diseases

These diseases are caused by insects which breed in standing or stagnant water. Some require only tiny amounts of water to breed in, for example the *Aedes* mosquito, which carries dengue fever. **Common urban diseases spread in this way include dengue fever (rapidly increasing in many cities), and malaria. Some forms of filariasis, and urban yellow fever are other examples. The prevention of these diseases involves trying to remove areas of standing water and taking precautions to avoid being bitten.**

There are two ways of reducing water-related diseases. The first is to improve water and sanitation. The second is to bring about changes in personal hygiene, especially hand washing. While planning for the first we must work on the second: behavioural changes alone can greatly reduce the amount of water-related illness.

Poisonous chemicals are in the water supply

Industries often dump chemical waste into rivers This waste may find its way into surface or groundwater supplies. Slums are especially at risk because they are often located near industrial areas. In some cities in Central Asia and Eastern Europe there is poisoning through heavy metals, and in some cities in the Russian Federation through radioactive waste. Sometimes naturally occurring poisonous substances can contaminate water supplies especially when there are changes in land use. A serious case in point is contamination by arsenic of wells in Bangladesh.

What we need to do

Chapter 12 explains the broad principles for each of the phases that follows. In this chapter we will look at areas of special relevance to improving water supplies.

Phase 1: Prepare the community for action

Step 1. Increase the knowledge and awareness of community members

The community will need to know and understand about the following:

1. What makes an adequate, accessible, reliable and safe water supply.
2. How an inadequate and/or unsafe water supply is related to illness.
3. What water sources are available in the community; which sources are used for which purpose; differences in access between different sectors of the population.
4. How surface water and groundwater can become contaminated with human excreta.
5. The names of government agencies and officials that deal with water supply issues.
6. What legal responsibilities the government has in providing citizens with civic services, including:
   - water supplies,
   - sanitary removal of excreta,
   - mosquito control measures,
   - garbage collection,
   - drainage systems,
   - regular cleaning of streets and drains.

Step 2. Motivate the community

All slum communities want a better water supply. Residents want more water of a better quality closer to their homes. But it may still be difficult to motivate the community. This is often because of the lack of hope that anything useful can be done to tackle such a huge problem.

Community members usually don't realise how many diseases are related to water. By raising their awareness two things can change. First, they will become more motivated to improve their water supply. Second, they will be willing to take more care with personal hygiene so as to reduce the amount of illness in their families.

> An improvement in the water supply will only be effective if individuals and families change their behaviours. For example, if children still don't wash their hands before eating, providing more water is not going to help much in preventing diarrhoea.

Step 3. Channel motivation through organising the community: the Community Action Group

Because most water sources are shared, any improvements to the water supply should involve the whole community. Women are usually the most motivated community members when it comes to improving the water supply: after all it is usually they, or their children who suffer most if the supply is poor. They fetch the water, cook, do the washing and need more privacy when bathing. When the water supply improves, their daily workload decreases. Women therefore must play a key role in planning and implementing change. They will need to be strongly represented on the Community Action Group or similar organisation empowered by the community to organise improvements.

The CAG will guide the community through the water improvement process. **The issue of water supply can be very controversial**. This is most clearly seen when deciding where water points will be located.

> Throughout the world, women and minority groups often suffer most from a poor water supply. They should be directly involved in deciding:
>
> - where to locate new houses in terms of nearness to the closest water source;
> - the amount of family income spent on water-related improvements such as buying from vendors, installing a gutter system to capture rainwater or contributing to a community-wide water project;
> - whether to make the need for a better water supply a priority for the community.

Phase 2: Help the community choose which problems to solve

Step 1. Gather information about present water supplies

'Making a community diagnosis' in Chapter 3 (page 39) gives further information on this.

Existing water points in the community

Before making decisions about how to improve the water supply, the community must first answer questions about the existing supply:

① **What types of water source** currently exist in the community?

② For each source, **is the water supply adequate, accessible, reliable and safe** to those who use it? (Table 14.1 gives a guide for helping to answer these questions.)

③ Is there **sanitary disposal of human excreta**? (For details on this see Chapter 15.)

The best way to answer these questions is to walk systematically through the community. While doing this we can observe, talk to community members and record on a map the location of all water points. The CAG and CHDP staff can divide the slum into different areas with two people carefully briefed beforehand, responsible for gathering information from each area. We should note the location of each water point and record the following details about each:

① whether it is public or private;

② whether it is household or communal;

③ the source of the water (municipal supply, well, municipal tanker, etc.);

④ the type of delivery system (handpump, tap, etc.);

⑤ whether the source is functioning or in disuse;

⑥ the quality (adequate, accessible, reliable, safe) for the people who use it, according to Table 14.1.

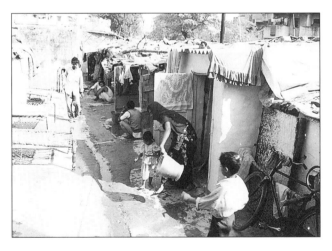

Use the questions listed in Table 14.1 to gather the information needed. On a separate piece of paper, answer questions listed in the table both for **each type of water supply**, and where relevant for **each separate water source**.

Figure 14.5 When thinking about the water supply, we must also think about how household waste water is disposed. (Beverley Booth)

Table 14.1 Helpful questions to ask about water supply that tells us if it is adequate, accessible, reliable and safe

Source of water	Is it adequate/accessible /reliable?	Is it safe?
For all types of water supply	Is the supply regular? Is supply affected during dry season? Does it provide enough water for everyone who uses it? How far away (in time or metres) is the farthest household that uses this water point? Is there a charge for the water? Per use or per household?	Is the water used for drinking? Does the community think the water is safe to drink? Do none, some, most or all of the households treat the water at home before drinking? If treated, how do they treat the water?
Municipal piped supply	How many times and hours per day does the tap run? How many times a week does the water not come as scheduled? Is theft (of tap) or vandalism a problem? What is the usual wait (in line and for filling)? Does it run fast, or slowly at low pressure? Does it run out before all are served?	What is the original source? (river, lake, etc.) Does the municipality treat the water before distributing it? Is the water regularly tested for contamination? Are there any known significant leakages? Is there drainage to carry spilled water to soakage pits or larger drains? Is there a storage tank located within the community?
Municipal supply by tanker	How often does the tanker come, how long does it stay and does it come on time? How many times a week does the tanker not come as scheduled?	What is the original source? (river, lake, etc.) Does the municipality treat the water before distributing it?
Surface water	Is the supply available year-round?	Does surface water drain areas where people defecate in the open? Are pit latrines, aqua privies or septic tanks nearby (closer than 15 metres)?
Water vendor	How often do vendors come, how long do they stay and do they come on time? How many times a week does the vendor not come as scheduled? How much does the water cost?	What is the original source? (river, lake, etc.) Does the vendor treat the water before distributing it?

Source of water	Is it adequate/accessible /reliable?	Is it safe?
Table 14.1 Helpful questions to ask about water supply that tells us if it is adequate, accessible, reliable and safe (continued)		
Well	For hand and electric pumps: • Is it in working order? • How often does it break? • How long does it stay broken? • Who maintains it (community, municipality, other)? • Does any community member know how to repair hand-pumps? If yes, do they know where they can get parts?	Is well deep or shallow? Is the water considered safe to drink? Is water treated? If so, how and how often? Is it a sanitary well? • More than 15 metres away from latrine/defecation area? • Covered? • Brick or stone lining? • Lining extends above ground level? • Cement platform around well? • One special well bucket and rope used by all users? • Drainage to carry spilled water to soakage pit or larger drain?

When important structures (wells, latrines, etc.) are identified, place each structure on the map. Use symbols or colours to represent important information (especially type of water source and whether it is functional). Also note any areas of standing water and poor drainage as well as the location of all places used for defecation (latrines, areas formally or informally set aside for open defecation).

For water sources that are used by more than one household, estimate the area each source serves. Ask household members where they most often get their water. Start by asking households that are about equal distance between two different water points, then work back towards a source untill finding the point where one water source takes over from another. On the map, lightly shade in areas served by each water point, using different colours or patterns. This way we can determine which households have the longest trip to the source they normally use.

Powerful people in the community often pressurise the community to place water points just outside their houses. Mapping gives a factual and objective way for the community to understand unfairness in distribution.

If wells are already in use or likely to become so, we will need to know more about the groundwater supply. Technical experts, such as government or private sanitation engineers can help us to learn the following:

• the depth of any existing wells;

- the height and variation of the water-table during the driest and wettest seasons;
- the direction of flow of groundwater;
- the make-up of the rock or soil and whether drilling would be possible;
- the depth of the nearest safe groundwater level where surface contamination is no longer a risk;
- the distance of septic tanks, defecation areas, drains or other surface water from any proposed well site;
- advice about the best site and depth for future wells.

Relevant health problems in the community

We should list the cause and frequency of any illness likely to be linked with problems in the water supply (or sanitation). This will help us to encourage the community to make changes and to provide solid evidence to support any improvement plans or applications. We may be surprised at the amount of illness.

Social and cultural factors

Water supplies and sanitation practices are often strongly wrapped up in tradition. This makes it difficult to bring in change unless we take great care not to cause offence by breaking traditions or taboos. Before making any major plans, we should consider calling on the help of an anthropologist who fully understands local customs and beliefs, and can advise about the best way of making changes without causing offence. Sometimes anthropology students from local universities can study the community and provide advice as part of a class project.

Consider for example the bathing of women. Is a separate, enclosed communal space a felt need? Take the washing of clothes: a community area, near a water point and served with good drainage would reduce the amount of excess wastewater produced by each house. It would probably reduce the frequency of dengue fever, or malaria. But would women use it? Take the concepts of 'clean' and 'dirty'. We may have one idea about what these terms mean: the community may have entirely different ideas.

Before making any improvements we need to fully understand the knowledge, attitudes and practices for each segment of the community involved in future change. Then we can build on sound community beliefs and gently try to change those attitudes that stand in the way of essential improvements. We start from where the people are and help move them towards healthier behaviours.

From the field: In a resettlement community in Fortaleza, Brazil, a health team interviewed mothers of infants and they also observed hygiene practices at home. They found that 95% of the mothers did not wash their hands before preparing and giving infants food even though all households had soap and water. They were also surprised to note that water was stored overnight in unhygienic conditions and not boiled before preparing milk formulas or gruel.

The results were shared with the mothers who decided that they would have a one-month trial of washing hands before preparing and giving food, and of boiling water for mixing with the powdered milk. At the end of the month trial period, the mothers felt that these new practices were definitely feasible.

The mothers held on to their belief that the water must be stored overnight 'to release the sun's heat'. The project did not try to change this belief, but instead encouraged mothers to boil water for mixing with powdered milk.

Lessons learned: The team's conclusion:

❶ Mothers know best what is feasible. They know what goes on in their homes and are good judges of which changes will work.

❷ Rather than trying to change practices associated with strong beliefs, look for an acceptable alternative or addition.

Source: Monte and Nations, 1994.

Step 2. Discover the government's willingness and capacity to take action

For any major improvements the government will need to be involved in one way or another. The first thing to do is to find out what water services the government is supposed to provide to city residents. Check with other communities to see what answers they have been given or any assistance they have received.

From the field: On the outskirts of Tegucigalpa, the capital of Honduras, some marginalized communities discovered that they were not included in the city's plans for upgrading the water supply. Community residents, mainly women, demanded change. Through their action, the government provided water, and the community agreed to supply the labour, some materials, and eventually to repay investment costs. The government agency and UNICEF provided most of the materials and technical assistance. The community operates the system and performs simple repairs. The very low user fees help to cover operating costs and repay the original investment.

Lesson learned: The voice of the community can be heard outside its walls (this is one definition of empowerment).

Source: UNICEF Annual Report, 1997.

We should find out if the government is able to provide any of the following forms of assistance:

❶ technical information and advice;

❷ special equipment to bore wells, etc.;

❸ handpumps and parts, either free or at subsidised rates;

❹ connections or extensions to the municipal supply;

❺ assistance with testing water for contamination or pollution;

❻ funding or revolving loans;

❼ help with major maintenance and repairs which the community cannot manage itself, either financially or technically.

Step 3. Obtain technical advice

Because water supply is a complex and technical subject experts will be needed for any major changes or improvements.

There are two periods when we are likely to call on their help. The first is in carrying out assessments such as analysing soil and water samples, and advising about the most effective improvements to the water supply and the siting of wells. The second period is when the community moves ahead with an agreed improvement. They can provide information, help draw up workable plans, and offer special training and skills for specific tasks. Technical experts can come from government, specialised NGOs, universities and the private sector.

Steps 4 and 5. Consider various cost options and their sustainability

Many improvements to a community's water supply will cost a great deal in terms of effort, time and money. Any option chosen must be good value for money, and be likely to work for a number of years with the level of maintenance that can easily be provided.

In practice water supplies will either be largely under community control, e.g. wells and handpumps, or under municipal control, e.g. taps and water tankers. Sometimes it will be a mixture of both.

> **From the field**: During the Decade of Water Supply and Sanitation from 1980 to 1990, billions of dollars were spent to improve the water and sanitation infrastructure in Africa. Many cities upgraded their water and sewer systems. However, many of these systems operate at less than 50% of their capacity. The major problems have been lack of technical expertise, spare parts and organisational capacity.
>
> **Lessons learned**:
>
> ❶ We should help the community to organise a group to be responsible for maintenance and repair of community improvements in the water supply.
>
> ❷ We should choose equipment that can be maintained by community members.
>
> ❸ We should make sure that community members know how to repair and maintain the equipment.
>
> ❹ We should make sure that spare parts are readily available and affordable.
>
> **Source**: Kirkwood, 1998.

For those under community control

The level of community involvement in operating and looking after the water supply is crucial. Without regular maintenance the system will rapidly deteriorate. Vandalism can make this worse and is more likely if the community is not responsible for keeping the system in working order. Ask these questions:

1. Is there a Community Action Group or other committee to monitor the water supply?

2. Is there a system in place for dealing with minor repairs, and knowing where and how to report more major problems?

3. Are there community members (preferably women) who specifically know how to make simple repairs to handpumps?

4. Is there income, e.g. from user fees, to cover the costs of maintenance and repair, including a contingency fund for major repairs (especially if an electric pump is being used)?

For those under government control

How effectively does the government maintain the supplies it is responsible for?

The CAG will need to keep in regular touch with officials, to report any problems and to ensure that action is taken to repair or replace faulty parts of the system with the least delay possible.

From the field: In a low-income community in Kerala, India, broken and vandalised handpumps were a serious problem. Using community mapping, it became clear that the non-functioning pumps were in public spaces where no one felt responsibility for looking after them. Taps were relocated at sites chosen by the community, which then committed itself to keep the taps in working order.

Lesson learned: If the community feels no responsibility for a public facility, it is likely to break down and be destroyed by vandals.

Source: Narayan, 1993.

Step 6. Choose the best way forwards

We must remember that there are many ways that families can protect themselves from water-related diseases at the household level at little expense. They can:

1. Obtain water from the safest possible source.

2. Remove disease-causing organisms from drinking water by sunlight: store water in a clear plastic bottle exposed to sunlight, perhaps on the roof.

3. Store water in clean, closed containers with a lid and provided with a scoop so that water can be taken out without hands touching the water.

4. Treat drinking water with chlorine tablets.

5. Wash hands before food preparation and eating, and after defecation.

6. Keep fingernails, especially of children, closely trimmed.

7. Bathe as often as possible, preferably at least once a day.

8. Cook food immediately before serving; do not keep cooked food without refrigeration.

9. Keep food covered, safe from flies.

10. Wash cooking utensils and dishes promptly, and allow to dry in a rack.

11. Do not bottle-feed infants. It is best to breastfeed. If animal milk is given, feed from cup with spoon.

12. Remove household garbage promptly, especially food refuse.

13. Use netting on windows.

14. Ensure that there are no vessels for standing water (empty cans, tyres, etc.).

It is now time for the community to decide which problem to work on, and the best way of going about it. In coming to this decision it is helpful to use a SWOT analysis (Strengths, Weaknesses, Opportunities and Threats) for each of the options being considered. See page 62.

In coming to our decisions we will need to look both at the obvious problems with the water supply and also at the local patterns of disease. Usually, of course, the two are related.

Problems with the existing water supply
Here is a list of common problems and preferred solutions

❶ **The water supply is inadequate.**

The commonest reasons for **inadequate water supply** include:
- There are not enough water points.
- Water flow is slow, unreliable or for too limited a number of hours.
- The water source is too far away.
- Water from vendors is too expensive.
- Handpumps or electric pumps are not in working order.

The **technical options** to reduce these problems include:
- Organise a system to fix leaks and repair broken pumps as soon as they occur.
- Provide more taps (if a piped municipal supply exists). If water pressure is low, providing more taps will not help. In this situation encourage the municipality to supply water for more hours a day or at a greater pressure (when more taps can then be added).

The more taps there are, the fewer households will use each tap. This means that families are more likely to start considering the tap as 'theirs', and take better care of it. This reduces breakage and vandalism.

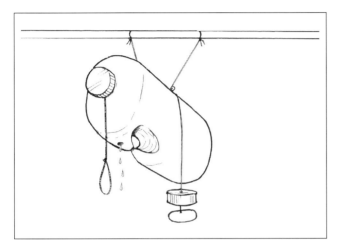

Figure 14.6   The Tippy Tap. (see Footsteps, No.30, March 1997, p. 20: an easy way to conserve water.

- Install overhead tanks (if water flow from existing taps is continuous but slow).
- Sink deep wells: when there is risk of faecal contamination (almost always), a deep well is far superior to a shallow well. Costs for sinking a deep well can be high but vary according to depth and type of rock. If the trend of the water-table is downward as is often the case, it is probably more cost-effective to sink a deeper well. Special grants may be available for well-drilling, or we might find support from a specialist NGO.

In many slums, dense housing coupled with narrow access roads limits the options for well sites. Trucks and equipment may only reach the outer areas of the slum.

② **The water supply is unsafe because of faecal contamination**.

The **water source** is usually:
- A shallow well that is contaminated by surface water draining from an area of open defecation: or a well close to soil contaminated by latrines, septic tanks, etc.
- An inadequately treated municipal supply from a contaminated body of water, or contaminated en route from faulty pipes or connections letting in sewage or contaminated surface water.
- Surface water (river, ditch, drain, etc.) that is inevitably contaminated.

The **technical options** to reduce these problems are:
- Improve the water supply by sinking a deep well, or establishing connections to a treated, well-maintained municipal water supply.
- In some communities people have to pay for well water. During the rainy season, they will use unsafe surface water because it is available and free. If

that is happening, we can develop rainwater harvesting, such as collecting roof water through guttering, then storing it in a protected tank or container.

- Set up an improved sanitation system (See Chapter 15).
- Chlorinate water in open wells or in the home.

Another system to make contaminated water safer to drink is to fill carefully cleaned water containers with the cleanest water available, seal them carefully and place them on the roof or by the side of the house in full sun for a day. This effectively makes the water safe to drink. A study among school-aged children in Kenya reported fewer diarrhoea episodes in children who drank sun-treated water compared with control children who drank water that was kept indoors. (Conroy *et al.*, 1996)

③ **Standing water provides breeding sites for mosquitoes and other insects.**

Common causes of **standing water** include:
- slow flowing or blocked drains,
- ponds,
- low-lying areas (below the water-table level),
- garbage: bottles, cans, tyres, etc. (Slums are often located near garbage dumps and scavenging is a common source of income and requires piling of sorted recyclable items, e.g. bottles, plastic containers.)
- flat rooftops, water coolers.

The **technical options** to this problem include:
- eliminate sites of standing water in the community (See Chapter 16);
- use personal protection agents mosquitoes including bed nets.

The local patterns of disease

We have probably already listed the common diseases in the community, as part of the community diagnosis. We can prioritise these illnesses according to the four categories described on page 61: How common they are, How serious they are, How much the community sees them as a priority (after education and awareness raising) and How easy they are to deal with.

We can use Table 14.2 below to help guide the best actions to take. For example, if diarrhoea is a serious problem in the community, then we should improve personal hygiene, prevent faecal contamination of water, e.g. by improving defecation options and/or improving the water supply.

Provide choices

We will now have a good understanding of problems with the water supply in the community we are involved with, and also with the pattern of disease. We will have worked with the community in discussing plans, costings and maintenance. We will have contacted the government and received help from technical experts.

The best options are probably becoming obvious. However within the community there may well be differing opinions depending on the level of education and understanding, the degree of poverty and how much certain segments of the community stick to traditional practices. A good compromise is to decide on one or two main improvements but to try and offer choices within those main areas. Here are some examples:

- If the municipality is willing to provide a certain number of communal water taps, then households may have the option of paying more and obtaining an individual tap. (This option should only be available when the amount of water is adequate and the household has a soak pit or is connected to an adequate drainage system that carries away wastewater.)

- If the basic source is to be a well, then, where possible, the community should have the option of using a handpump or an electric pump.

- Another choice is to install an overhead tank at the water point. This is especially useful when water flow is continuous or slow or when the municipality is prepared to turn on the water during the night. Where an electric pump is installed a tank can be extremely helpful. When the electricity is on the tank can be filled, making the community less dependent on a regular electric supply. People can then draw water at any time.

Phase 3: Carry out the improvements

Step 1. Mobilise skills

From within the community

As far as possible both skilled and unskilled labour should come from the community. Residents can be trained to make simple repairs of hand pumps. We will need to work out ways to obtain any special equipment or spare parts. The logistics of this is a skill in itself and community members or the CAG should be trained and empowered in this area. This could be combined with management and accounting skills.

From specialised NGOs, the private sector and universities

Some NGOs specialise in water supplies. In addition to providing expertise, they may have special equipment to bore wells or be able to provide spare parts for handpumps or handpump repair kits. They may be able to train community members to make ferrocement water tanks and know where to obtain the materials.

Step 2. Approach government officials

The community needs to keep in regular touch with government agencies:

- To obtain help which was agreed to earlier, such as equipment for boring wells, and connections or extensions to the municipal water supply.

- To participate in funding and loan schemes.

- To obtain necessary licenses or permits.

A few members from the CAG and CHDP should keep in regular touch with government agencies. Local politicians can be helpful. Consider inviting them to visit the community for a programme or to inaugurate an improvement. Give them credit and help them to feel personally affirmed by being involved.

Step 3. Mobilise funding

The government, international agencies and donor NGOs may provide loans or outright grants for major improvements to the water supply. Wells are an important example. Loans can then be paid back through user fees. User fees should be high enough to cover the costs of maintaining and repairing equipment such as handpumps and electric pumps, but we must ensure that the poorest households are still able to pay.

It can be very helpful when approaching government authorities or outside funding agencies to know how our community compares with other slums in the city or with the standards that have been set by the municipal authorities. For example if we find out how many households are sharing a single water point in our community, we can compare that with the situation in other slums, or with government targets.

From the field: In a Black homeland near Praetoria, South Africa, the major source of water was from the wells of people in the area who charged for water taken those who did not own wells. People had to pay much more for water than those living in more affluent areas who received the municipal supply. In addition, the water was heavily contaminated and unsafe to drink. The government wanted to provide municipal water connections but most of the land was privately owned. The owners refused to allow connections to be made for several reasons:

● They would have to pay for a connection fee.

● They would have to pay for the water used by the tenants and then arrange for the tenants to pay them back.

● Most important they owned the wells that were currently being used and if connections were made would lose that income.

But the government owned some plots of land in the area. It was proposed that connections should be installed on those plots and the water provided through kiosks. The community accepted this solution and helped to design the kiosks. Contractors from the community supervised the construction, which was done with community labour. Community members run the kiosk.

Initially, the government was going to charge the same price as the private vendors. But the community complained, now the community is getting safe water from the municipal supply at one-third of the cost of the water obtained from the private wells.

Source: Ratnam, CH in Pickford et al., 1996.

Step 4. Provide health education to the community

Health education should be part of any programme that wants to reduce water-related diseases in the community. **Changes in behaviour are more effective at reducing the**

spread of water-related diseases than improving the water supply. Some members of the community should be trained as motivators and educators to increase knowledge and awareness among all community members. In Table 14.2 specific activities are mentioned which will help to reduce common water-related diseases.

> The most effective way to reduce water-related illnesses is to use an integrated approach that includes health education as well as improving the water supply, sanitation and drainage.

Step 5. Set up the improvements or build the facility

To keep the process moving forward, it is helpful to make a plan that is broken down by specific task with deadlines for completion, responsible parties, etc. documented as described in Chapter 12. When this is done, progress can be monitored with rapid detection of obstacles.

Table 14.2 Water-related diseases and their prevention	
Water-related diseases	**Prevention activities**
Diarrhoeal diseases, including cholera, typhoid/paratyphoid, dysentery Ascariasis (roundworm) Giardiasis Hepatitis A and E	Educate community about: ● How diseases are spread ● Hand-washing, especially after defecating and before preparing or eating food ● Keeping fingernails short ● Breastfeeding ● Using sanitary latrines Ensure adequate water supply to encourage good personal hygiene and washing of utensils Ensure sanitary disposal of excreta Ensure safe drinking water Control flies by screening and rapid disposal of garbage Treat young children for intestinal worms every 4 months with albendazole
Conjunctivitis, skin infections Tinea Scabies Trachoma Flea-, louse-, and mite-borne typhus Yaws	Educate community about: ● How diseases are spread ● Importance of good personal hygiene, including daily shower/bath; hand-washing, especially after defecating and before preparing or eating food; keeping fingernails short and frequently changing and washing clothes. Keeping face clean where trachoma is prevalent ● Using sanitary latrines

Table 14.2   Water-related diseases and their prevention (continued)

Water-related diseases	Prevention activities
	Increase quantity and availability of water
	Reduce overcrowding
	Detect and treat infected cases to reduce spread
Clonorchiasis (oriental fluke disease)	Educate community about:
Diphyllobothriasis (fish tapeworm)	• How diseases are spread
Fasciolopsiasis (liver fluke disease)	• Not eating undercooked fish, shellfish, molluscs or water plants
Paragonimiasis (lung fluke disease)	
	Ensure sanitary disposal of excreta so that it does not reach body of fresh water
Schistosomiasis	Educate community about:
	• How disease is spread
	• Avoiding contact with water that may contain disease-causing organisms
	Ensure sanitary disposal of excreta so that it does not reach body of fresh water
Malaria	Educate community about:
Dengue	• How diseases are transmitted
Yellow fever	• Importance of personal protective measures such as wearing long-sleeved shirts and long trousers/skirt, using mosquito nets impregnated with insecticides such as permethrin
Filariasis	
Sleeping sickness (African trypanosomiasis)	
	• Netting on windows
Chagas' disease (American trypanosomiasis)	• Nightly spraying of sleeping quarters with pyrethroid sprays or use of insecticide mats or coils
Onchocerciasis	• Avoid going near breeding sites
	Eliminate breeding sites of standing water, especially water coolers (when not being used) and garbage that has containers that could hold water, such as tin cans, glass or plastic containers, tyres etc.
	Treat infected patients to reduce spread
Chemical toxicity due to organic chemicals, nitrates, acids, heavy metals.	Lobby for enacting and enforcing anti-pollution laws.
	Find out (perhaps from local environmental activist groups) the common chemical toxins that local industries are likely to dump.
	Survey the community for signs and symptoms of chemical poisoning from those toxins.
	Identify industries that are discharging chemicals that cause contamination into a body of water
	If facts are available, find out details of any toxicological examination of the water supply

Phase 4: Maintain and evaluate the changes

Maintenance

There are many tasks we need to do to make sure that water supplies continue to flow and supplies remain clean. The CAG or other committee should take on these management tasks. They include the following:

1 **Setting up a monitoring and reporting system**. The purpose of this is to make sure breakdowns, vandalism or leaks are reported promptly. A women's group or youth group can be given this task but two people should be responsible for monitoring each water point.

Various problems commonly arise:
- Taps are stolen, especially those made of metal (plastic ones are less valuable).
- Handpumps break and need parts that are not easy to find.
- Unauthorised hook-ups to pipes are made, lessening the flow at authorised taps or stopping it altogether.
- Pipes are blocked intentionally to increase flow at other sites.
- Electric pumps break down, illegal tapping into electricity lines leads to overload.
- Vandalism occurs, with rocks and other objects being thrown into wells.

2 **Ensuring that repairs can be made quickly:**

In practice community water supplies often fail because they are poorly maintained and repairs are delayed. Typical causes include:
- No one takes responsibility for looking after the water points.
- There are no funds to pay for the repairs.
- No one is trained to make them.
- Spare parts are difficult to find.

We should ensure that:
- Community members (women are often appropriate) should be trained to make simple handpump repairs.
- Appropriate tools and spare parts are available, safely stored and accessible for those who neeed them.
- Any water points should be repaired urgently.
- Those who do the repairs are paid promptly.

The remedy for maintenance problems is always the same: **An effective trained Community Action Group, empowered by the community to maintain the system, with well managed accounts and supplies to enable quick repairs to be made.**

3 **Developing a system to pay for repairs and maintenance. Here are some common options which are used:**
- **Monthly fee per household.**
  Advantages:
  – Easy to manage.
  Disadvantages:
  – Someone has to collect the fees or see that they are paid.

- Payment is difficult to enforce: problem of households that do not pay their share.
- Not equitable: Households that use lots of water pay the same as those that use little water.
- Does not encourage conserving water.

- **Pay as you use (for each bucket/25 litres, etc.)**
  Advantages:
  - Encourages water conservation.
  - Fair because people pay for what they use.
  - Payment is encouraged: those who don't pay are denied use.

  Disadvantages:
  - Someone has to collect fees at each water point, requiring wage and supervision.
  - It is hard to protect against untrustworthy attendants who keep some of the money. (One way to prevent this is to issue tickets from a single source, but this still requires someone at each water point to collect the tickets.)

- **Pay when repairs are needed. Some communities have an agreement that households using a water source will pay for repairs when they are needed.**
  Advantages:
  - Easy to manage.

  Disadvantages:
  - A major repair may require a relatively large amount of payment from each household.
  - Some households refuse to pay their share, making collection of contributions difficult and time-consuming.

4 **Managing chlorination of wells**

If the water source is a shallow well, it should be tested regularly for faecal contamination. Wells can be treated with bleaching powder ($CaOCl_2$). The amount required depends on the amount of contamination and the size of the well (details for chlorination, including amount of bleaching powder required for wells of different depths and widths can be found in *Water Supply*, IT Publications, given at end of chapter). A simple inexpensive test (ortho-tolidine test) is available to determine if the correct amount has been used. Simple chlorination pots, which provide continuous chlorination, are commonly used.

These activities can be managed by the CAG through giving two people responsibility for monitoring each water point. They will need basic training and have access to supplies.

5 **Monitoring the prevalence of water-related diseases (especially diarrhoea and malaria).**

This can be done from records held by clinics and CHVs.

6 **Managing disputes over water issues equitably.**

Disputes are bound to arise. The CAG should be responsible for listening to each side and giving a fair judgement as quickly as possible before the dispute spreads or gets out of hand.

Water loss from leaking/broken water points wastes a large portion of a city's water supply. As water becomes even more scarce and costly, repair and maintenance will become increasingly key issues.

From the field: In parts of old Patan, Nepal, open wells remain the major source of water for many people. Following an outbreak of typhoid fever, an NGO held several mass meetings in the community. They discussed how typhoid fever and diarrhoeal disease were spread, how wells got contaminated and what action they could take. The range of options for improvements was discussed.

The community was already divided into Well Groups. Each was invited to submit an application. The project then evaluated the state of the well and the quality of its water. Well Groups discussed various options and decided together which one(s) to follow. Each group contributed 10% of the financial costs, and another 10–40% as labour. Each Well Group is responsible for maintaining its own well, and for organising its chlorination. So far the project has helped 86 different Well Groups improve the quality of their water.

Source: C Preston, Yala Urban Health Programme, 1999.

Evaluation

After a period of time, we must evaluate the programme to make sure our objectives are being met. At an early stage the CAG and CHDP should choose some simple indicators to assess how well the programme activities are going (process indicators) and whether the activities are having an effect on the health and lives of people living in the community (impact indicators) (see Chapter 4, page 67).

For example a community's overall goal might be to reduce the frequency of water-related diseases by providing safe and adequate amounts of water for all. An objective towards fulfilling that goal might be to have at least eight of the ten community wells functioning when checked each week. The proportion of functioning wells would be the process indicator. The CAG could monitor those wells, or designate ten women, one from each well to report weekly to the women's group. At the end of 1, or 3, years each well can be inspected during a more formal evaluation and the weekly reports of the monitors can be inspected.

To assess the overall impact of the programme we could look at disease incidence, such as a reduction in the number of cases of diarrhoea. This would be the impact indicator. The disease chosen should be one that was a significant problem before the programme started. Frequency of illness can be calculated before and after the programme using clinic and CHV records or from quick sample surveys.

Chapter summary

A good quality water supply is one that is adequate, accessible and reliable, and that is free from disease-causing organisms or chemical pollutants. Common water supply systems include piped supplies through communal taps, tanker trucks, surface water (including ponds and rivers), water vendors, and wells, both shallow or deep, either open or covered and fixed with hand or electric pumps. Water-related diseases include diseases caused by lack of hygiene because of inadequate supplies for bathing and washing; diseases caused by organisms that are ingested in contaminated water; diseases caused by organisms living in water used for bathing and washing; mosquito borne diseases carried by insects which breed in standing water; and diseases caused by water polluted with poisonous chemicals.

In setting up a programme we need to follow four phases: preparing the community through education, and deciding which water supply problems to solve. We then work with the Community Action Group to implement the changes, gathering information, contacting government officials and setting up community action plans. We choose improvements that are both important to do, and within reach of community resources helped by loans, grants and expertise from outside sources. Finally we make sure that any changes are monitored and maintained through an active community group, and that the programme is regularly evaluated to make sure it is permanently effective. Helping the community to change its behaviours through adopting better personal hygiene is just as effective as improving the water supplies.

Resources

1. *Hygiene Evaluation Procedures: Approaches and Methods for Assessing Water- and Sanitation-related Hygiene Practices*. AM Almedom, U Blumenthal, L Manderson. International Nutrition Foundation for Developing Countries, 1997. Describes how to evaluate hygiene using participatory methods. There are many case studies. (Available from TALC.)

2. *Water Supply*. V Fernando. Intermediate Technology Publications, 1996. Many case studies and practical information, including details of chlorination.

3. *Sustainability of Water and Sanitation*. J Pickford, *et al*. Intermediate Technology Publications, 1996. A series of papers, many of them case studies, of what went well and what didn't with water and sanitation projects in developing countries. Very practical examples.

4. *Participatory Evaluation: Tools for Managing Change in Water and Sanitation*. D Narayan. The World Bank, 1993. Very good introduction to participatory evaluation with many examples. Helps communities to measure sustainability and impact of interventions.

15 Improvements in sanitation

> *In this chapter, we shall consider*:
>
> **What we need to know**:
>
> What is meant by effective sanitation?
>
> Why is sanitation in slum communities ineffective?
>
> What diseases occur because of ineffective sanitation?
>
> What are the various options for effective sanitation?
>
> **What we need to do**:
>
> Phase 1: Prepare the community for action
>
> Phase 2: Help the community choose what problems to solve
>
> Phase 3: Carry out the improvements
>
> Phase 4: Maintain and evaluate the changes

What we need to know

The problem of how to dispose of human waste is one of the most obvious problems in slum communities. It contributes greatly to illness, especially diarrhoea and intestinal worms in children. Open defecation seriously harms the environment, resulting in unpleasant sights and smells. For residents themselves the main problem is often the inconvenience and humiliation of having to defecate with no privacy or protection. All these reasons make improvements in sanitation a priority for everyone concerned.

What is meant by effective sanitation?

The word '**sanitation**' is sometimes used in a broad, inclusive way, encompassing the disposal methods for all kinds of waste, including human faeces, other solid waste, such as rubbish, and liquid waste such as kitchen and bathing wastewater. In this book, the word 'sanitation' is used in a more limited way, and refers to the way that human faeces (and urine) are disposed of. **Sanitation is effective when human faeces (and urine) are disposed of in such a way that organisms that cause disease are prevented from contaminating food, the water supply, and general environment.** Looked at in more detail, excreta must be prevented from contaminating each of the following:

❶ surface and ground water,

❷ the soil,

❸ paths, streets, homes and walkways,

❹ excreta must also be protected from flies and rodents.

Why is sanitation in slum communities ineffective?

Several factors contribute to poor sanitation in slums:

- **Government services are poor or non-existent.** The city government is reluctant to provide sewage disposal for slum communities. Most slum communities are illegal and unrecognised. The government rarely has the funds to do it. As a result sewerage services are usually limited to the city centre and wealthier residential areas.

- **Slums are often located in low-lying areas.** This makes it impossible to use pit latrines and septic tanks because there is nowhere for them to drain away. Surface water is often present, quickly becomes contaminated, and during heavy rains or floods spreads throughout the community. In addition, surface water is used for bathing, washing and as a childrens' play area.

- **Slums are crowded with little space for defecation and play.** This means that the area used for defecation is also used for other activities: walking, keeping animals and as a place for recreation.

- **Public latrines themselves spread disease-causing organisms.** Latrines quickly become filthy and offensive. Many residents will prefer to defecate in the open, unless latrines are strictly maintained.

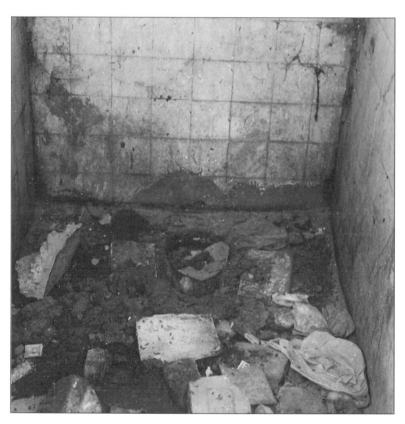

Figure 15.1   It's easy to see (and smell) why community latrines will not be used if they are not kept clean. (Godfrey Martin/ASHA)

What diseases occur because of ineffective sanitation?

Disease caused by poor sanitation can spread in four main ways:

Through direct exposure to contaminated soil

Intestinal worms are spread when people are exposed to faeces from an infected person. Worm eggs (ova) which are shed in faeces, remain in the soil and mature over days or weeks into an infective stage. Children are especially at risk because they may play in areas contaminated by faeces.

- In **roundworm (ascariasis) and whipworm (trichuriasis)**, eggs are passed with faeces into the soil, take time to mature and are then unknowingly taken in by mouth. When children play in the earth, eggs are transferred to their hands and then to their mouth. Eggs are often stored under long, unwashed fingernails.
- In **hookworm (caused by *Ancylostoma*, *Necator* or *Strongyloides*)**, eggs again pass from faeces into the soil, then gradually turn into larvae, which enter the body through the skin, often the foot. Children are at most risk when they play barefoot in areas used for defecation.

Through skin contact from contaminated water

Schistosomiasis (bilharzia) occurs when eggs in the faeces or urine of an infected person reach fresh water where certain species of snails live. The eggs develop into infective forms in the snail hosts and escape back into the water. The tiny infectious form called cercaria then passes through the skin when people bathe, wash, swim or play in infected water.

Through drinking contaminated water (or eating food contaminated by this water)

Many serious diseases are spread through this route. They include diarrhoeal diseases, including cholera and typhoid, giardiasis, amoebiasis and hepatitis A and E. All these occur when a person drinks water that has been contaminated with faeces from those who are infectious. Foods that have been washed or prepared in contaminated water, especially fruit and vegetables, also spread these diseases.

Through eating contaminated water animals or plants

When water is contaminated by faeces from an infected person, certain animals and plants that live in that water can become infectious. People become infected by eating those plants or animals. Most of these diseases are limited to certain parts of the world. This is because their complicated life cycles usually require other animal hosts that only live in certain places. Some of the more common illnesses are listed in Table 15.1. Cholera and hepatitis are more commonly spread directly through contaminated water.

Table 15.1 Diseases transmitted through contaminated water animals and plants		
Disease	**Location**	**Contaminated food source**
Hepatitis A	Worldwide	Raw or partially cooked shellfish
Cholera	Asia, Africa, Latin America	Raw or partially cooked seafood
Clonorchis infection (oriental liver fluke disease)	South-east Asia, China	Undercooked freshwater fish
Diphyllobothriasis (fish tapeworm)	Lake regions in tropical, temperate and arctic areas	Raw or partially cooked fish
Fasciola infection (liver fluke disease)	South-east Asia, South China, and scattered worldwide	Certain vegetables, especially watercress
Paragonimiasis (lung fluke disease)	Asia, Central and West Africa, Central and South America	Freshwater crabs and crayfish

What are the various options for effective sanitation?

Closed piped sewerage system

Ideally, each urban household should be connected to a closed piped, water-borne municipal sewerage system. This is only rarely possible for reasons we have stated before: vast populations, bankrupt city governments, illegal settlements and poor quality housing. However there have been some cases where this ideal solution has been possible. Usually a few key conditions are present:

➊ A **community that**:
- Is permanent or has a long-term lease or agreement.
- Is highly motivated with active participation from most of the residents.
- Participates in all levels of management, including decisions on what improvements to make.
- Contributes substantially in cash and labour.
- Takes responsibility for operating and maintaining the improvements.

➋ A **CHDP or individual who can**:
- Increase awareness, motivate and organise the community.
- Motivate the municipal authorities.
- Facilitate and link community and municipal efforts.
- Arrange for outside funding or loans.

➌ A **municipal authority that is**:
- Open to new or bold ideas.
- Relatively efficient and politically stable.
- Not overwhelmed by civil unrest, high levels of debt and rampant corruption.

➍ An **improvement that**:
- Is based on low-cost, innovative and often unorthodox technology, that depends heavily on community input and suggestions.
- Is based on providing a toilet for each individual household.

- Provides residents with a range of options at varying costs, enabling households to choose according to their own changing needs and priorities.

Although a piped sewerage system has many advantages, there are serious drawbacks which must be considered:

1. It is very expensive to build and maintain.

2. It requires an efficient maintenance system.

3. Sewage must be treated before being released into a body of water. Because of expense this is usually ignored, causing pollution of lakes, rivers and seas.

4. It requires large amounts of water, meaning it is an impossible option for many cities.

5. It does not recycle human waste into fuel or fertiliser.

There are low-cost alternatives to a closed piped sewerage system that greatly reduce the hazards caused by open defecation. Some of them, which are most appropriate in the settings of the urban poor, are described below.

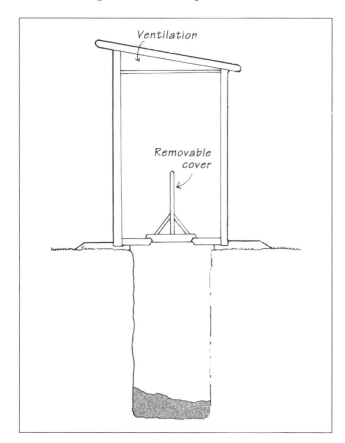

Simple pit latrine

Human waste falls into a pit that is directly below a slab that has a hole and squat plate or seat. Some decomposition occurs in the pit. Liquids seep from the pit into the surrounding soil. If the pit sides are likely to cave in, they can be reinforced, still allowing fluid to leak out. A tight-fitting cover over the hole helps to reduce flies, mosquitoes and smell. The addition of oil or very small polystyrene (styrofoam) balls to the pit helps to reduce breeding flies and mosquitoes.

Figure 15.2   Simple pit latrine.

Advantages	Disadvantages
• Low cost	• Flies
• Needs no water	• Mosquitoes
• Appropriate for people using dry bulky materials for anal cleansing (most of Africa)	• Smell
	• Unhygienic unless kept strictly clean
• Can be built by household using local materials	• Fear of falling into pit may discourage use, especially by children

Ventilated Improved Pit (VIP) latrine

In a VIP latrine, the pit is ventilated by a pipe extending from the top of the pit to above the latrine roof, with fly-proof netting across the top of the pipe. The inside of the outhouse is kept dark and an open space for letting in air is placed near the top of the superstructure and covered with netting. The hole should not be covered. Air flows from the opening in the outhouse through the hole into the pit and out through the ventilation pipe. This air movement eliminates the bad smell. As long as the outhouse is kept dark, any flies that do enter the pit are attracted to the light coming from the top of the ventilation pipe. They enter the pipe but since they cannot escape they fall back dead into the pit.

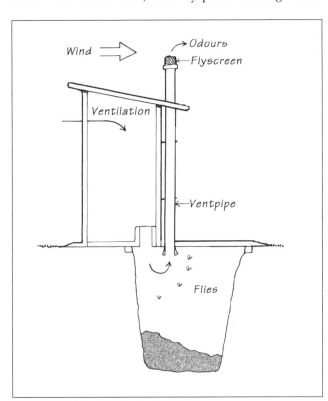

Figure 15.3   VIP latrine.

Advantages	Disadvantages
Same as for simple pit latrine plus:	• Mosquitoes are still attracted to the pit
• Controls flies and smell	• Extra cost of ventilation pipe
	• Interior of outhouse needs to be kept dark

Pour-flush pit latrine

This is the same as a pit latrine with a water trap built into the slab. Water is poured into the trap to clear the excreta and to replenish the water. The water seal prevents flies, mosquitoes and smell by separating the pit from the outhouse.

Advantages

- Low cost
- Controls flies, mosquitoes and smell
- Pit contents cannot be seen and causes less concern to children
- The pit can be located to the side, (an offset pit) and connected to the slab by a pipe. This enables the latrine to be inside the house while the pit is outside

Disadvantages

- Requires reliable water supply (1 litre per flush for direct, 3 litres per flush for offset pit)
- Only appropriate for people who use water for anal cleansing (most of Asia)

Any of the above designs can have two pits rather than one. The second pit can be dug near the first pit. When the first pit is nearly full, it is covered with earth, and the second pit is used. After about 2 years the first pit can be safely emptied, as disease-causing organisms will have died. Unfortunately space is seldom available in slums for twin pit latrines.

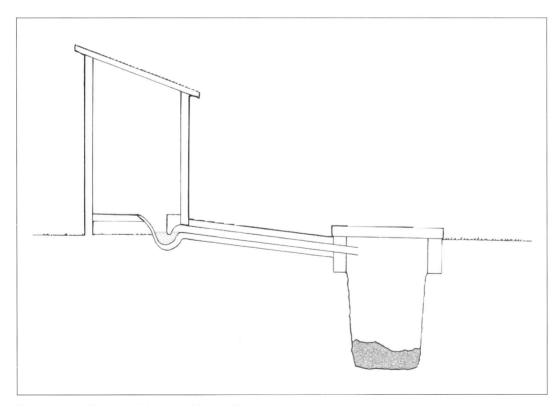

Figure 15.4   Water-seal in slab with an offset pit.

Advantages

- Gives greater flexibility and usage time, with one pit always in use
- Shallower pits can be dug which are easier to empty. Emptied contents can be used as fertiliser

Disadvantages

- Requires more space

Aqua privy

A watertight tank is placed directly below the slab with a hole. Excreta fall directly into the tank through a pipe that extends below the fluid level in the tank. This submerged pipe forms a water seal that prevents flies, mosquitoes and smell by separating the tank contents from the outhouse. Solid waste settles to the bottom of the tank and decomposes; fluid escapes through a pipe into the surrounding subsoil.

The low-lying location and lack of available land in slums often prevents the use of an aqua privy. However, a variant of the aqua privy in which the fluid pipe is connected to the municipal sewage system can be used.

Advantages

- Less expensive and requires less water than a septic tank

Disadvantages

- Expensive
- Usually needs to be connected to the municipal sewerage system
- Requires water to maintain the water seal: only appropriate for those using water for anal cleansing
- When the tank is cleaned out, the contents are infectious, and therefore dangerous to the cleaners and can contaminate the final destination unless treated

Septic tank

A watertight tank receives raw sewage from a pipe connected to a water seal toilet with overhead flush. It also receives household wastewater. Solids, including excreta, settle and decompose; liquids flow out through a pipe into the surrounding soil. As with the aqua privy, septic tanks in slums usually need to be connected to the municipal sewerage system.

Advantages

- Disposes of both human waste and household wastewater

Disadvantages

- Expensive
- Requires a large and reliable water supply
- Usually needs to be connected to the municipal sewerage system
- When the tank is cleaned out, the contents are infectious as with aqua privy above

Portable or permanent watertight tanks

A self-contained unit consisting of a squatting plate with or without water seal that is placed over a watertight tank. These can be single or multiple, permanent or portable. They are brought by truck and can be placed anywhere suitable. They need: an infrastructure that can ensure reliable, regular and frequent cleaning of tanks; and access for vacuum truck or special cleaning equipment.

Advantages	Disadvantages
• Can be used when ground is not suitable for pits or tanks	• Expensive to construct
• Minimises risk of contaminating ground water (unless tanks overflow)	• The need to use water for anal cleansing makes tank fill faster
• Can be installed quickly if need suddenly arises (e.g. during disasters or refugee situations)	• Requires vacuum truck to empty (or if removed by hand serious health risks to person emptying, and to residents if contents leak or are dumped nearby)

Methods of excreta removal

The various systems described, except a piped sewage system, all need periodic emptying of pits or tanks. If there is space to use a double pit system, the used pit can be covered over when full, meaning that emptying is relatively safe. The cleaning of all other systems is unsafe, as all are likely to contain disease-causing organisms. In addition to a piped sewerage system, the various methods of excreta removal include:

Manual removal

The pit or tank is cleaned out manually using scoops or shovels, or even bare hands. Sometimes people use latrines containing a small receptacle, such as a bucket or basket, which is then emptied by hand. This manual system is dangerous and demeaning to the cleaner. The community will be at risk if contents are dumped nearby.

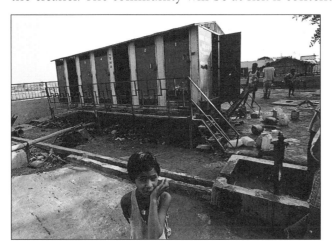

Vacuum truck removal

A vacuum truck with trained personnel can empty tanks or pits safely. In densely populated areas, trucks can rarely reach the tanks or pits. Special equipment has been developed which allows collection from tanks that the trucks themselves cannot reach.

Figure 15.5   Sometimes the only solutions are portable latrines with watertight tanks. If they are not emptied regularly, they will not be used. (ASHA)

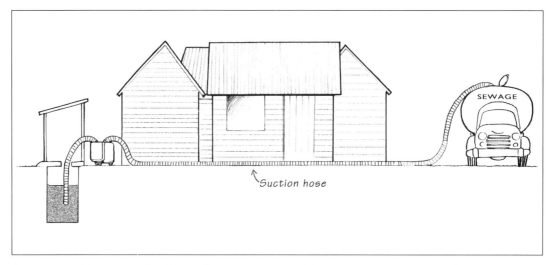

Figure 15.6   Vacuum trucks with auxiliary pumps are useful in slums when access is difficult.

Overhung latrine

People who live near or on a river or other body of water may build a latrine in which excreta falls directly into the body of water. Although the method is cheap and convenient it causes rapid and dangerous pollution of the water source, making diarrhoeal disease, including typhoid common. However those living in low-income housing over water have only two options: a slab over a watertight tank that is emptied when full, or an overhung latrine. The watertight tank is expensive to install and to operate. Therefore the overhung latrine is often the option chosen.

Reuse of excreta

The remains of excreta that have stayed in a sealed pit for 2 years are safe from disease-causing organisms. Untreated excreta from all other sources must be considered contaminated. Composting converts disease-carrying excreta into excellent fertiliser for crops. But this may not be practical in urban slums because of lack of space or lack of demand.

If overhung latrines have to be used it is worth trying to meet certain conditions:

- The water should not be used as a source of drinking water or used for swimming.
- The water should be deep enough so that the bottom is never exposed the dry season or low tide.
- The site should be in a place where floating solids will be quickly carried away from the community.

A more promising use of excreta in urban areas is in the production of biogas. Excreta are fermented to produce gas that has a high methane content and can be used as a fuel. It is more effective when the excreta of domestic animals such as cattle or pigs are also added. This technology is still being developed.

In most cities in developing countries, water is in short supply. Therefore it is unrealistic to have as a goal to provide all households connection to the municipal sewerage system, which requires large amounts of water. Research must continue to find low-cost, practical and low technology alternatives.

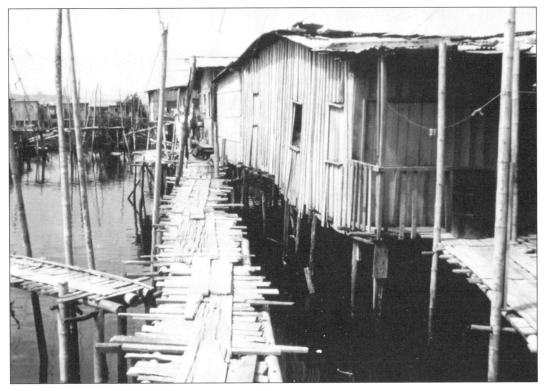

Figure 15.7   Slum communities that are situated over a body of water make it difficult to provide a safe sanitation system. (Tearfund)

What we need to do

Chapter 12 on Environmental Improvements contains the broad outlines for each of the four phases mentioned below. This chapter concentrates on specific issues related to safer sanitation.

Phase 1: Prepare the community for action

Step 1. Increase the knowledge and awareness of community members

Slum residents must decide on the best ways to improve their sanitation based on informed choices. We should help them understand each of the following:

- the meaning and importance of effective sanitation;
- why effective sanitation is so difficult in slum communities;
- the range of common diseases caused by faecal contamination;
- details of various improvements including advantages, disadvantages and costs;
- details of possible funding sources for capital costs, operation and maintenance;
- any legal obligations the government has to provide sanitary improvements;
- the names of government agencies and officials responsible for sanitation;
- the names of NGOs and other agencies that can provide financial support or technical advice.

Step 2. Motivate the community for action

Slum residents are all too aware of their need for better facilities. This is usually because of the inconvenience of their present arrangements rather than because they understand the dangers to health. We will need to raise their awareness about health and wider issues for two main reasons:

❶ To help them work for community-wide improvements:

We should emphasise the following advantages for them:
- **less illness**, especially diarrhoea and worm infestations in their children;
- **no more inconvenience or embarrassment** from open defecation;

From the field: In Lesotho, a government programme helps individual households to build a VIP latrine. The government:

- provides basic information, including cost and plans;
- helps to find a trained builder;
- offers a loan for 60% of the cost if the client can't pay the total cost at once;
- provides a technical expert who visits the house and advises where to put the latrine;
- provides technical experts who visit during the construction to make sure that it is built well, and then when the construction of the VIP latrine is finished to explain how to use, clean and maintain it.

The two main reasons that people choose to built the latrines are:

❶ They have learned that improved sanitation is good for their health.

❷ The latrine brings status to their house, and is easy and convenient to use.

Source: Isobel Blackett, 1994.

- **potential financial gain** because their property will be worth more for sale or rent;
- **increase in status** because their neighbourhood will improve.

② To help them change their own hygiene practices

We saw in the last chapter how important it is to improve personal hygiene as well as the water supplies. The same applies for sanitation. We must explain to the commuity why their health will improve if they change certain behaviours:

These are the key areas for behavioural change needed for effective sanitation:

- washing hands after defecation, and after cleaning children, and before eating or preparing food;

- keeping children's fingernails clean and short;

- covering prepared food to protect it from flies;

- protecting food stores from rodents and dogs;

- preventing children from defecating on paths or in roadside drains;

- breastfeeding for at least one year, and taking special care that supplementary foods added from 6 months of age are hygienically prepared;

- if animal milk is given, feed from cup with spoon.

Step 3. Channel motivation through organising the community

Poor sanitation affects the entire community. If one family builds a pit latrine a few feet away from a water source, all who use that water source may suffer. Therefore the community as a whole must be involved in choosing and implementing any improvements.

A Community Action Group should be formed, trained and empowered by the community, with women strongly represented. If the slum is large, divide the community into geographical areas. Each area can have its own working committee with a representative on the CAG. This is especially helpful when planning a piped sewerage system. Small committees are a useful means for choosing options and for organising work teams.

Phase 2: Help the community choose which improvements to make

As with other ways of improving the environment, the Community Action Group should take a leading role in co-ordinating this phase of the project. They will need frequent and regular discussions with a wide range of community members.

Step 1: Gather information about sanitary practices

Layout and facilities in the community

We should always look at excreta disposal, water supply and wastewater management together. The best way of doing this will be to organise a systematic walk through the community and carefully map anything relevant. The CAG should organise this but the more people involved the better – women, youth, students, and anyone with a particular interest. Because so much information needs to be gathered this process needs careful organising and briefing of those involved.

During the survey walk we should identify and map the following:

- **All water points**: public and private: by type (handpump, tap, etc.), by source (well, municipal supply, river, etc.).
- For all wells find out their approximate **depth**. Note whether the well, especially if shallow, is within 15 metres of any structure that could contaminate groundwater such as a pit latrine, septic tank, drainage ditch or other body of surface water.
- For all water points that come from a piped supply, check **pipes for leaks** and potential sources of contamination, such as pipes passing through standing water or next to sewage pipes.
- **All latrines** by type (pit, VIP, pour-flush, double or single pit, septic tank, etc.).
- For all latrines, check for **over-flowing septic tanks**, broken sewerage pipes, cleanliness, whether it is used or not, if not why not, etc.
- **Areas of open defecation**, or for dumping of excreta. Note the drainage route for that area.
- **Nearest municipal sewerage pipes**.
- **Areas of standing water** or that easily flood.
- **Natural drainage** routes.

Physical characteristics of the land

This is one of the main factors which helps us to decide which options are most appropriate – or even possible. We will need the help of technical experts to find out the following:

❶ **Suitability of the land for underground pits or tanks:**

What is the level of the water-table? In low-lying slum communities, the water-table is often very near ground level. This rules out the use of surface pit latrines. Watertight tanks can be used, or possibly pit latrines built on a raised up area.

❷ **What is the nature of the soil?**
- How easy is the soil to dig?
- Once the pit is dug are the sides likely to cave in? If so we will need to line the pit with bricks or blocks. Alternatively an oil drum could be used.

❸ **Availability of absorbent subsoil:**
- How large an area is available?

- Is the soil absorbent? How easily will water drain away? Latrines cannot be used if there is sold rock and non-absorbent soil.

④ The potential for contaminating water supplies
  - Which areas regularly or occasionally flood during the rainy season?
  - In which direction does the groundwater flow?
  - How deep is the groundwater level?

Answers to these questions will help us decide what sanitary improvements are possible. But we will need technical advice to interpret the findings and understand how they will influence our choices.

Health patterns in the community

This will give us a clear idea of how poor sanitation is affecting the health of the community. The number of cases of diarrhoea, including typhoid, and the frequency and type of worm infestations will be good indicators of how serious the problems are: so will recent or periodic outbreaks of cholera.

When a community improves its sanitation or its hygienic practices there can be dramatic falls in the cases of diarrhoea. Also with fewer worm infestations the overall health of children improves. They may become less anaemic and perform better in school.

Social and cultural factors

In almost all cultures, there are strong beliefs and practices about defecation. In some cultures faeces are believed to be polluting, often more in a spiritual sense than in terms of spreading infectious disease. In some cultures people are expected to defecate in a different place each day. In others, a person must not urinate or defecate facing a certain direction. We need to understand these beliefs and practices when planning improvements. Here are some questions that need to be answered:

- What is the method of anal cleansing? Some latrine systems need water and are only appropriate if water is used (most of Asia, Latin America). In many African cultures, dry pit latrines are the best option as sold materials such as leaves and corn husks are used for cleaning.

- Do people defecate squatting or sitting? Will they prefer a squat plate or a seat?

- How much privacy is needed?

- Are families prepared to share latrine facilities? In parts of East Africa daughters are forbidden to use the same latrine as their fathers.

- Are communities prepared to use a centralised latrine complex?

- Can men and women use the same latrine? In some cultures where there is open defecation, men and women traditionally defecate in separate areas or at different times. Is the community willing to change that practice?

- Will women be able to use the latrine while menstruating?

> **From the field**: In Bangladesh, the end of the sari, the normal female outer garment, is a handy cloth, towel, and handkerchief. Project staff noted that mothers sometimes used the end of their sari to clean their baby's bottoms. When project staff discussed with women how diarrhoeal diseases were spread, mothers came to understand that the practice was unsafe, they changed their behaviours and passed this information on to new mothers. Diarrhoea in the community has since become less common.
>
> **Lesson learned**: It is important to understand the community's traditional ideas of what is 'clean' and what is 'dirty'. Only then can we start to motivate and educate people about healthy behaviour.
>
> **Source**: Author visit.

When we understand local culture and beliefs, we will realise which practices are dangerous and need to be changed, which practices don't matter and can be left alone, and which practices are helpful and ought to be encouraged.

Step 2. Discover the government's willingness and capacity to take action

It is nearly impossible to improve sanitation without government help. This may include periodic emptying of watertight tanks, or connection of a community latrine complex to the municipal sewerage system.

Widespread building of latrines or the use of watertight tanks will often require loans. Any connection of individual houses to a municipal system is a major undertaking that will need prolonged and careful co-ordination.

The Community Action Group will need to discover just how much the government is prepared to help with loans, technical assistance and new installations. This will require a patient, firm and persistent attitude.

Step 3. Obtain technical advice

Technical advisors will be needed to advise about soil, the types of improvement or facilities that are possible, locations, costs and methods of installation. Unless good advice is sought at an early stage wrong ideas can cause a huge amount of wasted time and money. There are many worldwide examples of sanitation improvements that have been expensive and discouraging failures.

As well as technical advice we may also need the help of an anthropologist if we are undertaking major community-wide improvements. Anthropology students from a nearby university may assist to gain experience.

Steps 4 and 5. Consider the cost and sustainability of various options

The broad choice of which improvement to make has to be a community decision. However success is more likely if within any system agreed upon, individual households have a range of costed options. Then they can choose what is best for their particular situation and the money they have available.

For each option we should carry out a SWOT analysis, page 62 (see Chapter 4), looking at the Strengths, Weaknesses, Opportunities and Threats for each possible improvement. This will help us be informed about our choices.

Examples of choices include:

- pit latrine or VIP latrine;
- water seal or no water seal;
- pit directly under the latrine or set to the side (which allows latrine to be inside house, but is more expensive);
- hook-up to municipal sewerage system, and if so, now or as an option in the future.

> The use of innovative technology and local community labour can dramatically reduce costs. WITH EACH REDUCTION IN COST, MORE PEOPLE WILL HAVE MORE OPTIONS.

From the field: In Kumasi, Ghana, 75% of the population had no household sanitary facilities. Local officials did a 'willingness-to-pay' survey amongst city residents. They found that the poorest people paid more in fees to use public latrines than those with household systems paid for their sanitation service. They also found that people would be willing to pay for household latrines. Based on that survey, the government set up a revolving loan scheme in three pilot areas. Four thousand people ended up with improved, sanitary household latrines.

Lessons learned: When costs are analysed and the situation explained residents are often willing to pay for sanitary household latrines. Governments can move from *providing* services to *promoting* services.

Source: Narayan, 1993.

Long-term maintenance is most likely to work when the community is involved in choosing and installing the various options. The balance between who holds this responsibility – individual or community – will vary according to the type of improvement. For example, if the decision is made to install pit latrines for individual households then obviously each household looks after its own system. But if the decision is to have a community latrine/bathing complex, then the community as a whole will be responsible. The CAG will need to appoint and supervise those who clean and maintain the facility. Without careful management the system will rapidly deteriorate and people will stop using it.

Occasionally municipal governments will provide latrines without the community being involved in decision or planning. This nearly always leads to failure. Community latrine complexes will only be widely used if we take very careful precautions to make sure they are kept clean and well repaired. This will involve:

- a CAG or other committee to manage the operation and maintenance of the facility;
- a monitoring system to detect breakdowns;
- regular supervision and payment of cleaners;
- income, usually from user fees to cover costs;
- a good relationship with the government agency to make major repairs and ensure connection to the city sewerage system functions properly.

> Almost any improvement in sanitation will require regular removal of excreta from the community. The government must play the main role in this. The keys to success will be strong links with the government department, and community pressure if action is delayed.

Step 6. Choose the best way forwards

Lack of space, lack of funds and the reluctance of the government to be involved means we will only be successful if we are very determined and come up with imaginative ideas. We will need an approach that is innovative, cost-effective and above all depends on a high degree of self-help within the community.

Slum residents will need to decide on two linked questions:

1. Does the community want an individual, group or community system of latrines?
2. What type of excreta disposal system does the community prefer?

We will look at each in turn:

Does the community want an individual, group or community system of latrines?

A **community latrine complex** provides a number of latrines for the entire community at one site. Often a bathing/clothes washing area is included in the complex. In a **group latrine option**, units each containing a number of latrines and possibly a bathing area, are sited throughout the community, each unit serving the surrounding households. **Individual household latrines** provide the most dignity but are often impossible in crowded areas.

1. **Community latrine option.** Because of the huge amount of sewage formed this option is only possible if the complex can be linked to the municipal piped system or drained to a large septic tank. In some cases, the government is willing to respond to persistent requests by a community to provide latrines connected to the municipal system. Large amounts of water will be needed, especially if flush systems are used. If the water supply is unreliable the latrines will not be used. In

practice a tube well with an electric pump is needed as part of the complex, with a raised storage tank because of frequent electricity cuts.

At times, the only possible site for the complex is so far away from the nearest sewerage system that the connection is too costly to construct. In that case a septic tank will need to be built. This however requires plenty of space and good subsoil drainage, which may not be available in a crowded slum.

The complex must be sited so that most community members can reach it quickly and safely or again it will not be used.

A major challenge with community latrines is to keep them clean and to maintain them in working order. As we have seen, community latrines work best when the community operates and maintains them.

Life in a slum

Naomi used to bathe at the community latrine/bathing complex very early in the morning while it was still dark. The complex was quite far from where she lived, but it was the only place where she could bathe in privacy. One morning about 4 am she was walking to the complex when three men, all drunk, jumped her, dragged her behind a rubbish bin and raped her. She resisted and they beat her, hitting her so hard that she died. A few hours later her anxious parents found her body. She was 14 years old. (Uganda)

② **Group-latrine option**. Many of the above points apply to this. Large amounts of sewage again make a link to the city sewerage system, septic tank or aqua privy the only options, and a reliable water supply will be essential.

③ **Individual latrine option**. If there is no way to link into the municipal sewerage system, then individual latrines will need to be used. Septic tanks and even aqua privies require an amount of land for drainage that is rarely available in slums.

In practice the best options for latrines will usually be as follows:

- **for those using water or soft paper for cleansing**: a water-seal latrine with direct or off-set pit, or a double pit latrine;
- **for those using dry bulky materials for cleansing**: a direct double pit VIP latrine.

Unfortunately, in most slum communities, there is rarely enough land for two pits so that single pit latrines are usually the option chosen.

When permission is given for slum residents to build individual latrines, the surrounding neighbourhood may assume that the slum is becoming permanent. This can raise opposition and we must be quick to explain the advantages: a better environment, less smell, reduced risk of diseases, and a rise in property values as the slum evolves into low income housing.

Table 15.2 below can be used to help residents decide between community, group and individual latrines.

Table 15.2 Community, group or household latrines: some factors for the community to consider	Community	Group	Household
Space required	Less	Less	Much more
Cost	Less per resident; the option that is most likely to be provided by municipality	Moderate per resident	High per resident; the option that community is most willing to pay for
Community maintains the facility	Least likely	Quite likely	Most likely
Spread of disease	Much less likely than no latrines, but still possible	Less likely than community latrine	Least likely
Type of sewage disposal	Municipal sewerage system or septic tank	Municipal sewerage system or septic tank	Pit latrine, septic tank, aqua privy, watertight tank
Other advantages (+) /disadvantages (–)	+ Connection to municipal water and sewerage system more likely + Can be a source of revenue for the community – Requires electricity and tube well if city water supply is inadequate – More likely to fall into disuse because of dirtiness or breakdowns	+ A group of households can choose this option without agreement of community at large	+ Convenient, time-saving + Individual families can choose this option without agreement of community at large + More likely to increase value of the property + Likely to be kept clean and maintained
Causes of failure	No person/group is given responsibility for care and maintenance, so quickly breaks down and becomes unusable	Same as for community latrine unless responsibility is well defined so that specific families use and are responsible for a particular latrine	Unused if water is not readily available

What type of disposal system does the community prefer?

Community members must first decide between community, group or individual latrines. That decision gives the broad answers for which methods of excreta removal

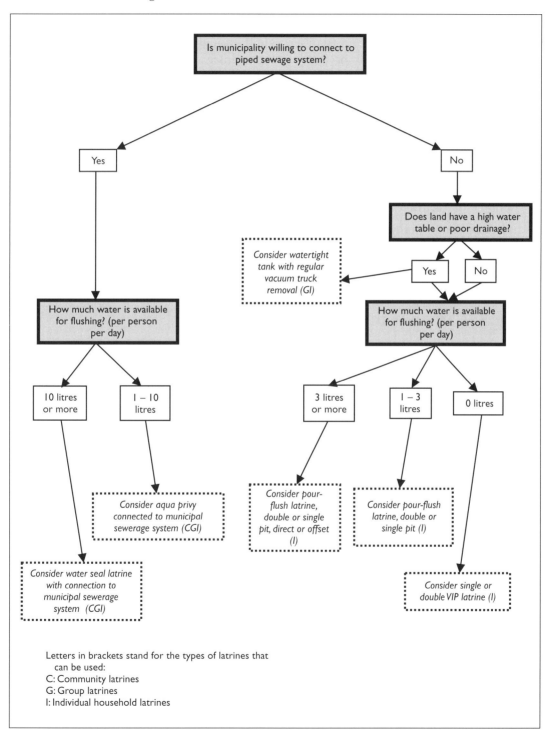

Figure 15.8 *Questions to ask when the community considers its options for sanitary removal of excreta.*

are possible. The flow chart (Figure 15.8), gives guidance about the best options for different situations.

A few other factors should also be borne in mind:

① **The amount of land available for pits or tanks**. If the preferred choice is a pit latrine, a double pit is better than a single **if** enough land is available. An extra large (deep) single pit may be the next best choice.

② **The absorbing quality of subsoil for pits or tanks (aqua privy and septic tank)**. Because septic tanks also receive household wastewater, the area of absorbing soil must be relatively larger. If soil cannot absorb, such as when the water-table is less than 2 metres below the surface, or the land is marshy or covered with water, then watertight tanks with regular emptying by vacuum truck should be considered.

③ **The availability of vacuum trucks to empty pits or tanks regularly**. If vacuum trucks (or empying machinery attached by pipe) are not available, consider a double pit latrine with composting.

④ **Costs** of each method and willingness of households to pay extra for a more convenient system.

⑤ **Cultural factors**, especially willingness of the community to use the system chosen.

Phase 3: Carry out the improvements

Step 1. Mobilise skills

From within the community

Most of the labour needed to build individual and group latrines can come from the community itself, with some training and guidance from technical experts. A community latrine complex may require outside contractors, but community members can do the building. Improving sanitation will give many chances to empower community members through developing their skills.

> **From the field**: As part of a community sanitation programme in Addis Ababa, community members provided the labour to construct communal (neighbourhood) latrines. The families that use the latrines organised a rota system to clean and maintain the latrines. The rota list is kept on the latrine door, which makes accountability easier. (Ethiopia)
>
> **Source**: Author visit.

From specialised NGOs, the private sector and universities

NGOs and other organisations that specialise in development may be able to provide technical assistance and advice. They may know where to obtain special materials such as slabs, water seals, ventilation pipes, etc. and to teach people how to make them.

We will already have made links with universities or other technical experts to advise about soil type and drainage and which improvements are most likely to work.

Step 2. Approach government officials

If the excreta disposal system is going to connect with the municipal sewerage system, intense discussions have already taken place by this stage. Now, however, very detailed plans need to be made in co-operation with government agencies. A few members from the CAG and the CHDP should interact regularly with officials to push the process forward.

The community also needs to follow up on any government loan or funding schemes, and to obtain necessary permits and approvals.

Step 3. Mobilise funding

The community should also seek help from NGOs that specialise in providing financial aid for upgrading sanitation. The need for capital to pay for improvements may lead to a community-run revolving savings and loan association. Community members deposit funds from which they receive some interest. This money is then available for others to borrow at low interest for buying materials for building latrines.

Step 4. Train people in skills and tasks

In addition to training craftsmen and other residents in how to construct latrines, we need to train community members, in the proper use of latrines.

> **From the field**: In Lesotho, southern Africa, young children were not using the latrines. Extension workers made two pictures of a mother encouraging her child to use the latrine and two more pictures of a mother refusing to let her child use the latrine. A set of both pictures was shown to a group of children and to a group of extension workers. Both groups were asked to discuss or draw why the mother did not allow her child to go into the latrine. They were then asked to make suggestions on how to persuade mothers to encourage their children to use the latrine.
>
> The drawings and discussions showed that most young children were not encouraged to use the latrine because of fear that they might fall in, fear of darkness, fear of snakes, or fear that the children might make the latrine dirty. The extension workers simply suggested; 'more health education'. But the children enthusiastically made suggestions on how to change the seat design, and make other changes so that both they and their mothers felt happy.
>
> **Lesson learned**: It is always helpful to consult users before implementation.
>
> **Source**: Narayan, 1993.

Steps 5 and 6. Carry out pilot studies and build demonstration unit(s)

If latrines have not been used before in the community, it is important to carry out pilot studies. If one type of latrine appears to be the most suitable, two or three homes can build one, use it and help others understand the advantages.

Often a few families in the community will have their own latrines. What design are they? Do they work well? Are they sanitary? Do family members, including children, regularly use them? These latrines can be considered a 'pilot study'. If they prove to have major faults, improved designs can be tried out.

The lining of the latrine is important. Is the ground sufficiently strong so that a lining is not needed, or should bricks or stones be used? Different types can be tried to see which is most suitable.

Several demonstration units can be constructed so that residents can see the variety of options. There should be enough designs of varying cost, so that householders with different levels of income can identify one which they can afford. The demonstration units should show two things: how the particular design can be used now and possible ways of upgrading the system in the future when family finances allow it.

It may seem a sensible idea to demonstrate a latrine in a school or health centre. However, the latrine may become so dirty so quickly that it actually discourages people from wanting to install their own.

Step 6. Choose the best way forwards

By now the community will have decided what options to go for and planning will be in hand. A key decision will be the exact siting of latrines and other facilities.

For **community or group latrines** the location will need:

1. **Sufficient land for the complex building.** If facilities for bathing and washing clothes are needed, much more land will be required. Some slum dwellings or other buildings may have to be relocated. If this is the case we must ensure that fair compensation is paid to displaced households and that this is incorporated into the total project budget.

2. **Easy connection to the piped municipal sewerage system** or sufficient subsoil for fluid that seeps from the septic tank.

3. **Sufficient water from a reliable supply** or tube well with reliable source of electricity.

4. **Reliable power supply.** In slums with no legal electricity supply a special power line may need to be sanctioned. This will need protection from illegal tapping by slum residents to prevent short circuits and burn-out of the pump motor.

For **individual pit latrines**, as well as septic tanks or septic tanks/aqua privies, the location must be downstream stream and more than 15 metres from any source of drinking water. There is an exception to this. If the municipality provides a piped water supply so that groundwater is not used, there can be more choice for siting of the latrine.

Sometimes another compromise has to be made. Even if pit latrines might threaten pollution to local wells, the benefits of building latrines may outweigh this risk, providing either that drinking water is brought from outside or that careful chlorination of wells takes place.

The selection of sites needs technical advice but the CAG can help to co-ordinate the building of latrines, and help distribute printed leaflets of instructions for each household.

It is helpful to have a 'building season', within which people can choose exact times for latrine construction which fits in with their family routines. This season should be at an appropriate time of year. The CAG can order supplies in advance, arrange training programmes and try to prevent noise and disruption continuing for too long a period.

Phase 4: Maintain and evaluate the changes

Maintenance
For improvements in sanitation, maintenance is as important as building the facilities. Because these two areas overlap many ideas on upkeep have already been included in this chapter. Here is a summary of what needs to be done:

Community complexes and group latrines
A community group, such as the CAG must be empowered by the community to monitor these facilities and supervise their upkeep and repair. Members of women's groups or youth groups can be involved in this process.

Here are the main tasks:

- **Keep the facility clean**. Cleaners should be supervised and trained. Fees must cover the costs of upkeep.
- **Monitor** the cleanliness of the facility and need for repairs.
- **Make repairs** promptly.

There are many reasons why repairs are delayed. Here is a common sequence: there is no monitoring system to report early breakdowns: no one has overall responsibility for making repairs: breakdowns are not reported: further breakdowns occur: filth and smells increase: residents stop using the facility.

The remedy is for a Community Action Group to take responsibility for the latrine complex, plus its water and electricity supply. They will ensure:

- regular checking for breakages;
- prompt repairs of minor problems through calling on skilled labourers who have materials available;
- quick contact with government if major repairs are needed;
- pressure is maintained if the government delays;
- collecting fees, managing accounts, paying cleaners and labourers and managing a contingency fund or agreement with the government for major repairs.

User fees: Each family can pay a certain amount each month, or individuals can pay as they use. Large sums of money will be handled. All those involved should be trustworthy individuals and be trained in the handling of money. Careful accounts must be kept. Those collecting fees per use or per household will need careful supervision.

Household latrines

Here the tasks will be slightly different. They will include:

- continuing to convince reluctant residents to invest in a latrine;
- teaching latrine maintenance;
- co-ordinating the emptying of pits;
- monitoring for poorly maintained latrines that pose hazards to the community.

Once latrines have been built the CAG will need to discourage open defecation, help solve disputes, and encourage new slum residents to build latrines or use the existing complexes.

Evaluation

With so much money, time and effort spent on improving sanitation, an evaluation will be of interest for all involved in the process.

Our overall aim will probably be to reduce the frequency of diarrhoeal illnesses, especially in children. Two main objectives to help bring this about will be to encourage as many households as possible to use or install latrines and for residents to improve their personal hygiene, especially hand washing.

From the field: In Reynosa, Mexico, the Puentes de Cristo project decided to address the problem of diarrhoea in one of the colonias, a poor urban community. When they began working in the community in 1995, diarrhoea was the cause of 28% of all clinic visits and the frequency of diarrhoea episodes was 8 per year per child. After studying the problem, the project decided that there were three major problems: mothers were not breastfeeding, mothers did not realise the importance of hand washing and the water supply was contaminated.

To tackle the problem, the project carried out the following:

1. held classes for pregnant women stressing the importance of breastfeeding and hand washing;

2. trained promotoras, women from the community, to educate pregnant women and mothers about personal hygiene and breastfeeding;

3. installed a water purification unit at the clinic. (Women from the community run the unit which sells safe drinking water to the community at a reasonable charge – just enough to cover expenses.)

Three years later, diarrhoea was the cause of only 1% of clinic visits and the frequency of episodes of diarrhoea had decreased to just 1.6 episodes per year per child.

Source: Author visit.

Process indicators could include: The precentage of individuals regularly using a latrine, or the percentage of households that install and use latrines over a 1-, 2- or 3-year period. Behavioural change could be measured by the number of children observed defecating in roadside drains.

The impact indicator will measure the effects of behavioural changes (i.e. improved personal hygiene) and latrine usage. Improved water supplies will also affect this. A useful indicator would be the frequency of diarrhoeal illness, especially in under-5 children, as shown from clinic and CHV records. This could be yearly over a 3-year period from the start of the programme, and could be compared with figures before the programme started (or if not available, figures obtained during the initial months of the programme).

We also need to evaluate the impact of change from the community's perspective. They may look at things very differently. For a teenage girl, not having to defecate in the open may far outweigh the reduced incidence of diarrhoea.

From the field: The IHAUDP project which works with very poor communities in Addis Ababa, Ethiopia helped the community set up neighbourhood committees responsible for managing improvements in water supply and sanitation. These have included constructing and maintaining group latrines and shower buildings. The privacy which this has brought has greatly improved the quality of life for community members, especially women. They no longer suffer from so many kidney infections and problems caused by poor personal hygiene, through lack of privacy for urination, defecation and bathing.

Lesson learned: The privacy that comes with latrines and improved bathing facilities improves health in many ways.

Source: Beall, 1997.

Chapter summary

Poor sanitation is a major health hazard in slums. Most people defecate in the open, meaning that germs quickly contaminate the water supply, and the hands and feet of residents, especially children who play in the open. Diarrhoeal diseases and worm infestations are the major health problems that occur.

Various improvements can be made. These include improving personal hygiene, especially hand washing, possibly the most important change of all. Designs for latrines include pit, VIP and water-flush latrines, each with either single or double pit. Aqua privies, septic tanks, and watertight tanks are other options. The ideal situation is to link excreta disposal to the municipal sewerage line, but alternatives include vaccuum removal by truck or soakaway into the subsoil if there is adequate space and drainage and the water-table is low enough. Latrines can either be designed for the community as a whole, for groups or for individual households.

We can help make improvements in four stages. First we must help the community understand the advantages of using latrines including increased convenience and improved health. Second the community will need to choose the best improvements both from the viewpoint of the community and from individual households. This will mean carefully looking at the advantages and costs of any options that are technically possible. Third we can help the community implement changes through training, obtaining funds and materials, and getting expert advice. Fourth we need to ensure all facilities are maintained in excellent working order. Otherwise residents will return to defecating in the open and all the effort will be wasted. We also need to set up systems for evaluating improvements both from the viewpoint of resident's health and their convenience. The Community Action Group will play a major part in all these activities.

Resources

1. *Solid Waste Management Directory*. A Coad. Swiss Centre for Development Cooperation, 1998. A directory of information sources in developing countries. (Available from SKAT.)

2. *Low-cost Sanitation: A Survey of Practical Experience*. J Pickford. Intermediate Technology Publications, 1995. A guide to providing sanitation coverage to urban (and rural) low-income communities, based on extensive experience, and outlining what is practical, appropriate and acceptable.

3. *Sustainable Sewerage: Guidelines for Community Schemes*. RA Reed. Intermediate Technology Publications, 1995. Describes how to build and maintain low-cost sewerage. Covers the various steps in planning, selection, design, management and maintenance of community schemes, as well as financial and technical guidance.

4. *Participatory Evaluation: Tools for Managing Change in Water and Sanitation*. D Narayan. World Bank, 1993.

5. *A Guide to the Development of On-site Sanitation*. R Franceys, J Pickford and R Reed. WHO, 1992. An excellent technical review of the options.

6. *Management of Solid and Liquid Wastes*. G N Nyang'echi. African Medical and Research Foundation, 1992. A good review of options.

7. *Community Health and Sanitation*. C Kerr (ed.) Intermediate Technology Publications, 1990. Deals with disease and problems of water in the house and at the source, waste disposal and education.

8. *Rural Water Supplies and Sanitation*. P Morgan. Macmillan, 1990. A simple practical manual. (Available from TALC.)

9. *Sanitation without Water*. U Winblad and W Kilama. Macmillan, 1985. Pactical information on how to design, build and operate compost and improved pit latrines. (Available from TALC.)

10. *Ecological Sanitation*. S Esrey *et al*. Sida, Stockholm, 1998. Advice on ecological sanitation systems, including dehydrating and composting systems, suitable for use in urban and other situations.

16 Improvements in wastewater disposal

In this chapter, we shall consider:

What we need to know:

Where does wastewater come from?

How does wastewater disappear?

Why is standing water a major problem in low-income communities?

How does standing water cause illness?

What we need to do:

Phase 1: Prepare the community for action

Phase 2: Help the community choose which problems to solve

Phase 3: Carry out the improvements

Phase 4: Maintain and evaluate the changes

What we need to know

Where does wastewater come from?

Muddy paths, puddles and pools of stagnant water are common sights in slums. This water accumulates when wastewater is produced at a faster rate than it can be eliminated. In slum communities the main sources of wastewater are as follows:

1. **Rainwater**, which is usually the biggest cause. Because there is often a rainy season or heavy downpours, large amounts can accumulate fast, often causing floods in low-lying slums. Pools of stagnant water can then remain for weeks.

2. **Household wastewater** from bathing and washing.

3. **Water run-off** from taps, hand pumps and leaking water pipes.

4. **Overflowing sewage** from septic tanks or blocked sewage systems.

How does wastewater disappear?

There are three main ways in which wastewater naturally disappears (see Figure 1.2):

Soaking into the ground
The speed at which water soaks into the ground depends on many factors (see Table 16.1).

Table 16.1 Factors affecting how fast water soaks into the ground	
Water soaks into the ground faster when:	Water soaks into the ground slowly when:
The water-table is deep	The water-table is close to the surface
The soil is sandy	The soil is rocky or is clay
The land is flat	The land is sloped
Open land is available	Land is covered with buildings, paths and concrete, etc.
There are many trees and plants	There is little vegetation

Soaking away through the existing drainage system

Urban drainage systems begin in the housing areas with small drains (called the **secondary drainage system**). These connect to larger drains (the **primary drainage system**) which carries the wastewater to the receiving body of water, usually a river, lake or sea. Each system must be higher than the one it drains into, otherwise water will fail to flow unless pumps are used.

Communities can make important improvements to the secondary system at relatively low cost. The primary drainage system is usually the responsibility of city authorities.

Drains should be large enough to drain away water during the rainy season and to cope with periodic flooding. If flooding occurs less than about once every 10 years, large drainage systems are probably not worth the cost.

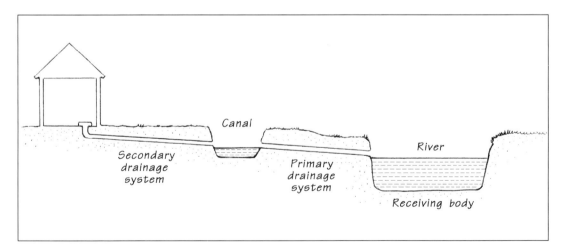

Figure 16.1   A typical community drainage system.

Evaporation into the air

The amount of water that evaporates depends on air temperature, humidity and wind speed. Hot, sunny weather causes water to evaporate very fast.

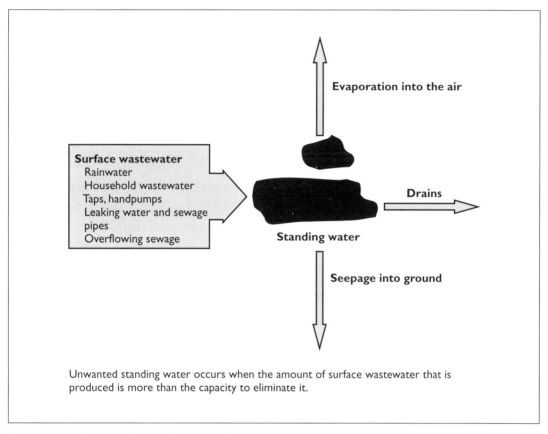

Unwanted standing water occurs when the amount of surface wastewater that is produced is more than the capacity to eliminate it.

Figure 16.2   Ways in which surface water is eliminated.

Why is standing water a major problem in low-income communities?

Slum communities usually have minimal means of eliminating wastewater. Water builds up in low-lying areas to form puddles, ponds, marshes, muddy areas or low-lying areas that flood. In richer communities, the piped sewerage system removes household wastewater, including excreta, and storm drains remove rainwater. This rarely happens in slum communities for the following reasons:

❶ **Slums have poor drainage systems or none at all**. These communities are usually considered illegal, meaning, as with water supplies and sanitation, the government often refuses to link the slum into the city's municipal drainage system. Drains that do exist in slums are usually unlined open trenches that have formed naturally or been dug by residents.

❷ **Slums are often located alongside large drains**, which overflow during the rainy season or when they become blocked downstream.

③ **Slums are often located in low-lying areas** that have no natural drainage. These areas are prone to flood during heavy rainfall.

④ **Slums may be located on steep hillsides** where lack of drainage causes fast flowing storm water to erode the land and cause landslides. Often buildings are damaged and shacks are washed away.

How does standing water cause illness?

Standing water can cause illness in the following ways:

① **It provides breeding sites for mosquitoes** that cause malaria, dengue fever, and filariasis.

② **It becomes contaminated with faeces** and causes diarrhoeal diseases, typhoid and hepatitis A and E if people drink contaminated surface water.

③ **It can seep through the ground and, if contaminated with human faeces, contaminate groundwater**, including shallow wells. The same diseases are caused.

④ **It provides a breeding place for snails** that carry the organism causing schistosomiasis. People bathing in the water can be infected through the skin, especially in Africa.

⑤ **It is a hazard that can cause drowning or injury**. Open drains are dangerous, especially for children who play near them.

⑥ When drainage is poor, **heavy rainfall causes flooding, landslides and collapsed buildings,** again leading to drowning and injury. This was seen on a huge scale in Nicaragua and Honduras in 1998 when Hurricane Mitch caused widespread devastation. A similar disaster occurred as a result of heavy rainfall in Venezuela in 1999.

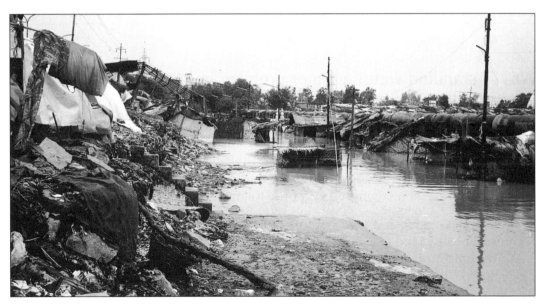

Figure 16.3   Many slum communities are located in low-lying areas and are often flooded during heavy rains. (ASHA)

Life in a slum

The Fernandez family, mother, father and 6-month-old baby boy, were asleep in their hut. They lived in a low-lying area that often flooded, especially after heavy rains. The water in their hut was about 15 cm deep, but the family decided it was probably safe to go to sleep. The next morning when they woke up, there was still only about 15 cm of water. But the baby was on the floor, dead. He had rolled off the bed during the night and drowned. (Ecuador)

What we need to do

Chapter 12, Environmental improvements, has broad outlines on each of the four phases described below. This chapter describes topics specifically related to wastewater.

Phase 1: Prepare the community for action

Step 1. Increase the knowledge and awareness of community members

Although communities dislike standing water – mainly because of its appearance and inconvenience, many residents do not realise it can cause serious disease. The community needs to know about:

1. Where surface wastewater comes from and how it is eliminated.
2. Why standing water is such a major problem in slums.
3. How standing water causes illnesses.
4. The government's legal responsibilities or targets (if any) to provide drainage services.
5. The names of government agencies and officials that deal with drainage issues.

In addition, community residents will need to develop a range of skills for any improvements decided on.

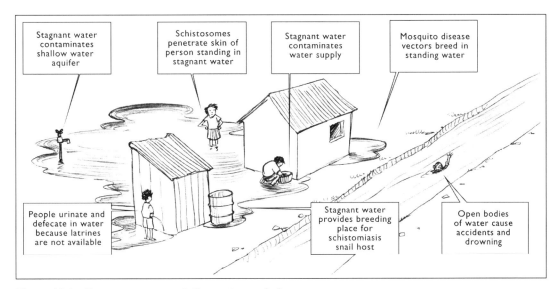

Figure 16.4   Stagnant water and disease transmission.

Step 2. Motivate the community to help solve the problem

When standing water is a serious problem, the community is often willing to help eliminate it. To further increase interest, we need to explain the full range of advantages:

① **It will make life more pleasant and convenient.** Residents won't have to wade through stagnant or stinking water. Bad smells will be less. The risk of landslides and floods will be reduced meaning less damage to houses.

② **Access will be easier** for vehicles, refuse collection and in case of emergencies such as fire.

③ **Mosquitoes will become less of a nuisance** and there will be less disease spread by them, especially dengue fever and malaria.

④ **Diarrhoea is likely to become less common.**

⑤ **House or rental values may improve.**

⑥ There will be **an increase in status** through living in a nicer environment.

Step 3. Channel action through organising the community

A Community Action Group or other committee needs to oversee changes. If an extensive system of drains is being considered, it can be helpful to form area groups based on each sector served by a common drain. A representative from each group can be seconded to the CAG while the programme is being carried out. Households in each group can make decisions that relate to their own area and be responsible for constructing and maintaining any improvements.

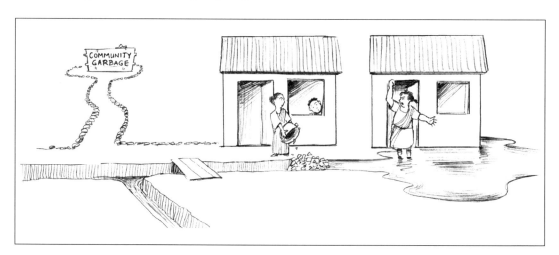

Figure 16.5   Keeping drains clean and functioning requires everyone's co-operation.

Phase 2: Help the community choose which problems to solve

Slum communities can do a great deal through their own efforts to reduce the problem of wastewater. They can even build or improve drainage systems with some technical help from outside. This can save large amounts of money.

Step 1. Gather information about the major problems with wastewater

Structures and problem areas in the community

When making the survey walk, we should ask the following questions:

❶ Where are the problem areas for standing water?

Identify and place on the map:

- All areas of standing water. Include those places where water only collects in the rainy season.
- The height water reaches during seasonal flooding – water lines may be visible on buildings or residents may remember the depth of the last flood.

❷ Where does the wastewater come from?

Identify and place on the map:

- All water points, public and private, by type (handpump, tap, etc.). Label on the map any which cause standing water (e.g. through leaks, poor drainage, major spills).
- All water pipes, tanks, and sewer pipes. Label on the map any leaks from pipes, overflowing septic tanks etc.
- Areas used for bathing and washing clothes. Label on the map areas where this normally causes standing water.
- Low-lying areas where rainwater collects.

❸ Why has the water not drained away?

Identify and label on the map:

- The direction of natural drainage and the flow paths of wastewater and floodwater.
- All man-made drains. Label where drains are blocked or broken.
- Areas of standing water with no drains.
- The places where drainage leaves the community.

> Although residents will not have a technical background, they can usually identify structures and problem areas, providing we give clear instructions. They may relate certain problems in the slum to construction work outside. For example a new road, large building or landfill site may have blocked a major drainage path.

What health problems could wastewater be causing?

If a major drainage system is being considered, an accurate map is essential. First try to obtain one from the municipal authorities or from another NGO. If none is available, architecture or engineering students from a local university, or private engineers might teach community members how to construct one. Mark on superimposed sheets, see page 199, all the items listed above.

Physical features of the land

Before planning a drainage system we will need to know about:

- the level of the water-table, see page 243,
- how often severe flooding occurs,
- the slope of the land,
- the type of soil.

The community will need technical help to discover these facts.

Relevant health problems in the community
We should find out about diseases that occur when there is standing water.

- Are diarrhoea, dengue fever, malaria or schistosomiasis common problems in the community?
- Is standing water obviously contaminated with human faeces?
- Label on the map the main areas for open defecation.
- Identify and label all latrines by type (see Chapter 15). Mark those where sewage is overflowing.
- Do people bathe, swim, wash clothes/dishes in areas of standing water? Label those places on the map.

For each illness that might be related to standing water, we will need to discover the frequency of that illness per season of the year. If a large colony is served by different clinics we need information for each separate area. When we know what illnesses are common, we can design our actions to have a maximum effect on reducing them. We will need to discover these from clinic and CHV records.

For example: in slums diarrhoea and intestinal worms are usually caused by a combination of poor sanitation, inadequate water supply, lack of personal hygiene and poor drainage. If these illnesses are common we should tackle each of these causes, starting with personal hygiene, especially hand washing.

If mosquito-borne illnesses are a problem our first priority will be to get rid of standing water. We will also encourage the use of mosquito nets and protective clothing.

Step 2. Discover the government's willingness and capacity to take action
The community will be able to make useful improvements without needing government help. For example it can repair leaking taps and install small drains to remove wastewater from bathing or washing areas. However, larger projects will require the help of government. This is true of any community-wide drainage system that must be connected to municipal drains or that leads to the discharge of large amounts of water. We will usually have to work hard to persuade the government to help with these improvements.

Step 3. Obtain technical advice
Drainage systems can be complex and mistakes can be costly. We will need technical advice from water engineers beginning at an early stage.

Steps 4 and 5. Consider the cost and sustainability of the various options

The community has many ways to reduce the amount of water standing outside each house and in communal areas of the colony. There are three broad categories of ways to reduce standing water:

❶ by decreasing the amount of wastewater that is produced;

❷ by increasing the amount of wastewater that seeps into the ground;

❸ by increasing the drainage of wastewater out of the community.

Within each broad category, the community has many options:

Decrease the amount of wastewater that is produced

❶ **Reduce the amount of water used by the household.** Rinse water can be used to water a garden. Hands can be washed using a water-saving can.

❷ **Repair leaking taps.**

❸ **Repair broken sewer and water lines.**

❹ **Clean out septic tanks and prevent them from overflowing.**

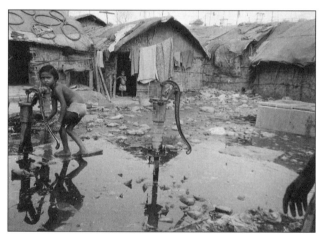

Figure 16.6   A water supply that is not properly drained can be a major source of standing water. (Godfrey Martin/ASHA)

In fact slum residents usually conserve water quite effectively at the household level because they have to carry or buy the water they need.

Increase the amount of wastewater that seeps into the ground

❶ **Add landfill to low-lying areas,** see illustration below.

❷ **Construct drains at water points** to prevent pooling of water.

❸ **Discourage the taking of mud from low-lying areas** for use in house building.

❹ **Encourage residents to plant kitchen gardens and other vegetation**, including trees when space is available.

❺ **Avoid covering the land surface with cement or other non-porous material** unless it is really needed.

Increase the drainage of wastewater out of the community
Special problems of flat areas

As we have seen, slums are often located on **flat areas** alongside streams or rivers because this land is available and has few other uses. Primary drainage systems often follow natural drainage channels such as streams and rivers. They are usually uncovered and often drain into these streams. Slum dwellers therefore have a double problem. They live alongside drains and streams full of polluted water, and their homes are sited on low-lying areas, which are difficult to drain, and frequently flood.

Flat areas are difficult to drain because:

❶ **The drainage gradient is low or non-existent**: When slums are located in low-lying flat areas, the land is almost as low as the body of water receiving the drainage, sometimes even lower. This limits the slope (or gradient) of the drains so that water drains away very slowly or not at all. This is especially true with underground drains, which are even lower than the land surface. Surface water therefore easily accumulates.

Solutions: A **temporary** solution, for example during the rainy season, is to use a water pump. The only **permanent** solution is landfill that raises the surface of the land well above the water-table, allowing drains to have a steeper gradient. The landfill must include the entire area, including land under the floors of the houses, otherwise houses will flood when the rest of the settlement remains dry. This means that dwellings will have to be rebuilt or modified.

> Before using a pump or depositing landfill, we need to make sure this will not cause a problem for other-low-lying areas nearby. Solving a problem for one area may create a problem for another.

❷ **Slow flow of water in the drains.** If drains have little or no gradient, silt builds up because the flow is so slow. Along with garbage thrown in higher up the system, this further blocks the drains.

Solution: Construct a small 'low-water' channel within the larger drain to channel water during drier periods of the year. Water will flow faster in this channel. This enables self-cleaning of the drain to take place, as the faster water speed carries silt downstream.

❸ **Tidal flooding**: In those cities near the sea, flooding into low-lying areas may be tidal. During the highest tides of the month or in stormy weather sea water flows into the colony.

Solution: It is possible, though expensive, to build a dyke to encircle the inhabited area. A sluice gate is installed through which all drainage from the settlement flows out. During high tide, the gate is closed to prevent sea water from entering the protected area.

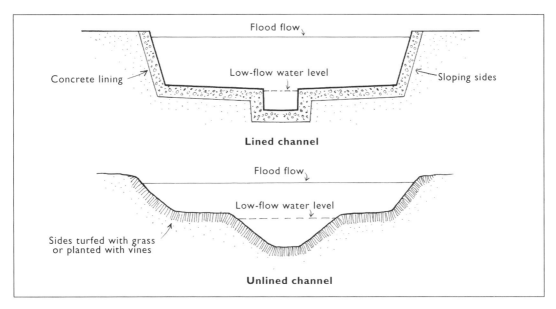

Figure 16.7 The use of low-flow channels helps to prevent blocked drains by increasing flow and removing silt.

Special problems of steep slopes

Steep slopes are another common site for slum communities. Sloped land is prone to soil erosion during heavy rainfall, especially when trees have been cut down and there is little vegetation. When hillsides are covered with dwellings little water can be absorbed by the soil. During heavy downpours rainwater pours through the settlement at great volume and speed, turning paths into gullies and undermining houses. Many slums in South America have grown up on slopes that are too steep for substantial buildings. Slopes of more than 5% are likely to have erosion problems, but many slums are on slopes with much higher gradients.

Solution: Water can sometimes be diverted laterally onto unused land, but this is only rarely available. Different types of drains and checkwalls can be built which help to decrease the flow of water.

Types of drain design

Building drains is the usual option to help remove wastewater. We need to choose whether these should be closed or open and whether or not they should be lined.

Open or closed drains? The main advantage of closed drains is that children are less likely to play or fall into polluted water (see Table 16.2). They also reduce mosquito breeding sites if drains are slow-flowing. A system that includes both open and closed drainage is the most difficult to keep clear: people throw garbage into the open section which then clogs up the closed section. A good compromise is to cover open drains with flat concrete covers that can be removed easily for cleaning. These prevent access to the polluted water and also provide space for footpaths. A grille should be placed at the entrance of any closed section of drain to capture garbage that can be removed easily.

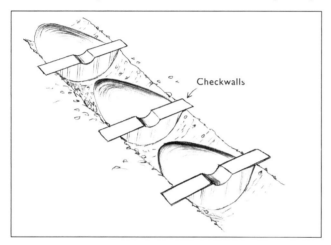

Checkwalls

Other design features: Drains can be unlined, partially lined or fully lined. Pre-fabricated drains are commonly used as they can be quickly laid. The type and size of drain chosen depends upon the gradient, rate of water flow including seasonal fluctuations, type of soil and cost. *Surface Water Drainage for Low-Income Communities* provides more information on this (see Resources).

Figure 16.8   Checkwalls can slow the rate of water flow on steep slopes.

Table 16.2 Some differences between closed and open drains	Closed	Open
Safety	More	Less
Mosquito breeding	More difficult to control, but fewer eggs laid	Easier to control, but more eggs laid
Flies, rats and other pests	Less	More
Gradient to receiving body	Tends to be less	Tends to be more
Space	Do not take up surface space (can be used as paths, etc.)	Take up surface space
Expertise required	More	Less
Maintenance	More difficult	Less difficult
Cost	More	Less

Step 6. Choose the best way forwards

As we have seen most communities have different areas of standing water, caused by varying factors and needing different solutions. A priority table can help a project and community decide which problems they should work on first, see page 62.

As much as possible, community residents should be given options, depending on the drainage problems of their house and relative costs. For example, some people may choose the more costly option of a drainage pipe running from inside the house direct to the drainage system. Others will choose the no-cost option of simply pouring their household waste into the drain that goes by their house.

Phase 3: Carry out the improvements

Although the Community Action Group or other committee will keep the process moving, plans should be developed in such a way that residents feel fully involved. For example, technical experts should share information with the whole community, not just with the committee. Community members with experience in sanitation and water supplies should be encouraged to share their opinions and be involved in construction.

Step 1. Mobilise skills

Community members can carry out most of the construction and maintenance tasks, even though engineers and other experts will need to advise on what changes to make and oversee any major changes. If members of the community do most of the construction work, large sums of money will be saved and the work will be of higher quality. With special training they can develop skills that will further improve their job opportunities in the future. Here are some of the tasks that can be done by community members:

- surveying and mapping,
- digging drains and septic tank,
- soil compacting,
- laying pipes,
- watering drain elements as they set,
- transporting supplies (sand, cement, pipes etc.),
- accounting,
- storing and guarding supplies.

Step 2. Approach government officials

If the community is thinking of installing an extensive drainage system, it will have to co-ordinate closely with the government to make sure that any solution is practical, and that the area can be effectively drained.

For drainage systems co-ordination with government is important for several reasons:

- **Permission** is usually required for new drainage systems, especially when located on government land, or if surrounding areas may be affected. As usual the government may be reluctant to give approval if there are plans to use the land differently in the future. Equally it will not be worth the community's trouble in making any changes.
- The government is often a good resource for **technical assistance, funding, loans, supplies and equipment**.
- **The community drainage system should complement the municipal system.** Even if the community funds and carries out its own drainage system, it will probably feed into the primary system or receiving body of water managed by the municipality (unless it can feed directly into a smaller river running alongside the community).

Step 3. Mobilise funding

Despite the example from Baroda (see below), most governments are very reluctant to expand their sewerage or drainage systems into new communities because of the high costs. Even if they help construct a system they are unlikely to maintain it, meaning it will quickly fall into disuse.

This means that slum communities themselves should plan, carry out and maintain low-cost improvements. They can contribute both in labour and cash. A properly prepared community can also see the wisdom of taking over the operation and maintenance of facilities which have previously been constructed by the government.

From the field: In Baroda, India, the concept of 'Slum Networking' has been developed in which slums are no longer seen as liabilities which drain resources. Instead they are seen as opportunities for improving the environment of the entire city. Slums are usually located in low-lying areas along natural drainage paths. These paths are the most appropriate for developing gravity-based drainage systems. An extensive city-wide drainage and sewerage system was created by incorporating these low-lying areas. New drains were placed to link up various low-lying areas as necessary. By providing a drainage system for the missing links within and between slums, it was possible to build up a city-wide system in a cost-effective manner. This system provides piped sewerage lines to each household, which also remove wastewater and stormwater. Because of the large number of families that could be connected to the system, including those living outside the slums, the scheme was affordable to most households, costing about the same as building a double pit latrine. The community paid for 50% of the cost of the work.

Lesson learned: When municipal authorities are enlightened, innovative improvements can upgrade the environment of an entire city.

Source: Author visit.

For all these options careful costings will need to be calculated. Outside loans or funding, from NGOs, government or industry, will be needed to make up the balance of any amounts the community is unable to afford.

From the field: A slum community in Karachi, Pakistan, whose streets were filled with standing water and excreta, constructed and maintained its own drainage system. An NGO, the Orangi Pilot Project, facilitated this by motivating the community to develop, construct and maintain the system, and by reducing costs to an affordable range through innovative technology. Using these means and removing the need for outside contractors, the costs of a household latrine, plot sewer and lane/street sewers and drains were kept down to less than $100 per household. The community was organised into lane groups (about 15 households on one lane), which managed the secondary sewers and drains. One representative from each group formed the neighbourhood committee (representing about 600 households) which managed the larger primary drains. Households were responsible for financing their share of the costs, helping with construction, and electing lane representatives. The committees maintain and operate the sewers within the zones they are responsible for. Money has always been managed by the community organisations. The NGO contributed less than 15% of the amount needed during the construction phase.

Lesson learned: Communities are willing to pay for and maintain a drainage system. Organisation into small lane groups enables improvements to take place.

Source: Serageldin Ismail, 1994.

Life in a slum

In a large Nairobi slum, part of the community is cut off by a small river of wastewater. Some enterprising young men have built and maintain a small footbridge over the smelly waters. People pay a small charge to use the bridge, which saves them much time when walking to their jobs.

Step 4. Train people in skills and tasks

We will need to make sure craftsmen are properly trained in construction. Also that the whole community understands about maintenance, how to keep the drains which run by their homes clear, and above all not to throw rubbish into the drains.

Step 5. Carry out pilot studies, build demonstration units and set up the improvement

Pilot studies can sometimes be useful in deciding which types of lining work best in different circumstances. Pilots studies can sometimes be avoided if community members, especially CAG members, visit neighbouring slums where improvements have been carried out. They can see which changes are most suitable in a range of circumstances.

In the case of a community-wide drainage system it is helpful to carry out work in one segment first where the problem of standing water is especially severe. Lessons can be learnt and benefits of the improvements will encourage other residents to start construction in their own areas.

Phase 4: Maintain and evaluate the changes

Maintenance

Dealing with surface water and making sure that drainage systems work is a continuing challenge to the community. Co-operation from all residents is important because only a small amount of garbage can block a main drain, causing great misery to those flooded by dirty water as a result. This list shows ways to help maintain the system:

1 Continue to educate the community:
  - not to throw garbage in drains,
  - not to allow children to defecate in drains,
  - that everyone must play their part in maintaining the system near their home.

2 Develop skills in community members:

  Some community members need to be trained in the technical skills of cleaning drains and making simple repairs.

3 Empower Community Action Group for the tasks of:
  - supervising and organising regular maintenance and repair work, especially if new drainage systems have been installed;
  - liaising with government to clean and repair drains that require special equipment and skills.

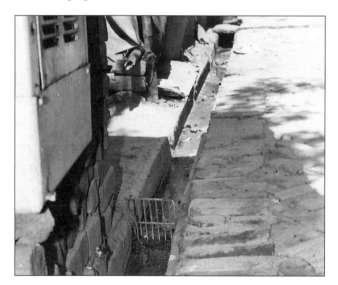

Figure 16.9   Grilles placed at stategic locations to hold back rubbish, can help to identify who is throwing rubbish into the drains. (Godfrey Martin/ASHA)

Maintaining the improvements

Even if the municipality is responsible for cleaning and maintaining drains, it is unlikely to do much in practice. This means the community itself should strongly consider taking over this responsibility. It is far more likely to do it effectively.

For a drainage system, the major task is to keep the drains clean. This has to be a community-wide responsibility, otherwise the whole system fails. The community must decide how to organise the regular cleaning of drains. Here are some possible arrangements:

1 **Each household** is responsible for the drains that run by the house.

2 Some **residents** are responsible for cleaning and are paid by monthly fees collected from the community by the CAG. The CAG in effect hires, supervises and pays the workers, and also supplies them with special equipment, including gloves, scrapers, brooms, shovels, wheelbarrows or carts.

③ A **youth (or other) group** is responsible for keeping the drains clean. There will need to be an incentive. For example residents could pay fees that help fund youth group activities, such as buying footballs or paying for football coaching.

④ **Rotating groups** of community members are responsible for cleaning.

> In some cultures, a particular caste or tribe traditionally does the cleaning tasks, including the disposal of human waste. A community-wide effort to maintain a drainage system is an opportunity of breaking down these degrading traditions.

Slums are often made up of people groups from different areas, traditions, practices and loyalties. It may be difficult to maintain drains because of the co-operation needed from different households. Here are some practical ways of helping this problem:

- Place grilles at regular intervals in the drainage system, for example where open sections become closed, or per fixed length of drain. This helps to show who is dumping rubbish, makes the task of cleaning simpler, and makes it easier to distribute the workload fairly.

- Pre-set sanctions with community agreement, so that pressure is brought on residents or sectors who do not do their share.

Cleaning drains can be made much easier when low-cost tools are used:

- Use shovels that exactly fit the width of the drain, and contain bore holes to let water drain through.

- Use wheelbarrows or carts which have holes in the bottom to let water drain out as the cart is being filled.

- Use agricultural hoes with extra long handles.

> For drains to work efficiently, a system for solid waste disposal must exist in the community. Otherwise residents will dump their rubbish into drains. In addition, If solid waste removed from drains is not disposed off-site, it will find its way back into the drainage system.

In addition to routine cleaning, the CAG should organise an intensive community-wide cleaning (and repair) of the secondary drains once a year. This should be at the end of any dry season when the smallest amount of water will be present in drains.

The community will also need to monitor the cleaning and de-silting, of larger, primary drains. If these drains become blocked, secondary drains will overflow.

Repairs

Drains may malfunction because they get blocked with garbage, vegetation, silt, or collapsed parts of the drain itself. Collapsed drains can be caused by soil erosion around the drains, the weight of vehicles driving over them or the effect of tree roots.

The CAG must organise a system to monitor the need for repairs and arrange for the supplies labour and payment. This should also include an annual inspection.

Evaluation

Our main objectives will be to remove the wastewater that accumulates in the slum and to reduce illnesses caused by standing water.

Process indicators could be the number of houses that have functional secondary drains, or the number of neighbourhood drainage committees that are functional.

Impact indicators could be:

1. The number and size of stagnant water areas, as estimated before and after the improvements. Community members can estimate or measure this.

2. The frequency of illness directly related to the amount of standing water. Dengue fever and malaria are probably the most widespread, and we can gather information from clinic and CHV records. The frequency of diarrhoea will indicate how effective environmental improvements have been in general, including sanitation, water supply and wastewater disposal.

Chapter summary

Standing water is usually a serious inconvenience and health hazard in slum communities. Its sources include rainwater, household wastewater, run-off from leaking water points, and overflowing sewage from septic tanks or blocked sewer pipes. Standing water can cause mosquito-borne diseases, such as malaria and dengue fever, and contribute towards diarrhoeal diseases. Open drains pose the risk of drowning or injury, especially for children. The removal of wastewater depends on the ability of water to soak into the ground, largely determined by the water level, evaporation and on the effectiveness of drainage systems. Buildings and paved surfaces decrease the amount of ground available to absorb water.

The first step is to understand the reasons why standing water collects, the diseases it can cause and any rights the community might have for drainage and related services, including water and sanitation. The next phase is to decide which approach is best for the community. Residents gather information about wastewater problems through a survey walk and mapping, and consider the physical aspects of the site, soil and drainage, usually with expert advice. They then estimate the cost of various options, and the ability of government or NGOs, to give loans or assistance. Further help from technical experts will be needed to guide the community in the best decisions.

Based on these findings, the community draws up a priority list, considers its options and makes its choices. The plan is implemented, ideally after a pilot study, especially if constructing drains is the option chosen. The community organises a system for cleaning and making regular repairs, and helps in evaluating the programme regularly.

Resources

1. *Surface Water Drainage for Low-Income Communities*. WHO, 1991. A very practical, step-wise approach laid out for communities interested in improving drainage.

17 Other environmental hazards

In this chapter, we shall consider:

What we need to know about the following hazards:

Solid waste

Flooding

Electricity and fire

Vehicles

The workplace

Air pollution

Noise pollution

What we need to do:

Phase 1: Prepare the community for action

Phase 2: Help the community to choose which problems to solve

Phase 3: Carry out the improvements

Phase 4: Maintain and evaluate the changes

What we need to know

The urban poor are at greater risk than others from illness or injury caused by environmental dangers. These are difficult to overcome. Most are beyond the resources of individuals to deal with, unless they develop a strong sense of community oganisation and advocacy. The government usually has little interest in enforcing or implementing health and safety regulations, including any laws to reduce pollution or enforce safety at work.

The CHDP can do a lot to help residents learn more about these hazards, take steps to lessen them and press for changes from the government.

Hazards from solid waste

Solid waste includes the whole range of rubbish, garbage and dirt that collects in a slum. Solid wastes are substances that result from human activities that are no longer wanted or needed by their users. In this chapter the term waste does not specifically refer to human waste and excreta.

Piles of rotting food, plastic bags, cans, bottles and other materials build up in the streets, sometimes making huge, dangerous and stinking piles. Even when household garbage reaches collection bins, problems still occur. It may overflow because the contents of the bin are not removed regularly. In addition, scavengers may spread garbage about as they look for items to resell, and animals may rummage through garbage for food.

What are the main sources of solid waste?

Household waste

The major human activity that produces solid waste is preparing food. This may include:

- ashes from a cooking fire;
- paper, plastic and tins from items that have been bought;
- inedible parts of fruit, vegetables and meat;
- uneaten food scraps.

Household waste can also contain dangerous substances such as medicines, batteries, paints and cleaning materials, needles and syringes, but these are usually less common than from richer neighbourhoods.

The urban poor produce less household waste per household than richer households because items that come in bottles, tins and plastic wrapping are usually too costly. But

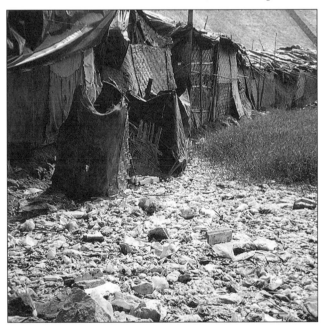

because of the high density of population, slum communities can generate a huge amount of solid waste each day.

Waste from streets and drains

Waste that accumulates in the streets and drains includes dirt and grit, paper and plastic bags, and other household garbage that is dumped into the drains. When latrines are not available or not used, people, usually children, defecate into drains. This means that in slums, waste on the streets and drains tends to be a mixture of household waste contaminated with human excreta.

Figure 17.1   Garbage often accumulates in slum communities.

Construction and industrial wastes

Slums are often located near (or on) construction sites. Typical examples of waste include metal, bricks, wood and other building materials. The urban poor often use these 'waste' materials to build their own houses.

Most industrial waste is not dangerous to health. However, some manufacturing processes produce acid or caustic materials, substances that can easily catch fire, or chemicals which are toxic to humans and animals. These materials are often discharged into nearby bodies of water, dumped on nearby land, or in the case of gases, discharged untreated into the air. Slums often become established near industries that provide low-paid employment. People living in these communities are at high risk of industrial diseases. A terrible example of this was the accidental release of methyl isocyanate gas from a factory in Bhopal, India in 1985, that killed over 3000 people living in slums near the factory, and injured more than 100,000 people.

Fruit or vegetable canneries may produce piles of rotting vegetables or fruit as waste products. Animal slaughterhouses can generate a large amount of solid waste that needs urgently disposal. Slums are often located near such areas because others find the sights and smells unbearable.

> **From the field**: In 1991 in a warehouse along the municipal port docks of Bangkok, Thailand, sacks containing chemicals exploded, presumably from the high mid-day temperatures. Nearby drums of alcohol, paint thinner and chemicals exploded soon afterwards. Klong Toey Slum is located just beyond the port docks and storage areas. This community bore the brunt of this chemical fire. Within minutes over 600 homes were destroyed. Even today, many people are still suffering from the effects of the toxic cloud that engulfed the community.
>
> **Lessons learned**: Low-income communities are often located in hazardous industrial or commercial areas and are therefore at risk of being affected by industrial accidents.
>
> **Source**: Human Resource Center, 1996

How is solid waste disposed of in slums?

At the household level

Household waste is usually dumped outside the house in a path-side drain. It should be placed in a bin or bag and then carried to a municipal garbage bin.

At the neighbourhood level

Slum communities seldom have government-paid street cleaners who keep the paths and drains clean. When cleaners are provided, they are often poorly supervised, frequently fail to attend and rarely do a good job. One main reason why street cleaners dislike working in slums is that human faeces contaminate the streets and paths. In practice therefore paths and drains are not usually cleaned unless the community organises its own system of cleaning.

At the community level

In developing countries, the municipal government rarely provides garbage collection for slum communities. As a result, garbage clutters the area, blocks drains, and gathers in piles on any open area that is informally selected as a place for dumping. In areas where garbage collection does take place it is often irregular and infrequent so that garbage overflows the bins.

What health problems are associated with solid waste?

People who live near solid waste have an increased risk of health problems. This is especially the case for young children who play in areas where garbage is thrown, and scavengers who earn their living by sorting through rubbish. Table 17.1 lists health problems that are frequently seen near solid waste.

Frequent, regular and reliable garbage collection reduces a wide variety of health risks.

Table 17.1 Health problems from solid waste	
Health problems	Cause
Dengue fever, malaria, filariasis and other mosquito-borne diseases	Standing water in tins, glass, barrels etc., and blocked drains provide breeding sites for mosquitoes
Rabies and plague, animal bites	Stray animals are attracted to garbage as a food source
Cuts, tetanus, hepatitis B and skin infections	Sharp objects, broken glass, etc. are buried in garbage
Diarrhoeal diseases	Drinking water supply is polluted by solid waste run-off
Chemical toxicity	Drinking water and food are contaminated by run-off from industrial waste piles

Hazards from flooding

Because slums are often situated in low-lying areas that drain poorly, they are prone to flooding. With houses at ground level there is no barrier to prevent water from sweeping through the shacks. Thus an entire community can be flooded in a very short time.

When a community is flooded, government and aid agencies will often provide urgent needs such as safe water, latrines and tents. The CHDP should not duplicate these efforts if they are coming from another source, but it should work closely with those providing emergency relief. The CHDP should also spend time with community members and give emotional support. When the government and aid agencies withdraw, the CHDP can provide tangible and co-ordinated support as the community rebuilds.

Life in a slum

Thokar is a large slum in Delhi that is located on the flood plain of the Jumuna River. Every 2 or 3 years, the monsoon is so heavy that the river overflows and the entire slum is under water. Often the flooding is very sudden because water has been released from a dam upriver. Usually when a release is going to happen, the police are notified and they inform the community to expect the flooding. One morning Laxmi was at home in Thokar. She was in labour with her second child. The community midwife was with her and the baby was delivered. But before the placenta was delivered, sudden flooding occurred. Laxmi and the midwife had to flee with the umbilical cord still attached to the undelivered placenta. They had to wade through the rising floodwaters. The police had forgotten to inform the community that water was going to be released upriver. The baby died of overwhelming infection.

What are the health risks from flooding?

Flooding itself can cause illness or injury (Table 17.2). But flooding can also cause illness and injury through the displacement it causes.

Hazards from electricity and fire

It is not surprising that catastrophic fires are common in slum communities. There are several reasons for this:

1. **Faulty electric wiring**. Electric power is seldom provided legally, and nearby electric power lines are often tapped illegally. Home-made connections hang down from cables into houses, overloading and short-circuiting the system. The supply is not earthed and fuses are not used. Residents have a variety of risks: burns from improper wiring, electric shocks or death from electrocution, and fires.

   Slum dwellers are usually willing to pay for electricity, as it can make such a huge difference to their standard of life. In tropical slums daylight lasts only about 12 hours meaning it becomes dark by early evening. It is also extremely hot, and people can become desperate for electric fans. Some home-based industries need electricity.

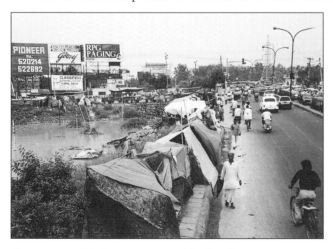

   However the government is usually not willing to provide connections, especially in cities where demand for electricity far outstrips the supply. This may be short-sighted since the slum dwellers (and many others) simply connect up illegally, and large amounts of money are lost through theft of electricity. By providing legal connections, some income would be generated for the electricity suppliers (government or private company) even if the supply was subsidised.

Figure 17.2   Displacement caused by flooding poses great difficulties, especially the lack of safe water and sanitation. (ASHA)

Table 17.2 Health problems from flooding related displacement	
Health problem	Cause
From flooding	
Drowning	High water, especially if rise in water level is sudden
Diarrhoeal diseases	Latrines overflow causing faecal contamination of the flood waters
Snake bite	Snakes, which are disturbed and displaced by flooding, seek land, where displaced people gather
Cuts, infections	Sharp objects deposited in silt (exposed during clean-up)
Leptospirosis (Weil's disease)	Water contaminated with rat urine
From displacement	
Diarrhoeal illnesses, typhoid and cholera	Latrines are not available so open defecation occurs
	Safe drinking water is not available.
Road-side accidents	The displaced remain as near their old homes as possible: no land is available so they settle on roadsides and by the edges of railways
Increasing poverty	Loss of household goods
	Theft and vandalism
	Cost of re-building

Life in a slum

During a hot spell, illegal tapping caused local overload and burned out the neighbourhood transformer on several occasions, leaving a slum community and its middle class neighbours without power. Repair of the transformer took hours or days. During one particularly long period without power, tension between slum dwellers and the affected middle class residents living nearby, erupted into a heated fist fight. (Pakistan)

❷ **Illegal tapping of natural gas lines**. In some cities with piped natural gas, the lines are tapped illegally. Accidental fire from a leaking gas line can be disastrous since the gas line continues to provide fuel as the fire progresses.

❸ **The use of open fires for cooking**. Open cooking fires, especially those using kerosene or gas are serious fire hazards. Gas cylinders sometimes leak and cause fires. In the usual slum dwelling, four or more people may be living in a single room that is only 2 by 2 metres in area. That allows no space to provide protection from an open cooking fire, especially with small children running about.

④ **Storage of materials that burn easily and/or emit toxic fumes while burning**. Materials used for work may be stored in or around the house. Garbage recyclers store their materials until they have enough to sell; much of this is plastic and paper that burns easily.

⑤ **High-density housing**. Slum housing is wall to wall, allowing fire to spread with terrifying speed.

⑥ **Lack of roads and narrow lanes**. Narrow lanes makes it hard to escape quickly especially when fire is already engulfing nearby houses. Narrow roads make it hard for fire engines and emergency vehicles to reach the affected area.

⑦ **Lack of water**. Limited access to water may make it very difficult for community members and fire fighters to put out the fire.

> Fires may be intentionally set; a frustrated landowner or even a government body may find arson the easiest way to clear the land.

What are health risks from fire?
Table 17.3 lists the main health risks from fire.

Table 17.3 Health risks from fire	
Health problem	**Cause**
Burns, smoke inhalation, death	Fire with no means of escape
Toxic burns or damage to lungs, eyes, etc.	Burning toxic materials
Road-side accidents	The displaced stay as near their homes as possible to guard their possessions: there is nowhere else to go so they camp by the side of the road and by railway lines
Increasing poverty	Loss of household goods
	Theft and vandalism
	Cost of re-building
Fear of fire in the future	Unresolved trauma from a previous bad experience

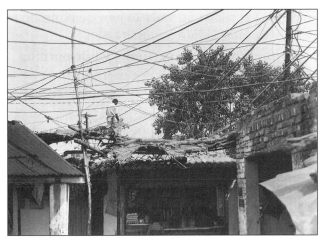

Figure 17.3 *Illegal tapping of electricity poses a serious fire hazard in most slums. (Godfrey Martin/ASHA)*

Hazards from vehicles

The urban poor are at risk of serious injury or death in road accidents for the following reasons:

- Poor residents often travel by foot or bicycle. When a collision occurs, they have no protection.
- Slums are often located alongside busy roads or railways. Young children may wander into the path of a vehicle or train.
- Mothers and children often beg on the streets or sell goods at traffic lights.

Life in a slum

A mother and her young son were asleep in their hut, which was located right next to a busy street. In the middle of the night, a drunk motorist lost control of his vehicle, which crashed into the hut killing her and her young son instantly. (Nigeria)

Hazards in the workplace

There is a huge range of occupational health problems that especially affect the poor. They are often involved in risky, unregulated work in manufacturing or construction. They may use dangerous tools and machinery that is old and not maintained in good working order. They may be exposed to toxic chemicals. They are often subjected to dangerous working conditions and long working hours. In developing countries, there are few laws that protect workers. And often laws that do exist are not obeyed or enforced.

What are health risks in the workplace?
Mechanical/physical
Injuries or illness due to:

- dangerous tools and equipment,
- unsafe structures,
- unshielded or broken machines, or machines with safety features removed,
- heavy manual labour,
- noise, vibration, and radiation,
- environment filled with dust or fumes,
- severe heat or cold.

Chemical/biological

Injuries or illnesses due to:

- heavy metals, solvents, pesticides and other toxic chemicals,

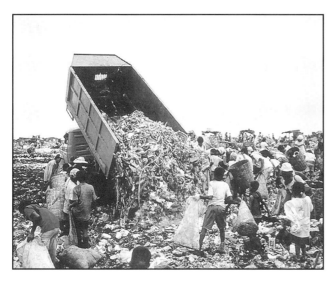

- viruses, bacteria, parasites, fungi and mould, including hepatitis B and HIV infection from hospital waste contaminated with blood.

Psychological/Social

Illnesses due to:

- work-related stress due to low pay, long or irregular working hours, strenuous labour,
- gender inequalities and harassment on the job,
- child labour.

Figure 17.4   Garbage recycling is hazardous work. (Greenleaf/Tearfund)

Reproductive (especially risky for women)

- infertility, fetal death or pregnancy-related problems from chemicals or excessive work or tiredness.

Hazards from air pollution

Indoor air pollution

There are two dangerous forms of indoor pollution in crowded slums. The first comes from the use of open fires with polluting fuels such as kerosene, coal or animal dung. Pollution by cooking fires may be so great that it can even seriously affect the outdoor air quality of the neighbourhood. The second is the effect of tobacco smoke. WHO describes cigarettes as follows: 'cleverly crafted products that deliver just the right amount of nicotine to keep their users addicted for life before killing them'. Unfortunately tobacco smoking by adults also kills children from the effects of inhaling the smoke (passive smoking) and causes them to start the habit themselves. Women and children are at greatest risk of being affected by indoor air pollution.

The rule of 1000: A pollutant that is released indoors is 1000 times more likely to reach someone's lung than a pollutant that is released outside (WHO).

Outdoor air pollution

Since the major causes of air pollution are motor vehicles, coal-burning power units and industry, it is no surprise that cities have major problems with air pollution. In developing countries the problem is made worse because:

- Vehicles are poorly maintained.
- A large proportion of vehicles are fuelled by diesel, which is more polluting than petrol.
- There are non-existent or poorly enforced vehicle anti-pollution laws.
- There is widespread use of polluting cooking fuels.
- There are are non-existent or poorly enforced industrial pollution laws. This is a growing and dangerous problem in many poor industrial cities in developing countries, China, Eastern Europe and parts of the former Soviet Union. In some of these cities there is an additional risk of nuclear radiation from reactors that generate electricity.

What are the health risks from air pollution?

Many pollutants are released into the atmosphere. Common ones include sulphur dioxide, nitrogen dioxide, carbon monoxide, lead and ozone. Many of these cause inflammation, which reduces the ability of the lungs and bronchial tubes to fight off infection. In turn, respiratory infection makes the lungs and bronchi more susceptible to air pollution. The cycle can repeat itself so many times that people end up with emphysema and chronic obstructive lung disease.

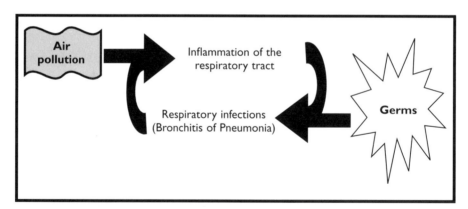

Figure 17.5   The vicious cycle of air pollution and respiratory infections.

In addition to these pollutants, 'greenhouse gases' such as excessive carbon dioxide caused by motor vehicles and from burning fuels such as wood and coal causes the environment to overheat with resultant changes in climate (global warming). This adds to climatic extremes such as the risk of flooding, drought or heat waves, depending on location.

Air pollution also contributes to conjunctivitis and also increases the risk of heart disease and lung cancer.

Hazards from noise

In cities, noise pollution comes from a variety of sources:

- road traffic, trains and aeroplanes,
- construction and other industries,
- loudspeakers broadcasting loud music, religious or political messages,
- loud personal music systems or 'ghetto-blasters',
- noisy parties or drunken residents.

Slums are frequently located alongside roads, near to factories and airports, and on land that cannot be developed for other use because of severe noise. In addition, slum dwellers often work on construction sites or in factories so they are exposed day and night, both at home and in the workplace.

What are the health risks from noise pollution?

High noise levels of noise frequently cause the following:

- sleep disturbances, especially if noise is present during the night – this in turn can cause tiredness, and reduce resistance to infections,
- mental stress,
- poor work performance,
- hearing loss.

What we need to do

Although the community alone may not be able to eliminate these hazards there are three useful things we can do to help lessen the problems:

1. Identify hazards that are present in the community.
2. Consider actions to eliminate those hazards.
3. If the hazard cannot be eliminated, encourage individuals and the community to take actions that will reduce their effects.

Phase 1: Prepare the community for action

Step 1. Increase the knowledge and awareness of community members

The community should learn about environmental hazards that are present within the slum or the workplace. In particular they should be aware of:

- the causes of the hazard,
- potential health problems that can result from the hazard,
- existing laws that may protect against the hazard,
- ways to eliminate the hazard or to minimise exposure to it (see Table 17.4).

Table 17.4   Ways of minimising risks from environmental hazards

Solid waste	• Educate community on ways to dispose of household waste and show them what should **not** be done
	• Organise a campaign to increase proper disposal of household waste
	• Install garbage bins that prevent entry by animals
	• Learn rights and laws about municipal cleaners, garbage bins, and garbage collection vehicles
	• Press municipality to collect garbage regularly from community collection sites
	• Hire and supervise street cleaners, ideally from the community, to keep streets and footpaths clean
	• Consider organising the collection of solid waste into three types: items for recycling, waste that generates fertiliser (composting), and unusable waste
	• Organise a campaign to remove mosquito-breeding sites in the community
	• Investigate possibility of whether there is chemical pollution from near-by industries
Flooding hazards	• Ensure that authorities inform slum when upriver dams are released
	• Weigh advantages and disadvantages of relocation
Electrical hazards	• Press for legal electrical connections for community households
	• Monitor existing wiring
Fire hazards	• Press for legal hook-ups to natural gas lines for the community
	• Check illegal hook-ups to gas line for leaks
	• Monitor homes for flammable chemicals
Vehicular accidents	• Avoid unnecessary risks when travelling on roads
	• Avoid travel during rush hour
	• Avoid begging/selling at traffic lights
	• Travel on less busy streets (unless a security risk)
Workplace hazards	• Avoid drinking alcohol before operating machinery or travelling
	• Obey safety rules when operating dangerous machinery
	• Advocate for safe working conditions in factories
Air pollution	• If possible, cook with clean fuel (natural gas or electricity)
	• If not possible, install smokeless cooking stove/chimney or cook outdoors
	• If not possible, provide ventilation if cooking indoors
	• Stop smoking tobacco inside the house and preferably stop completely
	• Avoid travel during rush hour
	• Take less travelled streets
Noise pollution	• Encourage setting radios, tape players at low volume
	• Advocate for ear protectors when working with loud equipment

Step 2. Motivate the community

There are several reasons it may be hard to motivate the community, unless a hazard is very obvious and disturbing:

- **Many harmful effects only take place gradually**. They may be slow to appear, lead to chronic illness and sometimes the problem and its cause may not even be linked in people's minds. For example many do not understand the long term effects of cigarette smoke or traffic pollution, nor realise that prolonged noise can lead to deafness. These facts make it hard to get support to bring about change.

- **The damage to health is not obvious because other factors also contribute to the illness** and are blamed for it. For example, air pollution does not cause a cold or flu, but it does weaken the respiratory tract so if a person gets flu it can easily lead to pneumonia.

- **The residents may feel powerless to do anything**. Hazards are often caused by events outside the community and beyond its control.

> Often, the precipitating event that moves a community to action is the death or serious injury of a resident, or a major catastrophe in the community. The CHDP should see this as an opportunity for change.

The CHDP can help to overcome fatalism and encourage people to act. As people understand how serious the hazards are and that there may be laws to protect them, they become more motivated to take action. The community needs convincing that they can, should and must work for change instead of passively accepting dangerous situations.

Phase 2: Help the community choose which problems to solve

Step 1. Gather information about environmental problems

Residents need to look at the situation in their own homes, community and workplace to determine what hazards are present. This can be done through a systematic walk and mapping, using a different transparent sheet to overlay the map for each type of hazard surveyed (see page 199).

Structures and hazards in the community
Solid waste hazards

❶ Find out about the complete process of garbage disposal. Trace garbage from when it is first produced in the household to when it is finally removed from the community. We can ask these questions about:

Inside the dwelling:
- Is the house clean?
- Are food scraps kept in a covered container?

- Is garbage disposed of daily?
- Where is household garbage disposed of?

Around the dwelling:
- Are paths/roads/drains clean?
- Who cleans them and how often/regularly?

From the community:
- Is garbage collected regularly?
- Is the garbage bin full and overflowing?
- Do scavengers scatter garbage?
- Do animals (dogs, cows, buffaloes, goats, pigs) rummage through garbage?

❷ Find out about defecation:
- Where do adults normally defecate? If outside what happens to the faeces?
- Where do children defacate? What happens to the faeces?

❸ Find out about neighbouring factories or other industries.
- Do they discharge any waste products into a body of water?
- Do they have a chimney (smokestack)? Does it discharge visible smoke?
- Do they have materials piled up outside? What are they?

❹ Find out about nearby animal slaughterhouses, food processing plants or large vegetable markets.
- How is the waste disposed of?
- How well does the disposal system work?

Flooding hazards

❶ Discover those areas of the community that are most prone to flooding: Look for high water marks on buildings, and map low-lying areas where standing water has gathered. Ask longer-term residents about previous floods – how often and how severe they are.

❷ Check drains for blockages.

Fire and electrical hazards

❶ Find out about electric power:
- Are there many illegal connections?
- Is wiring overloaded?
- Is wiring frayed and worn out?

❷ Is natural gas used as a a fuel?
- Are gas lines illegally tapped?

❸ Find out about the heat source for cooking
- What types of cooking stoves and fuels are used?
- Where is spare fuel stored?

❹ Find out if flammable materials are stored in the house.

❺ Indicate on the community map roads that are wide enough for emergency vehicles (if any).

Vehicle hazards

❶ Indicate major roads and railway tracks on the community map and walls or barriers between these and the community.

❷ Find out if cycle – or auto-rickshaw driving is a common occupation in the community.

Workplace hazards

❶ Find out the major types of employment of community members, including women and children.

❷ If many community members work in a factory or the slum is located near a factory, find out what the factory produces and what machinery and chemicals are used.

❸ Discover the cause of any road accidents or occupational health injuries, by asking community members, health workers or CHVs.
   ● Why did they happen?
   ● How could they have been prevented?

Air and noise pollution

❶ Identify the nearby roads, railway tracks and airports that generate air or noise pollution.

❷ Identify nearby factories, manufacturing units or power plants that generate air or noise pollution.

❸ Obtain an estimate of the number of adults and older children who smoke tobacco. This can be done by a survey. It may have been discovered when making the community diagnosis.

❹ Find out if conjunctivitis, 'flu', chronic coughs and asthma are common complaints.

❺ Does there seem to be an association between these illnesses and anyone in the household smoking tobacco, or using a polluting fuel for indoor cooking?

Social and cultural factors

We should look at traditional practices and determine which ones, if changed, might reduce a particular hazard. For example, traditional cooking practices may have to be changed so that cleaner fuels, such as natural gas, are used instead of kerosene or animal dung.

Step 2. Discover the government's willingness and capacity to take action

Government action will be needed for many improvements. One key area is the setting up of a reliable garbage disposal system. Another important area is to try to make factories and workplaces safer through enforcing any health and safety regulations.

Step 3. Obtain technical advice

Dealing with environmental hazards is a technically complex area, so we will need expert technical help. For example:

- **Building chimneys for cooking stoves and using cleaner fuel**. Although these changes are quite easy to make, the key skill is to help people follow designs which are culturally acceptable. Call in an expert to advise and to discuss options with women. Also to advise about cheap alternative sources of cooking fuel.
- **Health hazards of common jobs**. When the common types of employment are known we can ask experts with special knowledge about the hazards of those jobs.
- **Legal rights**. Lawyers with an interest in community affairs can help discover and explain legal rights to slum residents. This is especially helpful in improving conditions at work and to press for anti-pollution controls. They can guide on how best to lobby government officials or to mount a campaign.

Phase 3: Carry out the improvements

Step 1. Mobilise resources

There are strong worldwide movements to help protect the environment. This is a key issue for those living in slums, who suffer the worst effects, even if they don't understand the causes, and are relatively powerless to make changes.

Nearly every city will have groups that are interested in making a healthier environment. We should ask them for information and advice. They can often help with advocacy. Here are some groups that may help:

- NGOs and advocacy groups interested in cleaning up the environment,
- health-oriented groups like cancer or tuberculosis societies,
- tobacco-control groups,
- school children to do pollution checks and create awareness of the issues,
- helpful members of the local or national press, radio or television,
- labour unions.

From the field: The municipal government of Curitiba, Brazil has set up a programme in which garbage is exchanged for food. In these communities, conventional garbage trucks are unable to reach the community because roads are too narrow. Households separate recyclable materials such as metal, glass, paper and plastic from organic waste, placing these in different bags for recycling. Residents then bring the garbage in trolleys to the nearest collection points. The garbage is exchanged for fruits and vegetables, which are low cost surplus products from the surrounding agricultural area. In holiday seasons and at the beginning of the school year, the programme includes toys, fruitcakes and school supplies. The recyclable materials are sold and the remainder of the garbage is used for landfill. This Green Exchange Programme Serves 55 underprivileged communities in Curitiba. The efficient recycling has allowed Curitiba to expand the useful life of its landfill areas by reducing the amount of solid waste that must be dumped.

Source: Author visit.

Step 2. Approach government officials

Although it may seem futile to approach the government with large-scale demands, a great deal can be done when people join together to lobby for important changes. Sometimes demands for anti-pollution legislation can be effective when many people from different groups together press for the same changes. If there are motivated individuals with influence in the government, it may be possible to design innovative approaches at relatively low cost.

Step 3. Mobilise funding

Funding is generally not something that limits actions taken at individual level. Most useful actions are related to changes in behaviour. Supplies for installing smokeless cooking stoves with simple chimneys are usually fairly low cost. The government should be responsible for refuse collection. There are a variety of funding sources for projects involved in wider environmental improvements.

Step 4. Train community members

The most effective training is to help people change their behaviours. At community level a number of small changes can make large differences to health and safety. Examples include: reducing tobacco smoking, changing cooking patterns, disposing garbage more effectively, wearing helmets when cycling, which can dramatically reduce injuries on the roads.

Changes in behaviour do not come easily. We will need to arrange intensive training and promotional campaigns, helping people to understand **why it is worthwhile for them** to make these changes.

> We should invest a great deal of time and effort in school children. By training them in good practices a whole community can change its behaviours over a few years, especially if children demonstrate the value of changes to their parents and siblings.

Steps 5 and 6. Carry out pilot studies, build demonstration units and promote their use

If slum residents choose to carry out any community-wide improvements, it will be worth running a pilot project first. Take smokeless cooking stoves: the community should test out two or three different designs in different homes. This will help community members make sure that the stoves work well, and to choose which design they prefer. It will also help them see the advantages of having houses free of smoke.

The community may decide that keeping the streets clean from garbage is the top priority. They could then pilot a system in which cleaners are paid by the community to clean paths and drains each day. But within this system some may opt to pay an additional amount for the cleaners to remove their garbage to a collection site. If these options work well in one part of the community, they can be extended to another.

Step 7. Set up the improvements or build the facility

Phase 4: Maintain and evaluate the changes

Maintenance
For each activity we will need to make sure that behavioural change is sustained and that any improvements are cared for and repaired. For both of these there will need to be continuing reminders, reinforcement and education. Otherwise there could be a gradual return to the old ways of doing things.

Improvements in waste disposal will need monitoring and organising by the CAG. There should be regular inspections.

Evaluation
This cannot be easily summarised as it will depend on which of many activities have been carried out. For any major activity we should however select indicators and make sure that changes are evaluated.

One example is removing cooking smoke form inside houses. A **process indicator** could be the percentage of homes making a change to smokeless cooking fuel or improved ventilation. An **impact indicator** would be any change in the number of respiratory and eye infections occurring in household members. We could compare the frequency before any changes were made, and 1, 2 or 3 years later, or compare the frequency between those houses which have made the changes and a control group which have not.

We should also evaluate the level of satisfaction of community members for any changes that are made.

Chapter summary
Slum dwellers are at high risk from disease or injury caused by a number of environmental hazards. Solid waste in the form of household garbage is a particular problem since collection systems seldom exist in slums. Flooding, fire and electricity, danger from vehicles and air and noise pollution are further risks to physical and mental health. Slum dwellers also meet health and safety dangers in the workplace since they often work long hours in polluted, unsafe environments, with faulty equipment.

Many hazards can be reduced by behavioural change and relatively simple improvements. Two good examples are helping to set up regular street cleaning and rubbish disposal, and reducing indoor smoke pollution from cigarettes and smoky cooking fuels. More major changes can come about as residents link up with others, call in the help of experts and environmental pressure groups, and advocate for a less polluted environment and safer working practices.

Resources
1. *Health and Environment in Sustainable Development.* WHO, 1997. Excellent review of the effect of environment on health with some case studies.

Part 5

IMPORTANT PROJECT MANAGEMENT ISSUES

18 Co-operating with others

Community Health and Development Programmes can only be successful if they co-operate closely with all those they serve and come into regular contact with, in other words with all their 'stakeholders'. A stakeholder is any individual, agency or department that has its own particular reason for wanting to be associated with the CHDP. It has a stake or interest in its success. CHDPs need to make sure that they identify all their stakeholders, and build lasting and effective relationships with each of them. Some stakeholders will come from inside the community and some from outside. They will commonly include the following:

① From within the community:
- **slum leaders**: whether officially elected or self-appointed leaders and officials, landlords, religious leaders and schoolteachers;
- **health care providers**: doctors, practitioners, traditional healers, traditional birth attendants, government health workers and quacks;
- **community members**: women, men, youth, children;
- **community groups**: by ethnic, political or religious background or by working occupation.

② From outside the community:
- **neighbours**;
- **police**;
- **politicians**;
- **hospitals**;
- **government offices and agencies**: including the slum development wing, the water and sanitation agency, the land management department, etc.;
- **non-Governmental Organisations (NGOs)**: local grassroots, city-wide, national and international;
- **international agencies**: UNICEF, WHO, UNAIDS, UNDP, etc.

We will discuss issues that commonly arise as we co-operate with some of these stakeholders.

Co-operating with slum leaders

It is almost impossible to work in a community without the approval of the slum leadership. The typical slum leader is male and self-appointed. Usually he has created a powerful role as middleman or 'broker' between slum residents and those able to deliver the supplies, services and favours which slum dwellers need. He may negotiate with police to have someone released from jail. He may pay off government bureaucrats so that residents can continue the illegal tapping of power lines, then charge residents for electricity. He may organise political meetings so gaining votes for a particular candidate who in turn gives help or favours to the slum leader when some problem occurs.

Slum leaders usually become rich and powerful with strong connections into the community and with police and politicians. They can therefore be a great help to the CHDP, or alternatively make it impossible for the project to work in the community.

When we enter a slum for the first time, it is important to seek out slum leaders, introduce ourselves and explain why we are there. We will need to persuade the leader that the CHDP will bring benefits to the community and that this will indirectly be in the slum leader's interest. It often takes several informal discussions between the leader and CHDP to develop a valid relationship. We will need to take our time, get to know the leader's family and children, and accept his hospitality.

A dilemma occurs when the slum leader appears to be acting for his own benefit and not for that of the community. If CHDP staff members object to this or speak out against it, any co-operation will cease and the CHDP will probably have to move elsewhere. On the other hand, the CHDP will not want to condone the leader's actions, especially if they are illegal, dishonest or favour one group in the community at the expense of another. Each situation is different, and needs to be assessed.

Life in a slum

The government started a pre-school programme in a slum community. The slumlord managed the programme. The government paid him rent for a small hut that he provided for the programme (the hut was part of an illegal settlement on government land). The government also provided a nutritious midday snack for the children. But each month when the shipment came, half of it was delivered to the slumlord's house. He fed it to his pigs. The pre-school teacher knew what was happening, but there was little she could do. She knew if she complained, she would lose her job. (India)

One secret is to identify a particular interest or motivation a slum leader may have which will clearly have benefits for the community. This can then be encouraged and affirmed, both privately and where appropriate in public meetings. As the slum leader receives community support on account of these benefits, his public-spirited attitude is likely to grow at the expense of more dubious or illegal activities.

Co-operating with health care providers

People living in urban slums have access to a wide range of health care providers – both qualified and unqualified (Table 18.1). Doctors, traditional healers, government clinics, medicine shops and quacks work in or near most slum communities.

We should try to develop good relationships with each of these health-care providers, especially those who may think we are competing with them, or whose co-operation would benefit our programme. Here are some steps for building this co-operation:

1. Visit and meet them.
2. Explain the purpose of the project.
3. Learn from them as colleagues.
4. Offer medical educational opportunities for them.
5. Never speak poorly of them in public.

Table 18.1	Health-care providers in slums
Qualified doctors	• Interested in curative care
	• Prescribe expensive, western medicines
Traditional healers	• Often have special interests, e.g. bone-setting, acupuncture, traditional midwifery, mental illnesses and epilepsy
	• Generally have a more holistic approach
	• Dispense western and herbal medicines, and often give injections
	• Tend to charge lower rates and can often be paid in kind
Quacks	• Often dispense western medicines and give injections, frequently with unclean needles.
	• Usually untrained or self-taught
	• May make exaggerated claims

In practice, practitioners often feel threatened when a CHDP begins working in a slum. They are afraid of losing business. They fear their income will go down if the CHDP is offering curative services. They are unlikely to stop dangerous practices such as giving injections, since their livelihood depends on this. This may create a dilemma for the CHDP since our primary aim is to improve the health of the community. We may need to take time with practitioners, encouraging them to change or modify their practices and only as a last resort warning community members to avoid any forms of treatment which could be dangerous (Table 18.2)

Life in a slum

A woman had been in labour for many hours, but was not progressing. A local healer was called from his shop and gave an injection of oxytocin, which causes a strong contraction of the uterus.

The Community Health Volunteer knew that oxytocin was dangerous but was unable to convince the family. When the woman still failed to deliver, a quack gave her a second injection of oxytocin. Her uterus ruptured and she died soon afterwards. The Community Health Volunteer and the women's group reported the episode to the police: both healer and quack were arrested. On release they set up business in a different community. (Indonesia)

Co-operating with neighbours

Some slums are located near richer neighbourhoods that resent their existence. Richer residents object to the eyesore, smell, poor sanitation, petty crimes and negative effect on property prices. They often forget the advantages of unskilled labour immediately on their doorstep, such as house servants, guards and gardeners.

Table 18.2   Examples of dangerous health care practices
• Not referring patients to hospital until it is too late
• Giving unnecessary injections and intravenous drips
• Re-using syringes and needles without adequate sterilisation
• Giving antibiotics when they are not needed
• Giving inappropriate care for TB patients (both diagnosis and treatment)
• Giving many drugs at one time, when most are unnecessary (known as poly-pharmacy)

Life in a slum

A park separated a large slum from a middle class settlement. The slum dwellers had no place to defecate, so they used the park. Their middle class neighbours objected to this and obtained a court order forbidding the practice. A wall was built between the slum colony and the park. A short time later, a policeman spotted a slum dweller defecating in the park. The policeman beat the slum dweller so severely that he died. The slum community went on a rampage, and destroyed the park. The slum commissioner publicly supported the slum dwellers. He chastised the rich, accusing them of wanting cheap labour but not tolerating an eyesore. (India)

In practice CHDPs should work at developing relationships with richer neighbours, especially if major environmental changes are being planned. Even when a slum has existed for many years, neighbours may still hope the community will one day be demolished. We should discuss the planned improvements with neighbours ahead of time, emphasising the positive effect this will have on the neighbourhood, including property prices.

Co-operating with political parties and politicians

Political activity in slums is often cyclical, building up just before elections when politicians make all sorts of promises. Larger slums represent a huge voting block and political candidates are very eager for their votes. Unfortunately, promises are rarely kept, unless a community action group keeps pressing for them.

It is important to develop a good, working relationship with political leaders. They are usually happy for us to work within the community – **especially if they take credit for improvements that the CHDP has brought about**.

When working alongside political leaders we must avoid giving support to any one party and never be seen as having any political or party interests. Although difficult, this is essential. Our commission, like that of the Red Cross and Red Crescent, is to work impartially for all groups, solely according to their need. To do this effectively we will need to work with any or all of the political parties involved in the life of the slum.

Co-operating with hospitals

The problems

When slum dwellers become seriously ill the only option for most is to attend a government hospital. However most will be very reluctant to do this:

- **They cannot afford hospital care**. Although care is supposed to be free or subsidised, in practice bribes and enticements may have to be paid to hospital staff in order to be seen at all or to obtain a bed. Drugs should be available in the hospital, but in practice they often have to be bought from outside at exorbitant prices. The World Health Organization estimates that 2 billion people, one person in three, does not have access to essential medicines and that one course of antibiotics for pneumonia costs the average labourer one month's wages.

- **A relative or friend cannot afford time to go to hospital with the patient**. Most slum dwellers are paid wages for hours worked. Sparing an adult who could be working may plunge a family deeper into poverty.

- **Hospitals are confusing and overwhelming**. For slum dwellers, going to hospital is a frightening and traumatic experience. They do not know where to go and cannot read the signs. The whole process of queuing for each step of the process – registration, examination, lab tests, X-rays, drug supplies and payments is exhausting and humiliating.

- **Poor patients are badly treated by hospital staff**. They are often spoken too with harshness and impatience. Slum dwellers may prefer to go into debt in order to obtain better care from a private hospital.

- **Hospitals often have a poor reputation**. Many state-run or government hospitals have overworked staff with poor morale. Hygiene is often poor and equipment may be old, non-functioning or dangerous.

> It can be extremely frustrating when a preventable death occurs after project staff and Community Health Volunteers have finally persuaded the family of a very sick slum dweller to take their relative to hospital. Some deaths occur from neglect or inappropriate care and are beyond the control of the project staff or Community Health Volunteer.

Possible solutions

1. **Building relationships with hospital staff**. Sometimes CHDP members can get to know hospital staff who will then enable slum dwellers to be seen quickly and fairly. This 'door-opener' may be a doctor, a nurse in charge of outpatients, or a relatively junior but influential hospital official.

2. **Community Health Volunteers can accompany patients to hospital, acting as friend and advocate**. They can ensure patients are treated decently. The better trained and more assertive the CHVs the more effective they can be within the hospital. Sometimes it is possible to arrange for CHVs to have a training day in the hospital where they can get to know staff, understand how the hospital works

and then be more effective in helping community members in the future. Frequent turnover of hospital staff means that new relationships have to be continually re-established.

> One major reason for referral to hospital is for childbirth. During their training programme Traditional Birth Attendants (TBAs) from the community, can spend time in the labour rooms of the referring hospital, learning from the midwives and getting to know hospital staff. Later this can greatly increase the TBA's confidence when she accompanies a slum dweller to hospital. This process also promotes bonding between TBAs and delivery room staff making the referral of pregnant women or those in labour much easier.

❸ **Identifying sympathetic hospitals or clinics**. Sometimes NGOs, and religious or humanitarian groups run hospitals that may be more sympathetic to the needs of the poor. It is estimated that over half the hospital beds in Sub-Saharan Africa are provided by church-based institutions. Sometimes private hospitals can be persuaded to offer services at reduced rates – especially if senior staff are invited to visit the project and come to understand the needs of the poor. Small amounts of subsidy may be available from a contingency fund.

❹ **Building a polyclinic or small inpatient facility**. Larger NGOs are sometimes able to build their own 'First Referral Centre' where a large proportion of patients can be treated who would otherwise have to attend the government hospital.

Co-operating with government

The problems

Many improvements to the community cannot be done unless there is co-operation and support from the government, especially the municipal (city) authorities. This is especially true for environmental improvements and Chapter 12 describes ways of working on this type of project in more detail. Often the municipal government has a legal obligation or 'mandate' to provide certain services for its citizens such as:

- a safe and adequate water supply,
- sanitary disposal of human waste and garbage,
- drainage of rainwater and wastewater,
- electricity,
- basic preventive and curative medical services,
- schools.

Although government agencies may be legally required to provide these services, they are often unable to do so for some of the following reasons:

❶ The large number of people pouring into the city overwhelms the government's ability to cope.

❷ The government probably has higher priorities, often politically motivated.

③ Corruption drains off funds, meaning there is less money to provide services.

④ Government officials often have poor motivation and only co-operate if paid bribes or inducements.

⑤ The bureaucratic process is lengthy, time-consuming and inefficient, easily overwhelming the patience and tolerance of the community.

⑥ One government department may try to shift responsibility to another.

⑦ Government agencies may be unclear about the law, or the law itself may be unclear or unfair.

⑧ Services needed by the community may depend on active co-operation between different government departments. For example, when installing a tube well: the agency owning the land needs to grant permission, the agency responsible for electric power provides a line for the pump, the water department supplies pipes and the sanitation department provides drainage.

⑨ Mutual suspicion may exist between government and the community from previous experiences.

> Sometimes government schemes are administered through locally elected political representatives. If the community did not vote for them, permission for government programmes may be refused.

From the field: When a slum housing upgradation project was completed, a number of government officials were invited to the inauguration. As they walked down the reconstructed lanes with new houses on either side, one was heard to say to the other: 'Look! We've actually done something!' (Zambia)

Lesson learned: Many government officials are personally interested in working together to provide services, but are themselves victims of an inefficient and corrupt system. We can encourage such officials by inviting them to observe improvements made possible through their support.

Source: Authors.

Possible solutions

There are several ways that the CHDP can foster co-operation with the government:

① **Co-ordinate with government programmes**. The project should co-ordinate its activities with government programmes as far as possible. For example, the project should follow national immunisation schedules and guidelines for the national tuberculosis programme. CHDPs that work independently of the government are unlikely to be sustainable in the long run. Despite many obstacles, we must persist in working with government. Developing goodwill and good relationships is the basis for this and **perseverance is the key**. If we obtain support on major environmental improvements, this represents a huge financial input. The effort is worth it!

② **Keep government informed**. We must keep appropriate government agencies informed of the CHDP's activities and send in regular reports.

③ **Create awareness in the community**. The project should study government priorities and funding schemes for urban communities, keep the community informed and help them to put in successful applications.

④ **Claim rights**. The project should educate the community to understand which services the government is legally obliged to provide. Then we should help the community put in a robust application for these services.

⑤ **Develop personal relationships**. Within most government departments there are likely to be some officials who have a genuine concern for the poor, and who may be strategically placed to do something about it. It is worth spending time discovering who these people are and then getting to know them.

⑥ **Conduct education and advocacy with government agencies**. The project can help members of government agencies understand about the needs that exist, and the services they are legally obliged to provide.

⑦ **Promote legal justice**. When laws are unjust, the project can work with other NGOs to have the laws changed. If the government takes illegal actions such as evicting tenants, this can be challenged.

⑧ **Negotiate with government**. When technical standards are inappropriate and/or unreachable, the project may be able to work with the government to reach a compromise. For example, housing regulations may require a house to be of a certain minimum size, but slum dwellings may have to be built smaller than the minimum allowed. If compromises are not reached rebuilding or upgrading cannot take place.

In claiming government support we need to balance two approaches. The first is discussion, when HDP members and relevant government officials explore ways of working together or requesting government services. The second is community action, when residents press home their claim for improvements through united support and advocacy. In both situations the full community should be informed, but two or three selected representatives should carry through the negotiations in a firm but respectful manner.

Co-operating with NGOs

Reasons co-operation is necessary

In most cities, especially capitals, many NGOs are involved in working with the urban poor. All CHDPs should actively discover the names and main activities of other NGOs working in the same slum communities. There are several reasons for this:

- **To prevent duplication of effort**. Before deciding which community to work with, find out if other NGOs are already working there and doing similar work.

If they are, we should either find an unserved community, or define which areas or activities each NGO will be responsible for.

- **To work in co-operation and in a way where activities are complementary**. Different NGOs have different goals and areas of expertise. When there is need in our community for skills or services which our project cannot easily provide, we can invite an NGO with the needed expertise to work with the community. Many examples are given in this book.

- **To work together for advocacy**. One project alone may have little effect on government policies, but a council of organisations may help to change policy or bring in new labour laws. Join and support 'umbrella organisations', which are organisations that help NGOs to work together.

- **To know which organisations have appropriate programmes**. NGOs vary greatly in their approach to community health and development. Before linking up with others it is important for us to know whether the NGO is well respected, and has an approach which empowers communities rather than providing handouts and inappropriate aid.

From the field: A organisation was helping a slum community to improve its water supply. Many of the handpumps were broken and some had been vandalised. The community asked the project to arrange training for a group of women to learn basic handpump repairs. Before that happened, an international NGO came in and provided the community with new handpumps, and the women quickly lost interest in learning how to repair them. After several months, several of the new handpumps were already broken or vandalised. Within a year, the community's water supply was as bad as before the new pumps had been installed. The international NGO refused to provide more new pumps and considered its efforts a failure. The community then asked for help from the project that had originally offered to set up training. This duly occurred and pumps were repaired and maintained. Vandalism stopped as community members realised that maintaining the pumps in working order was their own responsibility. (Zimbabwe)

Lesson learned: When working with other NGOs, it is important to understand their approach to development. Different approaches may be incompatible.

Source: Authors.

Problems that may occur when more than one NGO is working in a community

- **Unhealthy competition**. Sometimes when more than one NGO is working in a community, jealousy, mistrust and a sense of competition develops. The NGOs may try to outdo each other, and the community ends up being caught in the middle and being pampered by both sides. This hinders self-reliance.

- **Staff snatching**. Good health and development workers who are willing to work in slums are not easy to find. Good, well-trained and experienced staff may be lured to another NGO that can offer a better salary. The original NGO loses a staff member, whose training has taken much time and effort.

- **Differing approach to development**. As the illustration from Zimbabwe shows NGOs who may be involved in similar fields such as health care or sanitation, may have such different approaches that they cannot work together. This book strongly supports a community development approach where communities are empowered to identify and solve their own problems. It will be difficult to work with NGOs that hand out free supplies and services as this will undermine the community's self-reliance, and work against our objectives.

Co-operating with donor partners

Problems that projects may have with donor agencies

- **Donors have a complicated funding process**. This often requires a lengthy and detailed proposal. Multiple copies must be made and deadlines have to be met.

- **Donors expect too many results too soon**. Service activities such as setting up clinics and generating statistics can be done quite quickly. But empowerment and capacity-building, i.e. key activities to bring about real and lasting improvements, take much longer. They involve changing people's attitudes, providing them with knowledge and skills, and then working with them as they carry out positive and permanent changes. The length of time needed for this varies greatly, but it usually takes at least 3–5 years before a community can progress on its own. Sometimes, especially when there is little or no government support, the CHDP may need funding for a long period of time.

- **Donors expect programmes to follow the time scales submitted with the proposal**. But if we are enabling the community to design and implement their own programme and march to their own drum-beat, the CHDP will not have control over the pace of progress. As a result we can get caught in the middle – between a community that makes decisions and a donor that expects compliance.

- **Donors want to see progress towards financial sustainability**. Some funding agencies set a goal for the community to self-finance its own health programmes. This is unrealistic. Slum communities are by definition very poor, and often have to pay for basic services that their richer neighbours often receive free of charge.

Problems that donor agencies may have with projects

- **Projects communicate poorly with donors**. Distance, coupled with poor telecommunications, despite improvements brought about by fax and e-mail.

- **Project proposals do not follow the requested format or are filled out incorrectly or incompletely**.

- **Finances are not transparent**. This opens the possibility that project funds could be embezzled or sums of money used for reasons other than their designated purpose.

Suggested solutions

1 **Help donors to understand** that it takes a number of years to change attitudes and to empower a community.

➋ **Make realistic timelines**. Set objectives that can be met. Allow for uncertainties and build in flexibility to the programme proposal.

➌ **Demonstrate sustainability**. One way of doing this is to reduce the input into original target areas, and reach out into new ones. But we must be sure to demonstrate the effect the programme has had in those original areas. For example we could show that community groups now enable residents to tackle problems effectively with little assistance from the project.

➍ **Supply all information requested by donor agencies in a timely fashion**. Start preparing the funding proposal early so that if questions are raised there is still time to obtain clarification.

➎ **Communicate regularly with the donor agency and provide case studies, stories and photographs of the project and its impact**. Donors depend upon their supporters. Stories and photographs help donors to 'sell' the project to their supporters.

➏ **Be frank about any problems**. Donors appreciate honesty and want to know about problems and how they are being solved.

➐ **Be financially accountable**. Set up a rigorous accounting system and submit independently audited accounts each year. Explain clearly any changes in the way money might be allocated, and if large sums are involved confirm with the donor agency that they have no objections.

➑ **Donors should visit the project for encouragement, training and mutual learning**. Many donor agencies are moving away from being primarily sources of funding towards training and empowerment. They want to build the capacity of their overseas partners so enabling them to become strong and self-reliant.

Chapter summary

Community health and development programmes will only achieve their objectives if they learn to work in close co-operation with other individuals, groups and agencies. This ability to work alongside others and to network widely is a basic principle of Community Health and Development Programmes (CHDPs). It also enables their programmes to be more effective. From within the community, CHDPs must work closely and impartially with slum leaders, health care practitioners and all community groups, including minority and marginalised segments.

Programmes also need to work in close co-operation with agencies based outside the slum. Most importantly this will include different government agencies, which will often provide essential permissions, supplies and finance. Other key groups include hospitals, other NGOs working in the same geographical area and donor agencies. The key to all co-operation is finding common ground, building relationships and sharing the fruits of success.

Aiming for sustainable development

As we work with communities to improve their health and environment, our aim is to empower those communities to become increasingly self-sufficient. Just how this comes about will vary greatly, depending upon the needs and resources of the community, and the approach and activities of the project.

What is sustainable development?

Sustainability is the ability to continue or to keep going.

Development is a positive change in people's health and environment. It depends on the ability of both individuals and the community to recognise problems standing in the way of healthy, fulfilled lifestyles and to take decisions to overcome those problems.

Sustainable development occurs when people can identify their own problems, come up with solutions, and work together in community to bring them about. They learn how to use outside ideas, skills and resources, but in doing so become less and less dependent on those resources.

Sustainable development does **not** mean that communities can solve their problems using only their own resources. We are working with the very poor and it is unrealistic to expect them to have the wide range of information, skills and finance to meet all their needs. But it **does** mean that communities learn how to call on and use resources both inside and outside their community without being dependent on others to do this for them.

A community that has learnt this secret has been empowered and has developed its capacity to own its own future. The main objective of programmes and outside agencies is to enable that to happen as quickly and effectively as possible.

Features needed in a community to bring about sustainable development

1. Motivation: The community understands and accepts responsibility for its own development

This starts the move towards self-reliance. A self-reliant community is likely to take the initiative to solve its own problems and to preserve the positive changes that occur. The role of the CHDP is to motivate the community to do this.

2. Community participation: there is increasing community ownership of all project activities

If a community is genuinely motivated it leads to participation. The sequence moves from motivation through participation to ownership. The role of the CHDP is to help bring this process about.

This is much easier when a community is united. If managed well, participation can help to bring harmony to slum communities. Progress is likely to occur because people will be willing to make compromises in order to achieve objectives that are seen to benefit all. Sometimes it is possible to help opposing groups understand that such a compromise will leave them better off than before, even though it may not be the ideal solution for either group. For example if two factions in a slum community each want a tube well in their own area, they can be helped to see that one well with equal access for both groups would be better than no well at all. The CHDP can sometimes act as negotiator and help to broker such agreements.

> Sustainable development does not require the participation or even co-operation of every member of the community. But the slum leadership, marginalised groups such as women, and ethnic minorities, must be included in the process.

3. An effective community group is organised

The vehicle that makes things happen is a group that represents the community and that has clear objectives. Without a cohesive group, activities if they happen at all, are haphazard and soon fizzle out.

4. Community management: community members are trained in leadership, communication and management skills

People from within the community need training in essential skills to lead the community through the development process. Projects often overlook this. For example skills such as how to run a meeting and how to keep simple accounts do not come naturally, they must be learned. Until these skills are mastered, the community will always depend on an outside agency to help them run their programmes. So we need to empower community members through training in a variety of practical management skills.

Here are some key examples:

- how to communicate effectively,
- how to run meetings fairly,
- how to organise community groups,
- how to motivate community members,
- how to do simple administration (keep accounts, write proposals and reports etc.).

> When we provide aid to a community without training them, we simply encourage dependency. We need to empower a community with basic skills in leadership and management so that it can own its own future and solve its own problems without dependency on outsiders.

5. Funding and resources: community leaders know how and where to access funds and resources

As we have seen throughout this book there are many sources of funds and expert help if only we can find them and use them. This is a skill which community members of the CHDP leadership team must learn. Sources of help include community members themselves, government, NGOs, universities and businesses.

CHDP leaders need to train community members how to find, approach and tap funding sources: also how to write letters, meet officials and write project proposals. This requires, skill, confidence and persistence. The project should identify appropriate people to train in these skills, and then spend time working together so that information and skills are transferred.

From the field. The Surkhet Project in Nepal supports marginalised communities. It raises awareness, trains groups how to make action skills and helps them to develop communication skills. Over a 30-month period these groups are formed and trained so they can then identify and solve their own problems. After that period the project reduces its input, and provides a different range of services:

- consultancy to groups when requested;
- networking between groups through a 3-monthly newsletter for mutual sharing;
- providing information about resources and funds that the groups can then access.

Source: Surkhet Project, United Mission to Nepal, Kathmandu.

---

6. Political will: The government must be willing to work with communities

Most successful urban health programmes have developed a close working relationship with government departments. This does not happen quickly even if a government has an enlightened attitude and resources to spend, which many of the poorest cities do not.

We can help the community identify government officials with a co-operative attitude, then build relationships more widely with other members of that department. After one successful venture, the government may be more willing to work with the community in the future, especially if the government is able to claim part of the credit.

Most governments are not prepared for the bottom-up approach needed for sustainable development. However, individuals within the government structure may understand and be committed to this approach.

7. Commitment of CHDP staff to empowering the communities

Training a community to take responsibility for its own future needs great skill and endless patience from members of the CHDP. They must be become good listeners and excellent communicators. Above all they need to be fully committed to the idea of transferring responsibility to the community, even if it means their own job may eventually change. They must be willing to give up power, so that the community can become empowered.

How can we monitor progress towards sustainable development?

As we work with a community we will need to have ways of measuring whether the processes needed for sustainability are actually occurring. We can do this by selecting indicators to monitor progress. Most of the indicators will be qualitative since we are monitoring changes in behaviour and attitudes. Indicators will obviously differ between projects. Table 19.1 gives a list of possible indicators to choose from. Examples are listed for each of the factors mentioned in the preceding section of the chapter. In each of the seven lists, the first indicator measures a very early stage of sustainability and could for example be used to monitor progress during the first 1 or 2 years of a project's life. Each list then gives measures of increasing degrees of sustainability. For any project it is worth choosing a level appropriate for where the project has reached, and then working down the list over the following months or years.

Features needed in a CHDP to bring about sustainable development

Certain key features need to be present in a CHDP for sustainability to 'happen'. Without these the project will not be able to guide the community through the seven activities listed and monitored in the previous section.

Before looking at these we must face up to the fact that a CHDP should not necessarily continue to exist year after year, simply because it is there, and gives employment. Its aim is to empower communities, leave a support network in place, then move on to a different underserved area or community. In order to know whether our CHDP is equipped to bring about sustainable development we need to ask these questions:

❶ **Does the CHDP seek EQUITY?** We start by looking at the people we serve. We are concerned about social justice and fairness. Therefore we focus on the marginalised – those people who are usually overlooked and are most in need.

Table 19.1 Possible indicators for key factors for sustainable change

Key factors for sustainable change	Possible indicators
1. **Motivation:** The community understands and accepts responsibility for its own development	• Community members attend and participate in meetings • The community discusses and prioritises its problems • Community members volunteer possible solutions • Community members volunteer time, materials and/or funds to solve community problems • The community selects and solves a problem without help of CHDP
2. **Community participation:** There is increasing community ownership of all project activities	• Members come to meetings without being reminded or encouraged by CHDP staff • The needs of marginalised groups, such as women and the very poor, are represented • Women speak up at meetings • The community prioritises problems and suggests solutions • The community monitors and evaluates the activities • The community manages the funds • The community obtains funds from outside agencies • The community develops ways of self-financing the project
3. **An effective community group** is organised	• Community leaders organise and conduct group meetings with minimum help of CHDP staff • The group identifies and prioritises problems, considers solutions, develops and implements an action plan with minimum help from CHDP staff • The group addresses the problems of the marginalised • The group develops its programme without the help of CHDP staff
4. **Community management:** Members are trained in leadership, communication and management skills	Community leaders can: • Lead and facilitate groups

Key factors for sustainable change	Possible indicators
	• Represent the community at meetings with outside agencies
	• Keep accurate accounts, maintain records and record minutes
	• Write letters and reports
5. **Funding and resources**: Community leaders know how and where to access funds and resources	• Community representatives meet with outside agencies and organisations
	• Community representatives make these contacts themselves
	• The community writes and submits funding proposals with CHDP assistance
	• The community writes and submits proposals without assistance from CHDP
6. **Political will**: The government must be willing to work with communities	• Community representatives meet with government agencies
	• Government officials visit the community
	• Government agency provides materials to the community
	• Government agency provides technical assistance and/or training materials to the community
	• Government agency provides funding to the community

7. **Commitment of CHDP staff** to empowering communities	• CHDP staff have specific training in:
	  – group dynamics
	  – motivation skills
	  – adult education skills
	  – facilitation and communication skills
	  – development cycle

	• Effective community groups are formed and functioning
	• CHDP members are increasingly willing to hand over control to the community
	• CHDP members are willing to move to other areas or projects as the community becomes empowered

② **Does the CHDP seek to EMPOWER?** Are its members able and willing to transfer skills and responsibility? Do they see this as the principle which must underline all project activities?

③ **Is the CHDP EFFECTIVE?** Has the CHDP accomplished what it set out to do? Is it likely to continue to do so? If a programme is ineffective it can never be sustainable. The quality and training of staff, including management skills are crucial to this success.

④ **Is the CHDP EFFICIENT?** Having made sure that the project is effective, we need to make sure it is also efficient. This means getting the job done effectively at the lowest possible cost, and without exploiting project or community members. This process can be helped by good management, careful accounting and the sensible use of computers with back-up and training.

The longer it takes a CHDP to make a community self-reliant, the less efficient it is. Therefore, if a CHDP takes too long to bring about change, sustainability may never happen. Some CHDPs work with the same communities, giving the same input for years – sometimes more than 10 years. This is usually inappropriate. It prevents development, and it encourages dependency. When a CHDP enters a community, it should calculate a time-line for various stages of the project, **including a provisional date for when it can reduce its input into the community**. Of course this length of time will vary, and the CHDP must not pull out too early, especially if there are unexpected factors which delay the time-line.

In most cases, urban communities should be ready to take a major responsibility for their own health and environment within 5 years of a CHDP starting work in the community.

⑤ **Is the CHDP ENVIRONMENTALLY sound?** When planning activities to meet the needs of the community, we must preserve the environment for future generations. When we make drains to remove surface water, where does the water go? Is it just moved to become someone else's problem? Do we tidy our community but dump garbage elsewhere? Do we encourage the use of fuels that pollute the environment?

⑥ **Is the CHDP committed to NETWORKING AND CO-OPERATION?** Do project members have the willingness to meet and share with other agencies involved in similar or complementary work? Is there a spirit of wanting to work together with others towards the common good?

Ways of assessing whether the CHDP is equipped for sustainable development

Table 19.2 gives a way of checking each of the factors we have just listed.

Practical examples of financial sustainability

We have seen that sustainability is much more than being financially self-sufficient. In practice however programmes rarely become sustainable unless they reduce costs and recover income. They cannot forever depend on outside support.

Table 19.2 Some ways to check if the CHDP is equipped for sustainable development	
Features of a sustainable CHDP	**Possible checks or indicators**
1. CHDP seeks **EQUITY**.	
● It works with under-served communities	Target population has few basic services or benefits
● It focuses on the marginalised	Target population is the most vulnerable in terms of income, gender or neglect
2. CHDP seeks to **EMPOWER**	
● It changes community members' attitudes and transfers skills	Community members gain confidence, learn new skills, develop leadership and share responsibilities
● It helps community members to make choices and solve problems	Community members actively participate, own and carry out the development process
3. CHDP is **EFFECTIVE**	
● Staff are well-trained and motivated	Staff receive regular training Staff contribute ideas and enthusiasm
● Leadership is visionary, well-trained and reassured	CDHP action plans are innovative and achievable
● Governing body is supportive, democratic and with diverse interests and competencies	Governing body neither rubber-stamps nor blocks initiatives, but acts in a constructive way
● CHDP provides quality services	Activities have measurable impact on community
4. CHDP is **EFFICIENT**	
● CHDP reduces input into the community within a planned length of time	Original target populations become self-reliant and project starts working in new areas/ communities
● Project is well managed	Materials, manpower and money are always available when needed, and utilised maximally
● Community volunteers share the workload	Significant numbers of community volunteers, give time and make valued contributions
● Project minimises costs of medicines and medical supplies	Project only dispenses drugs that are on the Essential Drugs List Project works according to government guidelines and obtains medicines and supplies from government

Features of a sustainable CHDP	Possible checks or indicators
	Project seeks out medicines that are lowest in cost, but maintains high quality
	Community contributes to funding
● Accounting is transparent and funds are carefully spent	Accounts are audited yearly by approved firm
	Financial statements are published and available
	Safeguards are in place to prevent misuse of funds
5. CHDP is **ENVIRONMENTALLY** sound	
● Its activities provide for current needs without harming the environment for future generations	Environmental impact is always an essential part of the planning process
	No adverse effects on the environment are observed or reported
6. CHDP is committed to **NETWORKING** and **CO-OPERATION**	
● It networks and has credibility with other communities, neighbours, government and agencies	Project meets/interacts with these groups
	Project invites outsiders to project/community functions and invitations are accepted
	Project activities are reported in press

Table 19.2 Continued

In practice, CHDPs will need both to **reduce expenditure and generate income**. Two of the highest programme costs are usually **medicines and salaries**. We will look at each in turn.

Medicines

1 The CHDP should only use medicines that are on the WHO Essential Drugs List, or a version that has been modified by the government. Sometimes lists for Primary Health centres are also drawn up – in which case we should use them.

2 CHDP should buy and use generic medicines rather than brand names provided that we can be sure that quality is assured. Generics are usually cheaper, sometimes much cheaper, than brand drugs.

3 Staff should be well-trained in the use of medicines so the minimum number of essential medicines are used. Specific treatment protocols based on the signs and symptoms of common illnesses should be used as guidelines for health workers. Patients will only rarely need as many as three medicines, some will need none at all – just an explanation. Antibiotic use should be strictly monitored. Most doctors overprescribe leading to wasted money – and the development of drug resistance.

4 The project should obtain free medicines to which it is entitled from other agencies, especially from the government. This usually includes vaccines, vitamin A, iron/folic acid, and anti-TB drugs.

But even if the CHDP has strict controls on the use of medicines it will still have a large drugs bill. We therefore have to consider one or more ways of introducing charges. This is known as cost recovery and always causes a great deal of discussion and argument. The dilemma is this: on the one hand programmes cannot be sustainable without user charges: on the other hand it is very easy for the poorest community members, the very ones we most want to help, to find our health care too expensive. Achieving the right balance is difficult and each project will need to work out the best way for its own particular situation.

A well known example of cost recovery is the Bamako Initiative, which was established by African Ministers of Health along with WHO and UNICEF. It calls for community participation in managing and funding health care, especially the supply of medicines, and it depends on user charges.

Here are some possible ways of charging for medicines:

● The full cost of the medicine is charged to the patient, but without profit, so that medicines are cheaper than in the market. The problem here is that the very poor cannot afford to pay for the medicines. Most NGOs will find using this method alone is unacceptable.

● The government or CHDP provides community health workers with simple medicines, free or at subsidised rates, which they can sell at a price slightly above cost, so providing them with a small amount of income. The problem is that this encourages the community health worker to concentrate on curative care and encourages the overuse of medicine.

One way NGOs can help communities to sustain their community health workers is through helping the CHVs to increase their incomes through development of micro-enterprises that **don't** involve selling medicines.

- The CHDP can introduce a sliding scale for services and medicines so that the poor pay less. In some projects, the health worker seeing the patient determines how much is to be paid and in others staff members are assigned to assess the ability to pay of all those attending the clinic.
- The best and most sustainable way, even though it takes more time to set up, is to train a community-based committee to decide on the socio-economic criteria for charging, according to agreed criteria. For example, the committee may decide to classify households according to how many High Risk Factors a household has for vulnerability (see page 186). This could work out as follows:
  - **Group 1** Those with five or more risk factors – the poorest. They pay a little or no fee.
  - **Group 2** Those with four risk factors. They pay a small fee.
  - **Group 3** Those with two to three risk factors. They pay a larger fee, e.g. half the price of the medicines
  - **Group 4** Those with one or no risk factors – the wealthiest. They pay the full cost of medicines.

- Some CHDPs set up an insurance scheme in which people (or households) pay a monthly or annual fee for medical care, including medicines. Then when they need health care, they receive this free or at reduced cost. Those without insurance pay the full rate. If well managed this idea can become popular, with increasing numbers signing on.

Whatever system is used, policies must be clear, categories clearly defined, and the community involved in the decision-making. All community members need to understand how the scheme works. All these plans must be drawn up **before** the health programme starts or the clinic opens.

From the field: The CHDP, Lalitpur is a large community health project based in Patan, Nepal. The project works in rural and semi-urban areas. For many years the project has used a medical insurance programme. There are significant differences in how well the programme works between rural and urban areas. Those living in the countryside have a high level of participation and are willing to pay a relatively high fee. The insurance programme is used by both rich and poor since there are few other options for obtaining health care or for getting medicines. In the urban setting, however, those who can afford private care opt out of the scheme meaning the poor only use it. With fewer subscribers, less income is generated and more subsidy has to be given. The project has adjusted to this lower income by careful prescribing and by limiting medicines to those that are simple and inexpensive.

Source: N Gurung, 1999. CHDP, Lalitpur, Patan, Nepal.

Guidelines for successful community-funded health care

1. Involve the community in all stages: in determining what services are needed, in planning, implementing, managing, monitoring and evaluating the activities.

2. Specifically help set up a community-based committee to manage the finances, and to calculate how much it costs to provide the services.

3. Decide on fees, based on a balance of:

- what people can afford to pay,

- the cost of providing the services,

- the balance which can be raised from other sources.

4. Ensure honest, transparent accounting, with all transactions clearly recorded.

5. Hire and train health staff who are competent, committed and courteous.

Salaries

The other major project cost is salaries. We can help to reduce this in several ways:

❶ Ensure that project morale is high, and that staff are well trained. They will then work more efficiently and achieve more.

❷ Train every staff member to be a multi-purpose worker. Drivers can weigh babies, clerks can make packets of iron/folate tablets, and nurses can drive vehicles. This reduces the amount of unproductive waiting around.

❸ Use community volunteers as much as possible. We should start this from the very beginning of our contact with a community. Make the options clear: if the community wants services, they will need to provide volunteers.

Other sources of income

Income generation: Some projects generate income through their project activities. In Delhi, an organisation that works with street children runs a restaurant in a large bus terminal. The street children run the restaurant, learning marketable skills such as cooking, waiting on tables, cashiering and accounting. The children are paid, and profits help to support other activities. One project in East Africa runs a petrol station, and another manages an out-of-town safari lodge for wildlife tourists.

Partnership with the private sector: Local industries, pharmaceutical companies and philanthropic organisations like Rotary International may be interested in providing funds or materials for project activities. Some organisations will sponsor fund-raising activities, such as concerts, plays or films, with proceeds going to the NGO, ideally a specific project. Networking by project leaders or board members is an important way to enlist the private sector.

From the field: In Nairobi, a church has taken the responsibility of running the pharmacy for a clinic that an NGO has set up in a nearby slum community. Some members of the church involved in the business community have organised an inventory system that minimises pilfering. Medicines are bought in bulk to reduce costs and are stored free at the church. Members of the church with appropriate training volunteer to staff the clinic pharmacy. The church's participation has greatly reduced the costs of running the clinic.

Source: Author visit.

Why will sustainability become an increasingly important issue in 2000 and beyond?

1. There will be less money available for health and development in the poorest communities because:

    ● Governments of developing countries have huge debt repayments to developed nations that siphon off funds that could be used for health and social development. Even if debts are written off this factor is likely to remain important.

    ● In an attempt to overcome poverty, The World Bank and International Monetary Fund introduced measures that reduce the amount countries spend on providing essential services for the very poor. This is known as Structural Readjustment.

    ● Western donors are experiencing 'donor fatigue'. There have been so many natural disasters and wars in the past 10 years that donors are sometimes less willing to give. Also funds are sometimes switched to emergency relief and away from longer term development.

    ● There will be increasing numbers of CHDPs and other NGOs competing for funds.

2. There will be ever greater needs for health and development because:

    ● The economic crisis in South-east Asia and in the former Soviet Union greatly adds to the number of people in severe need.

    ● The population in most developing countries is increasing.

    ● HIV/AIDS increases poverty and soaks up huge amounts of funding. The epidemic is spreading throughout Africa and Asia.

    ● There are increasing numbers of complex chronic emergencies where famine, civil war and human migration take large amounts of funding and make long term development more difficult.

Support from the government: As mentioned throughout this book, the government can assist projects and communities in many ways. It is important to find out what government schemes are available and to use them to the full. In recent years NGOs, government and international agencies have been increasingly working together. In some cases governments are 'contracting out' parts of health care to voluntary organisations and paying them to run the services.

Normal government programmes include the National Tuberculosis Programme and the Expanded Programme on Immunisation.

Chapter summary

Sustainable development occurs when people can identify their own problems, come up with solutions, and work together in community to bring them about. Sustainability does **not** mean that communities should be able to solve their problems using only their own resources. It means that communities should be self-reliant: they should be equipped to call on and use resources inside and outside their community without being dependent on others to do this for them. The aim of the CHDP should be to help the community to become self-reliant. Certain key factors are needed for community projects to become sustainable. The community must be motivated, participate in all aspects of the development process, and work through a community group as a vehicle for change. Community leaders must be trained in leadership, communications, and other skills, and the community must know where and how to access outside resources, especially from government. We can monitor the progress of the community towards self-reliance, by using a few simple indicators.

Certain factors have to be present in health and development programmes for them to lead communities through to self-reliance. They must be committed to social equity, and be effective and efficient. They need to be committed to sound policies on the environment and to networking with others. These features can also be monitored using simple indicators.

Finally projects must find ways of keeping expenditure on medicines and salaries as low as possible and creating ways of recovering costs through skilfully introducing user fees, being sure that the poor can always afford health care services. Generating income in a variety of ways can help the project to be less dependent on outside donors.

Resources

1. *Empowerment through Enterprise: A Training Manual for Non-government Organisations.* M Harper. Intermediate Technology Publications, 1996. An excellent series of training exercises to gain skills necessary for income generation through micro-enterprise.

2. *Community-Based Sustainable Human Development.* D Taylor-Ide, CE Taylor. UNICEF Environmental Section Discussion Paper Series. UNICEF New York, 1995. Discusses the critical factors necessary for sustainable development and how to scale up by training others.

3. *Health Financing and Sustainability.* A Lafond, P Smithson. Save the Children Fund, London, 1994. A review and case studies from five countries.

4. *Financing Health Care.* H Goodman, C Waddington. Oxfam, 1993. A practical manual with very useful information.

5. *Guidelines to Rational Drug Use.* R Korte, F von Massow, J Ndele. Provides information on the rational prescription of drugs in developing countries. It gives details on the use of a broad range of available drugs.

Appendix 1: References, publishers and resources

References

Bailey D, Hawes H, Bonati G. 1992. *Child-to-Child: A Resource Book: Part 1: Implementing the Child-to-Child aproach*. Child-to-Child Trust (available through TALC).

Beall J, ed. 1997. *A City for All: Valuing difference and working with diversity*. Zed Books.

Black M. 1991. *Philippines: Children of the runaway cities*. (Part Studies on the Urban Child in Difficult Circumstances) Innocenti.

Blackett IC 1994. *Low-Cost Urban Sanitation in Lesotho*. Water and Sanitation Discussion Paper Series No. 10. UNDP – World Bank Water and Sanitation Program.

Blinkhoff P, Bukanga E, Syamalevwe B, Williams G. 1999. *Under the Mupundu Tree: Volunteers in home care for people with HIV/AIDS TB in Zambia's Copperbelt*. Action Aid (available through TALC).

Conroy RM *et al*. 1996. Solar disinfection of drinking water and diarrhoea in Maasai children: a controlled field trial. *Lancet* 348(9043): 1695–7.

Department for Economic and Social Information and Policy Analysis, United Nations Statistics Division, 1996 figures

Harpham T, Lusty T, Vaughan P. 1988. *In the Shadow of the City: Community health and the urban poor*. Oxford University Press.

Harries A, Maher D, Uplekar M. 1997. *TB: A Clinical Manual for South East Asia*. WHO.

Jarman J. 1997 Water Supply and Sanitation. In: Beall J, ed. *A City for All: Valuing difference and working with diversity*. Zed Books.

Kirkwood A. Safe water for Africa. *Africa Health* 20(6):9–10.

Lwanga SK, Lemeshow S. 1991. *Sample Size Determination in Health Studies: A Practical Manual*. WHO.

Monte C, Nations, M. 1994. What changes are possible in practice. *Dialogue on Diarrhea* 56 (March–May):4. AHRTAG (now Healthlink).

Narayan D. 1993. *Participatory Evaluation: Tools for managing change in water and sanitation*. The World Bank.

Pickford J *et al*. 1996. *Sustainability of Water and Sanitation Systems*. IT Publications.

Serageldin Ismail. 1994. *Water Supply, Sanitation and Environmental Sustainability: The financing challenge*. The World Bank.

Shubert C. 1996. *Building Partnerships for Urban Poverty Alleviation*. United Nations Centre for Human Settlements (UNCHS).

Tabibzadeh I, Rossi-Espagnet A, Maxwell R. 1989. *Spotlight on the Cities*. WHO.

UNICEF Annual Report, 1997.

UNAIDS. 1998. *Partners in Prevention: International case studies of effective health promotion practice in HIV/AIDS.*

United Nations Centre for Human Settlements. 1996. *An Urbanizing World: Global report on human settlements.* Oxford University Press.

Wilkinson RG. 1994. The epidemiologic transition. From material security to social disadvantage? *Daedalus: Journal of the American Academy of Arts and Sciences* 123(4):67.

Williams G, Blibolo AD, Kerouedan D. 1995. *Filling the Gaps.* Action Aid.

Publishers

Action Aid
Hamlyn House,
Macdonald Road,
Archway,
London N19 5PG, UK

AHRTAG (See Healthlink)

Child-to-Child Trust
Institute of Education
20 Bedford Way
London WC1H 0AL, UK
Tel: +44 (0)20 7612-6650
Tel: +44 (0)20 7612-6645

Earthscan Publications Ltd
3 Endsleigh Street,
London WC1H 0DD, UK

Healthlink Worldwide (formerly AHRTAG)
Cityside
40 Adler Street
London E1 1EE, UK
Web: www.healthlink.org.uk
E-mail: info@healthlink.org.uk

The Hesperian Foundation
1919 Addison St, Suite 304,
Berkeley, CA 94704, USA

Innocenti (UNICEF)
International Child Development Centre,
Piazza S. S. Annunziata 12, 50122
Florence, Italy

Intermediate Technology Publications Ltd
103–105 Southampton Row,
London WC1B 4HH, UK
E-mail: order@itpubs.org.uk

Macmillan Education Ltd
Macmillan Oxford
Between Towns Road
Oxford OX4 3PP, UK

MAP International
PO Box 21663
Nairobi, Kenya

New Society Publishers
PO Bx 189
Gabriola Island, BC, VOR 1XO, Canada
E-mail: info@newsociety.com

Pact Publications
777 United Nations Plaza
New York, NY 10017, USA
Web: www.pactpub.com
E-mail: books@pactpub.org
Publishes education and training materials related to development.

TALC (Teaching Aids at Low Cost)
PO Box 49,
St Albans, Herts, AL1 4AX, UK
Web: www.talcuk.org
E-mail: talcuk@btinternet.com
(Under certain conditions, materials may be free)

Voluntary Health Association of India
Tong Swathya Bhavan,
40 Institutional Area,
Near Qutab Hotel,
New Delhi, India

The World Bank
Customer Service,
1818 H Street,
Washington, DC 20433, USA

World Health Organization
Distribution and Sales
World Health Organization
1211 Geneva 2Y, Switzerland
Web: www.who.org

Zed Books Ltd
7 Cynthia St.,
London N1 9JF, UK

Resources

Action Aid
Hamlyn House,
Macdonald Road,
Archway,
London N19 5PG, UK

AIDS Action: a newsletter about AIDS prevention, education and care. Free to readers in developing countries. Available from Healthlink.

The African Medical and Research Foundation
Wilson Airport,
PO Box 30125,
Nairobi, Kenya

Child Health Dialogue: A newsletter that provides a forum for exchange of information about the prevention and treatment of five key childhood illnesses: acute respiratory infections, diarrhoea, malaria, malnutrition and measles. Free to readers in developing countries. Available from Healthlink.

Child-to-Child Trust
Institute of Education,
20 Bedford Way,
London WC1H 0AL, UK
Publishes health education resources for use with children.

The Directory of Social Change
24 Stephenson Way
London NW1 2DP, UK
E-mail: info@d-s-c.demon.co.uk
Tel:+44 (0)20 7209 5151; Fax:+44 (0)20 7209 5049

ECHO
17430 Durrance Road,
North Fort Meyers,
FL 33917-2239, USA

Environment and Urbanization (journal)
IIED
3 Endsleigh Street
London WC1H 0DD, UK
Excellent journal with lots of case studies and examples of the status of the urban poor in developing countries, their problems and some solutions.

Footsteps (newsletter)
Tear Fund
100 Church Road
Teddington,
Middlesex TW11 8QE, UK

An excellent quarterly 16-page newsletter that is written in simple English and has many practical approaches to community health and development. Free of charge for those working in health and development in developing countries.

Future Generations
PO Box 10, Franklin,
WV 26807, USA

Health Action: A newsletter about implementing programmes in primary health care and related fields. Free to readers in developing countries. Available from Healthlink.

Institute for Development Training
212 E. Rosemary Street,
Chapel Hill, NC 27514, USA

International Institute for Environment and Development
3 Endsleigh Street,
London WC1H 0DD, UK
Fax: +44 (0)20 7388 2826

SKAT
Vadianstrasse 42,
CH-9000 St.,
Gallen, Switzerland

UNAIDS
CH-1211,
Geneva, 27, Switzerland
E-mail: info@unaids.org

UNICEF International Child Development Centre
Piazza S. S. Annunziata 12,
50122 Florence, Italy

The Urban Agricultural Network
1711 Lamont Street, NW,
Washington DC, 20010, USA
E-mail: 72144.3446@compuserve.com

Appendix 2: Approaching a donor agency

Before approaching overseas or international agencies think of every way possible for the project to become self-sustaining. Consider possible ways of generating income. Approach any local or national clubs, agencies or businesses that may have funds or resources available. Obtain as much support as possible from government departments, both national and municipal.

Even with these resources, CHDPs may often need funding from an outside donor agency. This appendix gives a few details on how to obtain this type of funding.

Step 1: Decide which agency to approach
What we should find out about the agency

What type of project does the donor like to support?

- General health and development?
- Training?
- Curative care?
- Water and sanitation?
- HIV/AIDS?

What development model does the donor agency follow?

- A **controlling model**, where the agencies decides how its funding should be used?
- A **top-down model**, where the agency provides goods, resources and cash to 'hand out' or provide?
- A **community empowering model** where the agency provides funds and resources that the CHDP can use as it and the community wish?

Does the agency believe in partnership?

- Will it be willing to share in our vision, planning, training and resourcing, in addition to providing funds?
- Will it be willing to help build the capacity of the CHDP so it can become increasingly self-reliant?

What is the size of grant the agency is likely to make available?

- It will need to be a substantial proportion of the priority needs of the project, after other sources have been taken into account.

By finding out about agencies it will make it less likely that we will waste our time and that of the agency by writing to those unlikely to help the project. In addition to time lost, it is de-moralising to have funding proposals repeatedly turned down.

One further advantage of knowing about a donor agency is that we can ask the agency to support those parts of our project in which it has a special interest. Then in our proposal we can draw attention to how the project fits in with the interests or development models of the agency.

Where do we find out about possible donors?

Information can be obtained:

- from other projects that are doing similar work;
- from government and international agencies;
- from community health and development newsletters, magazines and journals;
- at conferences and workshops;
- on the internet.

> One word of warning: This refers to the donor laying down conditions for funding, and trying to influence the way the project is run and the activities it carries out. Try to avoid being donor-driven: Programmes must be based on the needs of the community and solutions should arise from ideas that the community generates. Donors must not set the agenda, just because they have strong ideas of the way they wish their funds to be used.

Step 2: Submit a letter of enquiry
Contents of the letter

When we approach a donor agency for the first time, we should write a short letter of enquiry (less than two pages) that contains the following information:

- Name, position and details of any 'umbrella organisation' we work under or in association with such as a church, or NGO
- A brief background of the project, including aims, activities and target groups
- What funds are needed for
- Reasons why the project qualifies for funds
- A request for information and application form.

Points to remember when approaching a donor for the first time

- Be aware of laws that govern foreign contributions. Many countries have limitations, and/or require a special licence to receive foreign funds.
- Mention your contact or link with the donor organisation, especially if the agency is familiar with the contact.

- Mention previous donors, co-operative efforts with government or other points to give credibility to the project.
- Discover the name of the most appropriate senior person and direct the letter of enquiry to that person.

Step 3: Submit a project proposal

Most donor agencies have their own format and will explain how it should be completed. It usually covers some or all of the following:

Project details

- Name, address, telephone, fax and e-mail address of contact person
- Project name
- The overall aims or goals (see Chapter 4, Making an action plan)
- Date the proposal was written
- Inclusive funding dates (date project funding is to begin, and date it is to end – usually a number of years)
- The amount being requested from that donor

Situation Report

- General information about the project area
- Number of slum communities, total population
- Description of the people (by ethnic group, religion, language group, and any especially vulnerable or marginalised communities)
- Socio-economic situation: common occupations, literacy, school attendance, status of women
- Existing health and development services and providers
- Environmental situation: water, sanitation, solid waste, surface water
- (If available, include summary of any baseline or other surveys)
- Major problems in the community, ideally based on a community diagnosis (see Chapter 3, page 39, Making a community diagnosis). Explain how the community diagnosis was made. The project should not apply for funding until a community diagnosis or participatory appraisal has been made. This can be based on interviews, focus group discussions and a survey walk. None of these activities are expensive or time-consuming. Later on a survey may be wanted – the cost of that can be included in the funding proposal.

Project Action Plan

Many donors will ask for an action plan or development plan that will give a framework of how the money will be spent. Refer to Chapter 4 for details on making an action plan.

➊ List the problems that the community and the project have decided to work on together.

➋ State the objectives that the project intends to achieve during the funding period stated in the proposal. The objectives should be SMART (see Chapter 4, Making an action plan).

➌ For each objective, list the activities that are needed to accomplish the objective.

➍ For each major objective, select an indicator to monitor progress and explain when and how the monitoring will take place.

Some donor agencies ask that the action plan be prepared using a Logical Framework Analysis or Log Frame. This is described in Appendix 3.

Making a budget

When submitting a budget to donor agencies, consider the following guidelines:

- **Don't limit the budget to costs a single agency is being asked to cover**. The donor might falsely assume it is the sole funder of the project. Instead, include the entire budget for all project activities and highlight the costs being requested from the donor being approached.

- **Include a fair monetary estimate for community, government and other local contributions**. These contributions occur in different ways and are often unrecognised or underestimated. Calculate the monetary equivalent of services that are made available, free or at low cost, such as the provision of a rent-free clinic. This will help donors understand the true but often hidden contributions made by government and community; the donor agency will understand it is not providing the entire cost of the project.

- **Submit budgets on time and in the format that the agency requests**.

> Donors may be more willing to provide support when there is evidence of government contributions. When government provides this support, it signifies that the CHDP both has credibility and has taken steps to ensure it will be sustainable into the future.

Estimating income and expenditure

It is difficult to do this, especially for the first time, because it is so hard to estimate costs and expenses. Donor agencies do not like to be asked for extra funds in the middle of a funding cycle. Equally they do not like to see a large amount of unspent funds at the end of a cycle. But unforeseen circumstances do occur and estimates may be wrong. Explain this clearly to the agency if and when it happens.

In the sample budget that follows, income includes government, local and community contributions. In this example, if we submitted a budget that only included what we were requesting from one particular donor, that donor might think that it was being asked to cover all expenses. In reality, its is only being asked to supply one-third of the total project income.

CHDP expected expenses and income				
		Anticipated income		
	Anticipated expenses (Budget)	Government contribution	Local donations	Community contribution (cash, labour or materials)	Requested from donor
1. ADMINISTRATION					
Salaries	1,600				1,600
Supplies	200		20		180
Transportation	200				200
2. PROGRAMME COSTS					
LATRINE PROGRAMME	(Government is supplying half of the cost for materials; community members will pay for some of the materials and will provide all the labour. Donor is asked to pay for remaining materials)				
Salaries	1,000	200			800
Supplies	10,000	5,000		2,400	2,600
Labour	3,600			3,600	
HEALTH CLINIC	(Unpaid community volunteers assist in clinic; patients pay for half of the cost of their medicines)				
Salaries	2,000			400	1,600
Medicines	4,000	400		2,000	1,600
Other supplies	400	40			360
TB PROGRAMME	(Unpaid community volunteers act as observers and tracers in TB programme; Government hospital provides medicines and does sputum tests without charge)				
Salaries	2,000			600	1,400
Sputum tests	600	600			
Medicines	3,000	3,000			
COMMUNITY ORGANISATION ACTIVITIES	(Women provide tea and snacks on a rotating schedule. The CAG members come to project office once a month for training at their own expense (travel and lost wages).)				
Salaries	3,000			600	2400
Transportation	300			100	200
Supplies	1,000		100	200	700
Total	32,900	9,240	120	9,900	13,640

Sending off the proposal

Send this by post or courier well ahead of the deadline. Keep a spare copy. If the proposal was written on a computer and the project has access to e-mail, send the same document to the agency by e-mail as an attached file. Ask for confirmation that it has been received and whether any further information is required.

Appendix 3: Logical framework analysis (LogFrame or LFA)

Logical framework is a tool that helps projects plan and manage activities. It is a way of presenting objectives, activities, indicators and a SWOT analysis that are discussed in Chapter 4. In a LogFrame, these four components are set out in a special format that allows us to see clearly the links and interdependency between them: hence the term 'logical framework'. Many donor agencies are asking projects to provide LFA as part of their application for funds.

The LFA matrix

The framework is a table (also called a matrix). There are different ways of setting this out and many minor variations are possible, in order to help the LogFrame to be as useful and flexible as possible. Here is an example of how a LogFrame could be used for an urban health and development programme. The authors have made minor changes from the normal format.

1. Project design or structure	2. Indicators of progress	3. Means of following indicators	4. SWOT analysis
Project goal			
Project objectives			
Activities (Output)			
Resources (Input)			

Column 1: Project Structure

Our resources (inputs) enable us to carry out certain activities (outputs), so that we can reach our objectives, meaning we will ultimately meet our project goal.

$$\text{Input} \rightarrow \text{Output} \rightarrow \text{Project objectives} \rightarrow \text{Project goals}$$

This is what the terms mean:

- **Resources** (or Inputs): The manpower, materials and money needed to complete an activity.
- **Activities** (or Outputs): Results of completed project activities. These results enable us to meet project objectives.

- **Objectives**: The intended results of the activities on the target population. They must be SMART objectives (see Chapter 4, page 39).
- **Goal** (or aim): The overall purpose of the project.

As the table on the next page shows, when we are actually planning a project, we usually start from the other end, first deciding on our goals. Then we make specific objectives, decide on the activities we will need to meet the objectives and then finally decide on the resources we need to carry out these activities.

This is how we complete the first column:

Use one LogFrame Table for each major objective. For example a project has as its main goal, improving the status of women. One way to do this is to teach women to read and write. We complete one LogFrame for this objective (and others for any other objectives). We write in this column our goal, a SMART objective and the activities and resources needed.

Column 2: Indicators of Progress

This is how we complete the second column:

Here we enter indicators that allow us to monitor progress for each of the four boxes under Column 1, Project Design. We choose indicators which are easy to measure and collect, and give an accurate picture of progress and success.

Column 3: Means of following indicators

This is how we complete the third column:

In the third column, we must state how we are going to measure and collect the data required for each indicator. Sometimes this column is known as Means of Verification. We need to know who will collect the data, how it will be collected and the way it will be reported.

Column 4: Results of SWOT analysis

This is how we complete the fourth column:

In Column 4 we write down the findings from our SWOT analysis, emphasising threats, i.e. those factors which hinder us from achieving the objectives, and over which the project has little or no control.

1. Project design	2. Indicators of progress	3. Means of following indicators	4. SWOT analysis
Project goal: To improve the status of women	Female literacy rate in the community	Periodic (every 3–5 years) survey by staff and community as part of household survey	Heightened opposition to women's movement
Project objective: 150 women aged 15 and over (previously illiterate) to complete a literacy course successfully in one year	Number of illiterate women over 15 who complete a literacy course within one year	Registers kept by each CLA and reported monthly to literacy co-ordinator	In- and out-migration Men may not support Women may not want or be able to come
Project activities (Output): Train staff who will train community literacy animators (CLA) Train literate CLAs who will teach illiterate women Facilitate 15 classes of 10–15 women each	Number of staff trained as trainers to train CLAs Number of CLAs trained Number of classes offered/formed Number of women who successfully complete course	Register maintained by literacy co-ordinator and reported at monthly staff meeting	Riots or elections in slum may cause disruption Illness is common in rainy season CLAs may demand payment
Project resources (Input): Trainers to train staff facilitators. Literacy and training materials. A location large enough and with electricity	Number of staff attending government trainers programme Proportion of students that receive Government-supplied literacy material Proportion of staff trainers that have Government-supplied trainers' manual Proportion of class sessions that have location and electricity	Register maintained by literacy co-ordinator and reported at monthly staff meeting Women's group reports on whether meeting place is satisfactory	Depend upon government continuing the programme and willing and able to provide materials Meeting hall difficult to find in crowded slums Power supply is unreliable

Strengths and weaknesses of LFA

The strengths

- In a single document we can see the key components of a programme.
- We are forced to think about setting objectives, indicators and methods of monitoring. By building these into the programme from the start it makes it more likely each will happen, so strengthening the programme.
- We are forced to think about threats to success. This makes us consider feasibility, and have alternative strategies in reserve.

The weaknesses

- Creating and using LFA is complicated, time-consuming and requires training.
- It is beyond the reach of smaller projects.
- The structure can be rigid, locking us into activities and making it harder to change. This can undermine community involvement and give the impression that the programme is being imposed on the community.
- It stresses quantitative assessment rather than qualitative, making it hard to measure key achievements such as behavioural change and personal development.
- It is often difficult to reduce complex ideas into phrases that fit in a box. This is especially true for Column 4.

Index

Numbers in *italics* indicate Figures; those in **bold** indicate Tables.